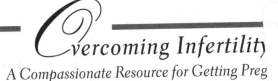
# Overcoming Infertility

*A Compassionate Resource for Getting Preg*

ROBERT JANSEN, M.D.

## INFERTILITY: MYTHS AND FACTS

**MYTH:** "You won't have any problems. It's easy to get pregnant."
**FACT:** More than five million people of childbearing age in the United States—or one in six couples—experience infertility. As Dr. Robert Jansen explains in *Overcoming Infertility*, "Getting pregnant is always a matter of chance and luck. The reason we have infertility medicine is to change the odds; the better the medicine, the better the odds."

**MYTH:** "Only women are infertile."
**FACT:** Infertility is a female problem in 35% of cases, a male problem in 35% of cases, a combined problem in 20% of cases, and unexplained in 10% of cases. It's essential that both the man and the woman be evaluated for infertility.

**MYTH:** "You're too stressed-out and impatient. If you relax, everything will be fine."
**FACT:** Infertility is a disease or condition of the reproductive system. Worrying is usually the result of infertility, not the cause of it.

**MYTH:** "Maybe you two are doing something wrong!"
**FACT:** Infertility is a medical condition, not a sexual disorder.

**MYTH:** "If you adopt, then you'll become pregnant."
**FACT:** The rate of achieving pregnancy after adopting is the same as for those who do not adopt.

**MYTH:** "Infertility is nature's way of controlling population."
**FACT:** Zero population growth is a worthy goal, but it still allows for couples to replace themselves with two children.

**MYTH:** "I feel depressed and anxious. No one understands. My life will never be the same because of infertility!"
**FACT:** Infertility is a life crisis—it affects all areas of your life. That's why *Overcoming Infertility* explores how those affected by infertility can best overcome it by relating to their partner, to their physician, to society, and to their own psychology and biology. Remember, infertility is not an uncommon problem. Stay informed about the wide range of options and connect with others facing similar experiences.

W. H. Freeman and Company
41 Madison Avenue
New York, NY 10010
Houndmills, Basingstoke RG21 6XS, England

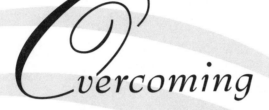

# Overcoming
# Infertility

## *A Compassionate Resource for Getting Pregrant*

*A Compassionate*
*Resource for Getting*
*Pregnant*

ROBERT JANSEN, M.D.

W. H. FREEMAN · NEW YORK

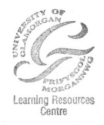

Learning Resources
Centre

Text and Cover Designer: *Blake Logan*
Illustrator: *Christopher Wikoff, CMI*

Library of Congress Cataloging–in–Publication Data

Jansen, Robert, 1946–
     Overcoming infertility : a compassionate resource for getting
 . pregnant / Robert Jansen.
               p.       cm.
     Includes bibliographical references and index.
     ISBN 0-7167-3055-3
     1. Infertility—Popular works.   2. Human reproductive technology—
Popular works.      I. Title.
RG201.J36   1996
618.1'78—dc21
                                                              96-46768
                                                              CIP

First printing, 1997

# Contents

# Part IV ASSISTED CONCEPTION 247

# Part V GETTING WHAT YOU DESERVE 319

# Foreword

*I*n *Overcoming Infertility*, Robert Jansen has provided an important and up-to-date resource for patients and clinicians alike. With infertility apparently on the rise, or at least more publicly discussed, and with fewer healthy babies available for adoption than in the past, many individuals and couples who are having trouble getting pregnant need both emotional support and scientific knowledge about the biomedical treatments for infertility that have been making such rapid progress in recent years.

*Overcoming Infertility* addresses all these issues and meets all these needs in a detailed but extremely readable style. Known internationally for his meticulous research in fertility treatments and their outcomes, Dr. Jansen brings to his text wit and learning, the empathy of years of clinical experience and an extraordinary depth of knowledge of scientific method. Dr. Jansen was a pioneer in using "evidence-based medicine"—that is, making decisions based on careful assessment of the probabilities of a good outcome, rather than clinical hunches that can often go astray. This approach gives the book a directness and honesty, including times when evidence doesn't exist for a choice, and patient and physician must rely on their best educated guesses.

From the very first chapter, "Pregnancy and Chance," it is clear that Dr. Jansen, unlike many other physicians writing for a general readership, is not going to talk down to his readers. Beginning with a general bird's-eye view of the history and current extent of infertility (in which he points out that very high fertility is probably historically rare), he goes on to discuss the many specific problems that can cause infertility nowadays, and to describe and evaluate the treatments that now exist, or that may exist soon. Dr. Jansen covers the full range of diseases associated with infertility, including male factors, ovulatory defects, endocrine phenomena and tubal diseases. He describes them in a direct and readable way, providing insight and reassurance. The confusing array of medications often prescribed for infertility is made clear—how they work, what their side effects are, and how effective they are likely to be. At every step he considers the psychological aspects with compassion and good sense.

Fertility treatments and technologies raise complex and controversial questions for society. Dr. Jansen tackles many difficult and controversial issues, including commercial surrogacy, lesbian motherhood, virgin births(!), and the great financial costs of infertility treatment. These prospects are important and should be discussed openly; Dr. Jansen does so with aplomb.

In short, *Overcoming Infertility* is a comprehensive text for a wide range of readers, from those who are first experiencing anxiety about what may be a problem for them, to those who spend their lives in research on infertility. I must confess that I learned a great deal from reading this book—most of all about an approach to infertility, and its effects on peoples' lives, that is warm, sympathetic, confident, knowledgeable and admirable.

Alan H. DeCherney, M.D.
*Chairman, Department of Obstetrics and Gynecology, UCLA*
*President, American Fertility Society*

# Preface

Our book—mine and, I hope, yours—has come about for four reasons. First, I want to build on the information we at Sydney IVF—our clinic in Australia—give our patients about how to get pregnant (naturally or with help) and to make it more widely available. Second, I want to explain how *normal* it is, biologically speaking, to have trouble getting pregnant. Taking a long time to get pregnant is as normal as getting pregnant almost immediately. Once you understand this, you can make sensible decisions about reproductive technologies and plan your life. Third, I want to relate to the more general reader what I've written on infertility and its treatment for specialists, not just on the medical and scientific aspects, but also on the morals, ethics, regulations and politics of infertility. Finally, I want to respond to the criticism of in vitro fertilization still being published by some commentators, whose apparent concern for the medical and social welfare of women in an infertile relationship is not always well placed.

The causes of infertility and the way it is treated need not be hard to explain. Important for understanding fertility, whether you are getting pregnant naturally or with help, is to appreciate that *no one* has a 100 percent chance of conceiving, or, if they've had a baby before, of conceiving again. Getting pregnant is *always* a matter of chance, of luck and, of course, sometimes bad luck. The reason we have infertility medicine is to change the odds; the better the medicine, the better the odds.

## Using this Book

Each chapter in the book is self-contained, so you can start anywhere you choose and continue reading chapters in any order. If you read the book from cover to cover, I trust that it will be a coherent, satisfying account of just about

## More Technical Elaborations Are Put in Boxes

The information contained in the boxes is more detailed and explains a subject further, if you are interested in learning more. They can be skipped without missing the point of the chapter. You might enter some of the boxes the second time you read a chapter.

everything that is happening in infertility medicine. Because each chapter is self-contained, you can also use it as a source of selective information that directly affects you or someone close to you.

I've dealt with the more difficult, technical aspects in several ways. The Glossary explains such abbreviations and acronyms as IVF and GIFT, as well as terms such as "mitosis" and "cleavage," which without explanation would either be jargon or possibly misunderstood. The first time one of these terms is used in a chapter it is printed in **boldface**, as are tests that can be ordered from a pathologist, radiologist or ultrasonologist, such as **serum follicle stimulating hormone** or **serum FSH** and **transvaginal ultrasound**. Such tests are explained in the text, and they are also included in the Glossary.

I've kept some of the most abstract and technical considerations on the arithmetic of getting pregnant separate, as Appendix A: The New Fertility and Infertility Math, and Appendix B: Results of Assisted Conception. The writing style in the boxes and appendixes lies between what I hope is the conversational style of the book itself and the way the subject can be read about in medical journals and textbooks. Some people will want to read further, and to help there is a list of References and a Further Reading section. As a scientific writer, I intuitively feel uncomfortable not supporting my assertions with references, so I've disproportionately listed my own publications in the References section, which in turn provide a thorough path to the medical and scientific literature.

## A Way Forward

This book presents infertility and assisting conception in a new and modern way. Most of the information comes from the answers I have given over the past fifteen years to questions from someone like you. I've learned what to say from your questions. Several of my patients read the manuscript and most of their suggestions are here. This a person-driven book, written for people I've gotten to know—people like you.

I hope you find it as illuminating to read as I found it to write. Let me know what you think of it; send me your comments on the Internet (http://www.jansen.com.au), by e-mail (robert@jansen.com.au), or by letter (c/o W. H. Freeman and Company, 41 Madison Avenue, New York, NY 10010), so that the book's next edition can grow and develop with us all. Write and tell me what needs to be included, what seems redundant and what might be hard to follow. I want the book to develop with you, with me and with the field of infertility as we all move further along.

I thank those of you who by reading the draft manuscript have helped me so far, particularly Rosemary Clarke, Debbie Dellazari, Carmel Nelson, Jennifer O'Connor, Trisha Sheehan, Jenny Wadwell and Coralie Younger. I also thank Jill Hickson of Hickson Associates for turning the manuscript into this book, the excellent people at W. H. Freeman and Company, especially Elizabeth Knoll, Allyson Siegel and Louise Ketz for their patient editing, and Christopher Wikoff for his careful illustrations.

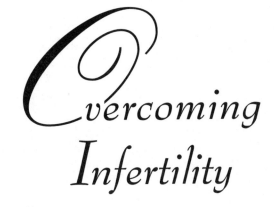

# Overcoming Infertility

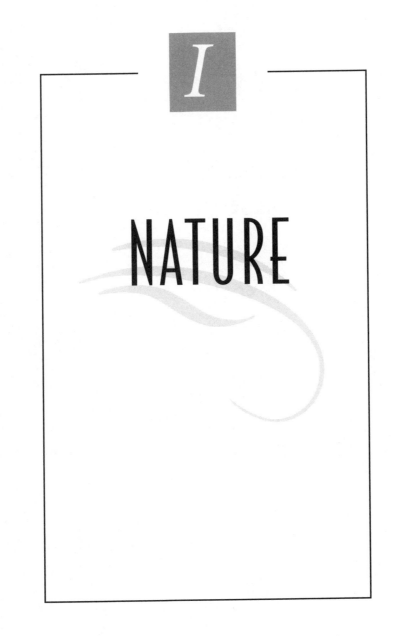

# I

# NATURE

# Pregnancy
# and Chance

*There was an old woman who lived in a shoe;*
*she had so many children, she knew not*
*what to do.*

—English nursery rhyme from about
the sixteenth century

At the best of times, and perhaps at the worst of times, pregnancy is a matter of chance. Normal fertility varies between couples, so the chance of getting pregnant if you have sex around the time an egg is produced can be high or low. If the chance of pregnancy is too low, we have the disability known as **infertility**. This book is about infertility, but, once upon a time, high fertility was also a curse.

# High Fertility–A Disability?

After about the year 1500 in England among the emerging wealthier classes, a boom began in the practice of wet-nursing (today we might call it surrogate breast-feeding). For these recent mothers, who were concerned more with preserving their figures than feeding their new infants, the social practice of wet-nursing put a stop to thousands of years of what is nature's best contraceptive—lactation, or the production of milk by the breasts.

Wet-nursing was at first restricted to the aristocracy and the gentry, but by the early 1700s many middle-class women were forgoing this natural brake on fertility, this natural way of spacing the birth of children. Mothers would send off their infants shortly after birth to women in the countryside who had recently lost their own infants in childbirth. This helped them conserve their bustlines, but it also meant they could be pregnant again within a few months of delivering their babies. Well-to-do English women of that time had anywhere from a dozen to 20 babies, and 30 babies was not unusual. Childhood mortality was high and the concern of parents about it was generally low, but with many surviving offspring who needed to be educated and either placed in a profession or married off, a family's wealth could be soon diminished. ("Making children a commodity" is a reproach we hear today from some critics of modern reproductive technology. But if ever children were a commodity, it was in England and places like it several hundred years ago, when they came by the dozen and nurturing them was contracted out commercially.) High fertility, at this unique time in history, was a stark disability. How envied were those who conceived only once every five years!

In modern societies an unplanned five-year wait between children means four years of anguish. Today we would call the couple's state infertility. Now that the misfortune of high fertility can be overcome easily by efficient contraception, it is less obvious that there is a very wide range that nature regards as normal.

# Normal Fertility

When it comes to fertility, how do we separate normal from abnormal? We are used to seeing what is normal spread across a wide range of possibilities. In nature there is the large with the small, the tall with the short, the high with the low. The normal and the abnormal blend, often with no clear separation between them. Attributes that have disadvantages in one context have advantages in others. In practice we loosely call something "abnormal" if our encounters with it are outside what we expect.

And what can a young couple embarking on a family expect? We need to get a bit closer to just what the chances are of getting pregnant each month—or what the chances are of conceiving in one **menstrual** or **ovarian cycle**. We can call this statistic **monthly fertility**. Nature gives **normal monthly fertility** a wide range.

The French demographer Henri Leridon has studied records from rural European societies from 100 years ago, when there was little or no effective contraception (except for breast-feeding). He calculated that the average normal chance of getting pregnant for a young couple living in the French countryside and embarking on a family was 20 percent per month. The normal range of this statistic, he found, was from about 7 percent per month to about 45 percent per month (more on what we mean by "normal range" later). Arithmetic shows that the expected time such normal couples took to achieve a pregnancy was thus in the range of two to 18 months.

But society has changed since the careful parish records of rural England and France were compiled in the 1800s. We now see couples starting their families at a much older age—in their thirties instead of their twenties or teen years. We also have the effects of the environment on fertility, particularly the social effects of sexually transmitted diseases and the effects of environmental pollutants, which are responsible it seems for a long-term trend downward in sperm counts (discussed in Chapter 9).

The result of these changes in society from 100 years ago is that because there are more older couples, we should halve the average monthly expectation of fertility from 20 percent to about 10 percent. This gives a normal range of monthly fertility in modern industrial societies of about 1.5 to 25 percent. The expected time it takes to achieve pregnancy will thus be in the range of three months to four years.

# Normal or Abnormal?

The art and science of medicine exists to render the abnormal normal. That is why our societies train physicians. But who's to say where the distinction lies between normal and abnormal? If fertility is like height or weight—with no sharp distinction between normal and abnormal—and if we were to represent it on a graph, we are left with calling, say, the middle 90 percent of the population normal and both the top 5 percent and the bottom 5 percent (with greatest and least fertility) abnormal. In this book we are not bothered by the top 5 percent of the population (these couples should no longer have a worry). The bottom 5 percent, however, is surely an underrepresentation of the infertility problem. There is the perfectly understandable pressure for everyone with below average fertility to be concerned and seek treatment. The concern that can result from the allocation of resources by society is not hard to appreciate. It is the arbitrariness and a capacity for exaggerating the medical extent of infertility that troubles administrators, politicians, radical feminists and others in Western society who are critics of modern technological medical practice. Public funding for overcoming childlessness is under close scrutiny everywhere. The most this book can hope to contribute to the public debate is to make the facts regarding difficulties in getting pregnant more available and accessible.

Meanwhile, most physicians tend sympathetically to define abnormal as something troublesome enough to draw a patient into the chair on the other side of the doctor's desk. To be sure, some physicians are also administrators and others are social scientists; they might argue with their patients about what is best for the community. But the doctor an infertile couple wants to see is one who puts their interests first, or who at least tells them when there are constraints that prevent that from happening. The infertility doctor and the patient become allies in securing what is wanted, which is usually a baby. This, of course, is the position I take in this book. (There is more on what to expect of your doctor and how to get it in Chapter 26.)

# Sterility, Relative Infertility and Unexplained Infertility

Most couples expect to get pregnant within about six months of trying. If pregnancy does not occur within a year, most will have at least thought of seeing a

## Medicine's Perennial Paradox

The slighter the variation from normal, the more trouble medicine has in correcting it. Returning a circumstance that is a departure from normal *back* toward normal (which, after all, is why medicine exists) is most likely to be successful when the departure from normal is major. Because any medical or surgical intervention risks introducing disturbances attributable to the intervention, the less the departure from normal, the less likely it is that the intervention will improve the situation and not make it worse.

The difficulty is exaggerated when there is more than one abnormality, and separate but simultaneously effective maneuvers need to be devised. Taking a mathematical approach to understanding infertility is essential to appreciating how a combination of separately mild disturbances malignantly thwarts getting pregnant (see Appendix A: The New Fertility and Infertility Math).

---

physician. The tests that are done on the doctor's recommendation lead generally to one of three conclusions.

First, a cause may be found for **sterility**, that is, for absolute infertility (the subject of Chapter 6). The cause can be a complete absence of sperm cells (**spermatozoa**) in the **ejaculate**. It can result from a complete absence of ovulation (**anovulation**), and in the worst case there may be no eggs left in the ovaries (**primary ovarian failure**). It also can result from a complete obstruction of the **fallopian tubes**, which prevents sperm from reaching and fertilizing an ovulated egg. In addition, the embryos that result from fertilization can repeatedly fail to develop, perhaps because the eggs are abnormal (the cause of sterility leading up to menopause) or, less commonly, because disease of the uterus ruins **implantation**.

Second, a cause may be found for **relative infertility**, by which we mean fertility that is low in relation to what we expect but is not zero. Examples include a low sperm count, irregular ovulation, a problem of anatomy or physiology that lowers the chance of sperm or egg arriving for fertilization at the right place at the right time, or some incomplete, unpredictable disturbance in embryo development. (Relative infertility is the subject of Chapter 7.)

Third, tests may show nothing wrong whatsoever, that is, there is **unexplained infertility** (a subject that has no special chapter but is discussed here and in Chapter 2). The temptations here are to try to discover new causes of infertility or, failing this, to think of the infertility as psychological. As it turns out, not one major new cause of infertility has been discovered. There are no diagnostic labels that have not been around for decades, despite the unprecedented opportunity that **in vitro fertilization** (IVF) technology has given us since 1978 for new insights into what might go wrong. Later on I will return to the temptation to explain the otherwise unexplainable as "psychological." Meanwhile, as researching physicians and informed patients, we are left with the conclusion that, biologically speaking, much infertility is not strictly abnormal.

We often hear calls for more research into the causes of infertility—into how we can stop infertility from happening. The real problem is that the chief culprits for the infertility prevalent in today's society are social ones. We have sexually transmitted diseases as causes of sterility. We have the probable but unproven possibility of environmental toxins as potentially important contributors to relative infertility. In addition to these two environmental threats, numerically as important is the modern social custom of normal women postponing getting pregnant until they are out of their most fertile years.

# Psychological Infertility

When time goes by without a pregnancy, mental stress is not far behind, but can it be the other way around? What part do psychological factors play in causing infertility or in causing infertility to persist? Does a romantic weekend or an ocean cruise really help? How valid are such well-meant comments as, "If you'd only stop trying so hard you'd get pregnant"? Is it useful to hear that if you could only relax, if you could only forget about infertility, everything would be all right? Should you avoid having sex before ovulation "to save up the sperm" but thereby add to the stress?

One reason the mistaken notion that stress causes infertility is so widespread is that everyone seems to have heard of couples who adopt a child and then promptly conceive one of their own, despite years of infertility. We refer to such evidence as being "anecdotal," relying on spectacular examples that bowl you over instead of relying on boring, painstaking studies to work out what actually happens. (It is the same technique that some critics of IVF use to frighten

## Stressed Rhesus Monkeys

Reid Norman works with rhesus monkeys at the Texas Tech University Health Sciences Center in Lubbock, Texas. Monkeys are among our close relatives in the animal kingdom and in many ways resemble us in their reproductive physiology, including their 28-day menstrual cycle. Dr. Norman has been investigating the effects of brief periods of mental stress on the process of ovulation. He and his colleagues have shown that six hours of physically constraining female monkeys closely—for example, the monkeys were strapped comfortably but irritatingly to a chair—interferes with levels of **luteinizing hormone** (LH), which causes the mature ovarian **follicle** to ovulate (discussed in detail in Chapter 3). The way this happens seems to be a result of an increase in cortisol, the main hormone of the adrenal gland and commonly increased by physical or mental stress. This inhibitory effect of cortisol on the monkeys' LH was noticeable in the first half of the menstrual cycle (the **follicular phase**) but not in the second half (the **luteal phase**).

In extreme cases, suppressing LH by stress-induced increases in cortisol (or possibly by other mental and neurological pathways in the brain that involve **gonadotropin-releasing hormone**, or **GnRH**, the hormone directly responsible for production of LH) may stop ovulation altogether, disturbing the menstrual cycle rather obviously. In less severe cases there may be enough LH to luteinize the mature follicle but not enough to cause it to open and release the egg, resulting in what is known as the **luteinized unruptured follicle** (see the box "Fake Ovulation" in Chapter 4).

couples away from what on balance can otherwise be a sensible approach.) Mark Twain said, "Get your facts first and then you can distort them as much as you please." The facts are that there are two good psychologically based reasons for not getting pregnant—not ovulating properly and not having sex.

In fact, there have been no fewer than five careful studies on the real chance of getting pregnant after adoption. These studies compared adopting couples with similar couples trying to conceive for just as long but who were not adopting. In every one of these studies, it was obvious that couples who kept trying to get pregnant instead of adopting had more chance of conceiving than those who adopted! When you think about it the reasons are plain: once you adopt a baby

A not-so-young couple, each with busy professional careers and having sex just once a week—and then with some stress and strain—might need to take more time off than just one week. A lower frequency of sexual intercourse is one of the best documented reasons for decreased fertility in older couples, whether on vacation or not.

### ... Especially in the Mornings

The beginning of the midcycle surge of LH, which 36 hours later will trigger ovulation (see Chapter 3), usually starts during sleep, at around three o'clock in the morning (according to research that IVF pioneers Robert Edwards and Patrick Steptoe did when they were developing in vitro fertilization and trying to anticipate when best to collect mature eggs). If this is true, it means that most ovulations take place *during the afternoon.* If it is best for sperm to get to the meeting place for fertilization a bit ahead of the egg, which we certainly believe is the case, then the best time to have sex may not be at night, but in the morning.

the pressure to have sex is off and you do it less often; you may even avoid it at midcycle on purpose. A crying baby, your own or adopted, does disturb your sex life.

Psychological stress needs to be extreme if it is to cause anovulation, that is, no ovulation, which is signaled by absent periods (**amenorrhea**). It is most unusual for the ordinary stresses of modern life to be enough to stop ovulation completely, but stress around the time of ovulation could make an ovulation less optimal than it might be (see the box "Stressed Rhesus Monkeys"). Nevertheless, exercising too much or losing weight are important causes for ovulation to fail and are discussed in Chapter 10.

The second psychologically related factor when it comes to trying to conceive is that you need to have sex at more or less the right time. This is an area where many couples get into a vicious circle; sex is postponed in the hope of saving up for a king-size hit that is meant to coincide with ovulation. Then the moment comes (or is thought to come) and stress or some other excuse gets in the way.

Is having sex often ever bad for getting pregnant? The answer is no. No one has ever shown that you can have sex too often for fertility. What *has* been shown in the laboratory is that frequent ejaculation decreases the sperm concentration in each ejaculate. But who cares? Research and common sense both suggest that the best place for sperm is not the laboratory but the vagina, or, more exactly, the mucus of the cervix, where sperm are nourished and stored over several days for steady release upward toward the fallopian tube. The more sperm that get there, and the fresher they are, the better. If this is two or three times a day, then terrific! And this will be true no matter what sperm count result you get from the laboratory.

If, as a young couple, you are living in a room at home with one or the other's parents or maybe with children and thin walls, having sex is going to be a stressful event, and almost certainly not as frequent or successful as it would be otherwise. A week away during ovulation will then work wonders. A small amount of wine does no harm either. I go into what can help in more detail in Chapter 19.

## Goodbye to the Do-Gooders

The evidence in this chapter should mean goodbye to the do-gooders who tell people to relax and then they'll get pregnant. There is just no evidence that this is true for most people. Certainly it is good for the chance of getting pregnant to have sex more often, but you can forget the myth that there is some mysterious, psychological link between the stress of not getting pregnant and continuing not to. Thinking about infertility does not stop someone from getting pregnant.

We leave this chapter with the conclusion that what we today call unexplained infertility, as well as much "not-well-explained" infertility, is a natural and often normal phenomenon.

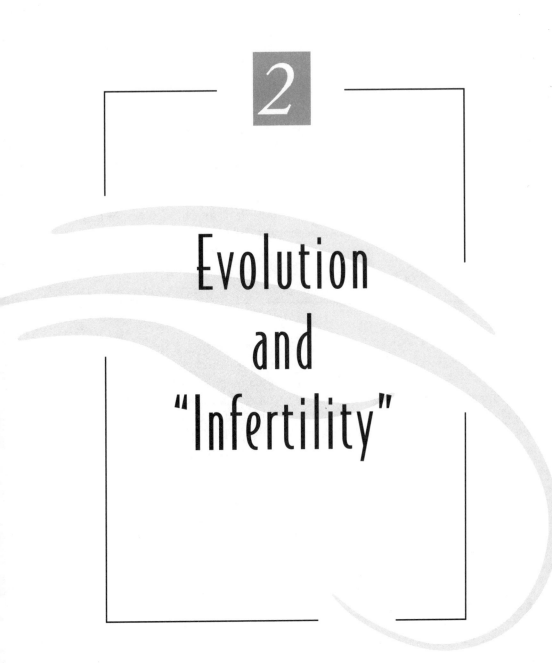

2

# Evolution
# and
# "Infertility"

Getting pregnant can be too easy. Let me explain why nature often seeks to limit fertility, and why evolution has produced so much genetically determined infertility among humans.

From single-celled animals, such as the amoeba, to man, successfully reproducing organisms that are part of expanding populations gather resources so that their progeny will outnumber their ancestors. In today's society, humans need to have an average of just over two children per couple to sustain the population; more than this will increase it. Back in the fourteenth century, however, six or more children were needed per couple to sustain the population because of the high likelihood of death, not just of the children within families but also of the adults before their dependent children were grown and able to have children of their own.

## Of Whales and Women

Population scientists talk of two general strategies for achieving reproductive fitness among animals. These two strategies are mutually exclusive. And they mean that all-out reproduction is not always the best way for a population to grow reliably and for a species to flourish.

The first reproductive strategy, called **r-selection**, shows rapid sexual maturity, superabundant production of eggs by the female, low survival rates of offspring and a short life for the parent. The r-selection strategy is typically favored by or forced on smaller species, whose numbers wax and wane with changes in the environment. When the environment turns bad, numbers decline drastically; when it improves again an explosive increase in numbers is needed for the species to exploit the opportunity. Reproductive growth is highly leveraged, but adult life is brittle and short. The father may not survive more than a few hours after copulation, all energy having been given to producing sperm; the mother may not survive more than a few hours after laying eggs. Think of insects, butterflies and all sorts of other small animals. Relatively speaking, small mammals such as mice also show features of r-selection, including large litters, short times to maturity and short adult life.

The second strategy, called **K-selection**, shows a slowly gained sexual maturity, limited production of eggs, high survival rates of (usually single) offspring and a longer life for the parents. The mother will experience several episodes of gestation. There is invariably a premium placed on parental care of the young, so that the offspring can reach first the size and then the sexual maturity they need for the genetic potential of their parents to be realized. In general, the larger the animal, the more it

For a species to succeed, it is not enough just to give birth to babies. For a human couple to be reproductively successful—for their reproductive strategy to triumph—they not only must have children, they must also survive long enough to rear their offspring to an age at which the children become fertile adults. Children need to be nurtured to the point of independence; otherwise the reproductive effort is wasted. This principle is behind the reproductive strategy of all large animals.

In the course of our evolution toward bigger and better brains, the time from birth to maturity has increased considerably. The anatomy of the female pelvis eventually limited the size the fetus's head could be at birth without getting stuck, so a lot of brain development had to occur after birth. This in turn meant that infants were born less and less mature, more and more vulnerable

## Of Whales and Women (concluded)

will rely on a *K*-selection strategy for reproductive success. For example, whales and elephants both have long gestation periods (15 months for sperm whales, 22 months for elephants), long periods from birth to adolescence and sexual maturity, and three- to five-year intervals between births, in order to protect the parent and the existing offspring from the ravages that frequent pregnancy would have on the mother.

Our species, *Homo sapiens*, has become just as extremely *K*-selected as the world's largest mammals, despite our being much smaller physically. This is because the time our young need to grow to be independent has, for different purposes, become the same. Our gestation periods are shorter at nine months, so that our large-headed babies do not get stuck too often during birth. Human infants are therefore much more dependent at birth

than whale or elephant calves, with large brains anticipating the learning that will follow. Add to this the time it takes for the human brain to mature and be educated and we have in our species the longest times of childhood dependency and maternal vulnerability seen on the planet.

In natural (say "prehistoric") circumstances, ungraced by the trappings of civilization, the interval between human births—the birth interval—is about the same as the three years or more found among whales and elephants. A lengthening birth interval for our prehistorically evolving hominoid ancestors depended on various natural ways—various biological devices—for spacing pregnancies. We need to understand the importance of long birth intervals and the nature of the devices for achieving the long intervals if we are to comprehend what we today call infertility.

and reliant on their mothers. Longer periods of time came to be devoted to dependent infancy and childhood. This long duration of childhood is needed for the brain to grow and for the person to learn living skills. In primitive human societies, **menarche**, the time of the first period (and pronounced "men-ar-kee"), occurs about age 16 and a half, and first pregnancy does not occur until about age 18.

Having many children is extremely detrimental to a woman's health, as is her ability to raise the children. Pregnancies and bearing children wear out a woman. Put simply, too many pregnancies can be bad for a woman and bad for the survival of her genes, especially if the environment is harsh and challenging, as it has probably been for most of human history and prehistory—indeed, as it has been right up to modern times.

Thus, interestingly, we have a reproductive strategy in which delaying sexual maturity among offspring turns out to be an advantage for our species. During this time it is important for the continuation of the species that childhood be secure, that parents in general, and mothers in particular, do not wear themselves out with too many pregnancies and children. As a result, we have experienced much evolutionary pressure for curbing fertility and for spacing the birth of children.

# Putting a Brake on Fertility

Spacing pregnancies in mammals—humans as well as the largest of them, whales and elephants— has come about in several ways. The first is lactational amenorrhea, or the inhibition of ovulation and, for humans, the inhibition of menstrual periods that is caused by suckling the young at the breast. This is the chief natural contraceptive of the great apes and humans. To be an effective contraceptive, however, breast-feeding should not be diluted by other feeding. The hunter-gatherer Kung nomads of the Kalahari Desert in southern Africa feed their babies several times an hour for the first two or three years of life, and sleep with them at the breast. As a result, the average birth interval among the Kung is more than four years, despite their natural, apparently high, fertility. There is no way of knowing, however, for what time in human history and prehistory such intensive suckling was usual. Modern but primitive societies such as the Kung may have evolved considerably from the early tribes we once had in common as ancestors.

## Twixt Sex and Reproduction

Reproductive function in women, which is dependent on production by the **hypothalamus** of **gonadotropin-releasing hormone** (see Chapter 3), is very sensitive to body weight. The physiological result of this sensitivity is that the improvement in human nutrition that has taken place in many societies in the past 100 years has produced an important lowering of the age at menarche from 15 or 16 in the mid-nineteenth century to 12 or 13 in Western societies today. At the same time, the need for enculturation of our young is raising even further the age at which emotional and educational maturity are reached. This counter-*K*-selective long-term trend in age at menarche has further increased the gap between the ages of physical and mental maturity for adolescents—a gap that has already had clear and deep social consequences. Biology seems to have always been destined to play havoc with nineteenth-century morals and twentieth-century ideals.

Seasonal breeding among mammals is also associated with a lack of ovulation in the off-season. It helps to space pregnancies among the lesser apes, such as the lar gibbon of the Malayan rain forest. Among humans, however, other than the observation that we have higher sperm concentrations in winter, seasonal changes in fertility are not conspicuous. (It is probable that men and women outside the tropics, through clothing, shelter and sometimes migration, have successfully adapted to the environment to provide rough constancy between the seasons.)

Environmental constraints on human fertility are seen, however, in the cessation of periods and ovulation when a woman's weight falls below that at which menstruation began during adolescence (this is explained further in Chapter 10). An intriguing exception to this occurs with **polycystic ovary syndrome** (PCOS), in which fertility in the past might have been best during times of famine (see the box "Polycystic Ovary Syndrome: Fertility in Famine").

Environmental and lactational **anovulation**, or lack of ovulation, may not however have been contraceptive enough over the past several hundred thousand years (in environments other than the Kalahari Desert), as flowering intelligence forced the evolution of longer childhoods. What was it then that nature could turn to for evolving early humans to extend their birth interval and to increase the number of young raised safely to maturity? How did evolving humans, pressed to reproduce, unconsciously slow down their fertility to achieve an ultimately successful reproductive strategy? Not by limiting sexuality. Not by getting rid of the pleasure of sex. Desmond Morris in his book *The Naked Ape* argues convincingly, as do others, that sexuality became (probably a million or more years ago), and remains today, the enjoyable cement required for durable human relationships. Predictable sexual reward was presumably important to help make sure that females had the food supplied by their mates for themselves and their dependent children.

Today, the lessons of medicine tell us that human fertility is not only rather low by the standards of other primates, but that a number of conditions that diminish fertility have a genetic—an evolutionary—cause. Any or all of the clinical conditions we can identify today might have acted to limit early human fertility and thus improved the reproductive success of the generations that followed. Any or all of the identifiable conditions we associate with clinical infertility might in fact be inseparable from the successful long-term reproductive strategy of our species.

## High Miscarriage Rates

A high chance of **miscarriage** can serve a useful purpose in long-childhood species, according to Roger Short, a reproductive biologist at Monash University in Melbourne. He draws attention to the advantages brought by "a sprinkling of genetically defective gametes [to produce] a measure of non-recurrent infertility through early embryonic death." Evidence of high rates of failure of early pregnancy among humans shows that no more than 25 to 50 percent of fertilizations will produce a healthy pregnancy—a lower proportion than among the other primates. It also compares with a similar evolutionary development among species with long childhoods because of the demands of huge adult size. Elephants also have high rates of embryonic death.

## Low Sperm Counts

The inheritance of low **sperm counts**, or **oligospermia** (see Chapter 9), has an effect similar to defective eggs in systematically diminishing fertility. Roger Short and others have shown that variation in sperm counts and in the size of the **testes** in primates is determined genetically.

Before I knew about Short's work, I had an exciting encounter with the American urologist Sherman Silber in an airport lounge in Singapore. I was explaining my theories of evolutionary causes for the high prevalence of **endometriosis** in modern women, when he drew my attention to the advantages that genetically determined oligospermia may paradoxically have for men (at least men in monogamous relationships). What we had in common—and, it turns out, in common with Roger Short—was that we all had independently reached the conclusion that, by limiting fertility without limiting sexuality, evolving humans (or more exactly groups of humans as societies) probably were able to achieve greater ultimate reproductive fitness.

# Endometriosis

Endometriosis (explained in detail in Chapter 15) is a condition in which tissue that is the same as the lining membrane of the uterus, the **endometrium**, develops in locations outside the uterus, changing the environment for a woman's pelvic organs and producing **relative infertility**. Endometriosis gets more common with age during the reproductive years, as the modern woman, generally neither pregnant nor breast-feeding (unlike her ancient predecessors), experiences an unprecedented number of ovulatory menstrual cycles, each one increasing the chance of new endometrium developing in the wrong place.

Endometriosis is rarely severe enough to be an undoubted cause of **sterility**, but several lines of evidence show that fertility is reduced even in mild endometriosis. Such information fits a theory that endometriosis reduces fertility in a manner that could be called "dose-dependent"—the more endometriosis, other things being equal, the greater the reduction of the chance each month of getting pregnant.

Endometriosis has been found in the other menstruating mammals, namely monkeys and apes, but it only occasionally obviously disables them. Endometriosis could possibly have evolved independently in early humans, but more probably nature seized on this mostly harmless consequence of menstruation in primates, opportunistically bestowing it with an added responsibility. This would mean that endometriosis might date from at least 14 million years ago (which is when the Old World monkeys separated from the line destined to become humans). Whether my exercise in theoretical anthropology is right or wrong, endometriosis is so common in women that, given its hereditary basis (see the section

## Polycystic Ovary Syndrome (PCOS): Fertility in Famine

With polycystic ovary syndrome (discussed in Chapter 10) we have another example of an at least partly inherited condition that diminishes fertility (by lengthening the menstrual cycle and reducing the frequency of ovulation), thus advantaging the evolution of reproductive success according to our thesis. But Dr. John Eden, a reproductive endocrinologist at the Royal Hospital for Women in Sydney, believes that PCOS may have had more direct evolutionary advantages in some special circumstances.

In times of starvation, most women's periods stop, and they become infertile as they lose weight. But would it be useful for *some* women to show the opposite? Say a famine went on for more than a generation: if all women stopped ovulating the population would be wiped out. One can imagine that at times of prolonged famine (and subnormal weight), some women—a minority, perhaps—would advantage the species by retaining their capacity to reproduce, even at the expense of decreased fertility in times of plenty. This is exactly what happens among women with PCOS, who can have irregular periods (and ovulations) at normal body weight (and who stop ovulating completely as they gain weight into the realms of obesity), but who will usually ovulate well if their weight falls considerably below what we call normal. This might explain why perhaps as many as one in five women have evidence of polycystic ovaries when this condition is looked for carefully.

"Inheriting Endometriosis" in Chapter 15), it is plausible that nature—at the cruel expense of significant symptoms for many modern sufferers—kept it and developed it for a purpose. That purpose may have been to improve reproductive fitness through diminishing fertility.

Oligospermia in the male and endometriosis in the female are a common combination among infertile couples. One often suspects that if these two conditions were isolated and mild there would be no serious difficulty with conception, and that it is their coming together by chance, or their chance genetic exaggeration to a more severe form, that pushes the once desirable restraint they put on fertility into the realm of serious infertility.

# Yesterday's Advantage

You can conclude from this chapter that low human fertility is the result of a long and generally positive evolutionary sequence. What today we call **unexplained infertility** is by no means necessarily abnormal; it is actually a highly evolved human condition. But that is not to say it should not be treated. Having to wait about five years to get pregnant is no longer considered the pinnacle of human reproductive achievement that it once was anthropologically. Just as we use contraception to minimize the social disadvantages of excessive fertility, we are also justified in employing **assisted conception** to cope with insufficient fertility. To appreciate the finer points of infertility and its effective treatment, Chapter 3 takes us into those normal workings of the body that lead to getting pregnant naturally.

3

# Behind a Successful Conception

When a girl has her first menstrual period her ovaries have been functioning since before she was born. The eggs in each ovary were made while she was a fetus in her mother's uterus, when her mother was between about 14 and 20 weeks pregnant. The most eggs a woman will ever have, or have had—about 7 million—is when there are still 20 weeks to go before birth. From this time on, there will be fewer and fewer eggs, and none will be replaced. By the time of birth there are about 2 million eggs left in the ovaries—a fraction of the original number.

## Ova and Follicles

As the eggs are made, they are surrounded by a thin layer of cells that form a **follicle**. The **follicle cells** will support the egg they enclose for up to 50 years or more, providing it with nourishment but stopping the egg from maturing. Eggs that are left bereft of a follicle soon die and disappear.

### Laying Down Eggs for the Future

The process by which the eggs, or ova, are formed is called **oogenesis**, and the multiplying forms of the eggs are the **oogonia**. The oogonia are all gone by birth. From then on the eggs are in the form of **primary oocytes**, which cannot divide except in a way called **meiosis**, by which the egg's genetic complement (the chromosomes) is halved. The equivalent of oogonia in males, the **spermatogonia**, persist in the testis throughout life, multiplying and replenishing themselves the way all other cells in the body do, by **mitosis** (see the box "Nuts and Bolts").

Why does nature insist that all the eggs be made before birth, whereas new sperm cells are usually made into old age? The reason must be important, because it seems to be true for much of the animal kingdom. Whether it be fish, frogs, reptiles, birds or mammals, the eggs are formed before the female of the species becomes fertile. For some speculation on why eggs need to be laid down fast and then kept in suspended animation while waiting for their owner to grow up and reproduce, see the box "How Eggs Get Their 'Use-by Date': Mishaps in the Mitochondria" in Chapter 7.

When follicles grow inside the ovary, it is because the follicle cells are multiplying, increasing in number from a handful to many thousands. The great majority of follicles, however, never grow to maturity and ovulate. They start to develop, but then conditions for them to keep growing are not right, and the egg they contain loses its nourishment and dies. The follicle cells themselves die, and the tissue from the follicle is absorbed back into the ovary. We call this process **atresia**. The egg undergoes atresia and so does the follicle.

Atresia continues until all the follicles are gone. The younger a woman is, the more follicles at any one time are starting to develop, and hence the more follicles will be undergoing atresia. Atresia starts in the fetus, continues through childhood, adolescence and the reproductive years and finishes after menopause, when finally there are no eggs left. Atresia marches on at the same rate, heedless of pregnancy, the use of the oral contraceptive pill and conditions in which the periods stop (**amenorrhea**). Only during ovarian stimulation for **assisted conception** is it, transiently, overcome. At the time of the first period, when reproduction first becomes technically possible, there are just 300,000 or so eggs left in the ovaries.

# The Pituitary Gland's Control of the Ovaries

The pituitary gland, lying under the brain behind the nose, produces two hormones that the ovary needs for ovulation: **follicle stimulating hormone** (FSH)

## Pituitary Hormones Depend on the Brain

Production of FSH and LH by the pituitary gland demands stimulation from nearby brain tissue—the **hypothalamus**. The hypothalamus does this by secreting **gonadotropin-releasing hormone** (GnRH) into special veins that go only to the pituitary gland. The pattern of this secretion is pulsatile, occurring as a spurt every 60 to 90 minutes, continuing from the beginning of the cycle right through the time of ovulation. (Chapter 10 describes the pulsatile use of GnRH intravenously to induce ovulation in women in whom the hypothalamus is not working properly.)

and **luteinizing hormone** (LH). The purpose of FSH, as the name indicates, is to keep follicles growing once they have started. What makes a particular follicle start to grow after so many years of rest? This is still a puzzle, but the number that will be getting started, say in one day, one week or one month (it is a continuous affair), depends on how many follicles are still in the ovaries. The purpose of LH (this hormone's name will be explained later) is to push a fully developed, large, preovulatory follicle into going further ahead and ovulating (which will also be discussed later).

A resting follicle, or **primordial follicle**, is about one-eighth of a millimeter in diameter— only a little bigger than the egg it contains. It starts to grow, for a reason that is still obscure, as the follicle cells begin to divide and increase in number. As the follicle grows, the follicle cells produce fluid, which forms an enlarging space, or **antrum**, among the cells, leaving the egg to one side, attached to the wall of the follicle and still surrounded by a layer of follicle cells (see Figure 3.1).

Figure 3.2 shows the changes in pituitary hormones and ovarian hormones during a typical ovarian cycle. Refer to it while we consider how a follicle grows and then ovulates.

For a follicle to have a chance of ovulating, it must already be growing in the month, or cycle, before the ovulation cycle we focus on. This follicle and its cohort of fellow follicles will have an antrum and be about two millimeters in diameter by the time the period starts. There is a small rise in FSH levels in the blood at this time—enough to get this group of similar follicles growing further

## Follicle Talk

The resting, unstimulated follicles are called primordial follicles; **primary follicles** have just one layer of (multiplying) follicle cells; **secondary follicles** have more than one layer of follicle cells, and a **tertiary follicle** has formed a fluid-filled space, or antrum, among the follicle cells. An early tertiary follicle is about one millimeter across. A preovulatory, or **Graafian follicle**, is a large, mature tertiary follicle, usually bigger than 1.5 centimeters in diameter, and is named after Reijnier de Graaf (1641–1673), a Dutch microscopist and the first person to observe and describe the ovarian follicle. An **atretic follicle** is a degenerating primary or tertiary follicle, representing the two stages or decision points at which either continued growth of the follicle or atresia can happen.

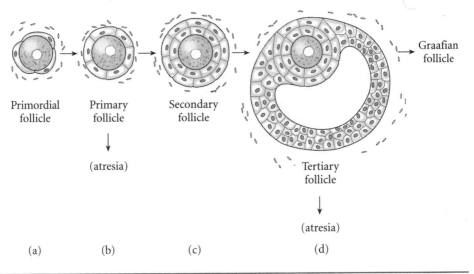

**Figure 3.1**  Stages of development of an ovarian follicle, showing the points at which atresia is likely: (a) a primordial follicle, with a thin layer of follicle cells, is the resting state for the egg over many years; (b) a primary follicle, with still just one layer of follicle cells, is the first step to development, but most follicles that start to develop quickly undergo atresia and are lost forever; (c) a secondary follicle has more than one layer of follicle cells, and most will go on to the next stage; (d) a tertiary follicle has formed an antrum, or space, filled with fluid (and hormones). At this stage the follicle is about one millimeter in diameter. Only follicles that reach this point near the beginning of a new ovarian cycle have a chance to grow much further. When they do grow, tissue around the follicles takes part in the function of the follicle and is called the theca interna. If the woman is not on the birth control pill and is not pregnant or breast-feeding, ultimately one (or sometimes more) tertiary follicle will ovulate each month after reaching the stage referred to as a preovulatory, or Graafian, follicle.

instead of immediately undergoing atresia. The number of follicles in the cohort (spread between the two ovaries) will depend inversely on the woman's age: at age 20 it could be about 50 or so; at age 30, perhaps 20 to 30; at 40 years, say 5 to 10, and at 45, maybe just one or two. This concept is important, because no amount of stimulating the ovaries can increase the number. The actual number at a particular age will be different in different women, and to a small extent it may be different in a woman from one cycle to the next, especially when she gets older.

The follicle becomes visible with ultrasound scanning of the ovaries when it is about four millimeters in size. As the follicle grows, it secretes **estrogen**, the ovary's important sex hormone. The rise of estrogen in the blood is slow at first, but after the first week it goes up quickly. In response to this estrogen, the

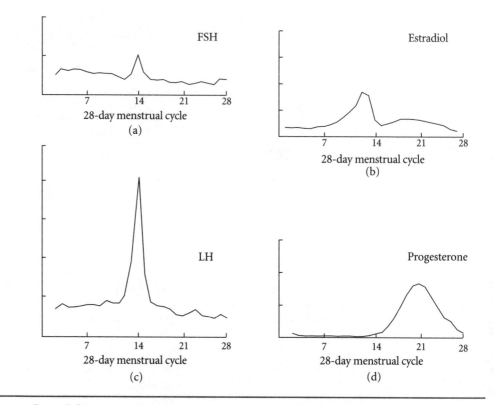

**Figure 3.2** Hormone changes during a typical 28-day menstrual cycle in the pituitary hormones LH and FSH and in the ovarian hormones estradiol and progesterone. There is a small rise in FSH (a) at the end of the cycle, to push early tertiary follicles into growth. As the follicles grow, estradiol starts to rise (b), especially once the dominant follicle has been selected. The high level of estradiol at midcycle triggers a surge of LH (c), which causes the follicle to ovulate (release the egg) and to begin to secrete progesterone. When progesterone (and estradiol) fall (d) at the end of the cycle, menstruation starts in the uterus, FSH rises a little again and a new cycle starts in the ovary.

pituitary gland cuts back its FSH production—and this soon sorts the sheep from the goats in the ovaries. One after the other, the follicles that by bad luck are slower than their fellows run out of steam (or FSH) and undergo atresia. By the end of the first week just one follicle is left—charged up with FSH and its own capacity for making estrogen. This **dominant follicle**, now about eight to ten millimeters in diameter, will keep growing, producing more and more estrogen, until it is mature and approaching two centimeters in size. (Remember

## Hormones in Follicles

In addition to follicle cells, the wall of the follicle is surrounded by a layer of special cells picked up from the ovary's substance as the follicle grows, known as the **theca interna**; its cells, the **thecal cells**, play an important part in the ovary's hormone manufacture. The thecal cells, under the influence of a tiny amount of LH, make the male sex hormone **androstenedione**, which diffuses in among the follicle cells, where, under the stimulus of FSH, it is converted to **estradiol**, the most potent and important of the estrogens. Estradiol directly stimulates the follicle cells to divide and increase in number, and the more follicle cells there are, the less the follicle needs to depend on FSH from the blood, and it is thus more likely to survive as falling FSH levels put on the squeeze. Measuring the hormones in a follicle's antrum can distinguish the three types of follicle: a healthy, still-growing follicle will be rich in estradiol; an atretic follicle will be dominated by androstenedione, and a preovulatory follicle will have loads of progesterone as well as estradiol.

that the follicle, although it now has many thousands of follicle cells, consists largely of fluid—it is, literally, a small cyst.)

## The Ovarian Cycle

The first half of the ovary's cycle, from menstruation to ovulation, is thus called the **follicular phase**. For the week before ovulation, the ovary (left or right) that contains the dominant follicle will become the sole producer of ovarian hormones for that cycle; the other ovary sleeps. If, for one reason or another, a woman has only one ovary, then that ovary will normally take over, providing a follicle for ovulation every month.

The length of the follicular phase is usually two weeks but it varies. In young teenagers, when follicular development may not be sustained, one follicle can take another's place without ovulation, resulting in cycles that can be long and irregular. Leading up to menopause, when there are few follicles left and those that develop seem to have a head start from higher FSH levels, the follicular phase can be short, sometimes so short that ovulation takes place before the period is finished.

As the dominant follicle matures to become preovulatory, its follicle cells switch their allegiance from FSH to LH. At the same time, the pituitary senses that the dominant follicle is ready to be ovulated by the high levels of estrogen now present in the blood (see Figure 3.2). The pituitary then releases a surge of LH, which causes the follicle cells to start to synthesize the ovary's second main hormone, **progesterone**—the hormone that prepares the body for pregnancy. Ovulation will take place 20 hours or so from the time LH levels peak in the blood, or about 36 hours after the start of the LH surge.

# Ovulation

During the hours leading up to ovulation, the follicle cells surrounding the egg secrete mucus, which causes them to space themselves more widely, forming an expanding surround, or "cumulus." Whereas the egg itself is too small to be seen by the naked eye, the structure that the follicle ovulates and presents to the fallopian tube is a millimeter or two in diameter—and it is very sticky. The **cumulus mass**, as the egg plus its surround is called, adheres resolutely to the opening of the tube when contact is made. (We will move on to discussion of the tube shortly.)

## Chromosomes in the Egg

A few hours before ovulation, the primary oocyte, which we met in the box "Laying Down Eggs for the Future" at the beginning of this chapter, undergoes the first division of meiosis, having first doubled its number of chromosomes the way a cell multiplying by mitosis does; the result is one **secondary oocyte** and one **polar body**—a tiny, discarded packet containing half the chromosomes. The ovulated secondary oocyte remains suspended in its second meiotic division until it is fertilized, when it will release a second polar body to expel half of its chromosomes again, bringing it from the **diploid** state with the full complement of 46 chromosomes to the **haploid** state of 23 chromosomes, the same chromosome status as that of the sperm cell that fertilizes it.

The corpus luteum is usually about two centimeters in diameter, like the follicle it springs from, but it can be a lot bigger if it gets cystic. A cystic corpus luteum usually functions normally—and grows still bigger if pregnancy happens. It can be painful, for a while, but otherwise a cystic corpus luteum has no medical importance, as long as it is left alone. Because the corpus luteum can have an astonishing range of appearances—some of them reminiscent of a malignant tumor—insufficiently trained surgeons sometimes remove them when they happen to see them during operations (or, worse, they may remove the whole ovary). The loss of a corpus luteum early in pregnancy deprives the uterus of progesterone, causing miscarriage.

As the follicle opens to release its fluid and its cumulus mass (which contains the egg), there is usually some bleeding from the ovary into the abdomen. (In rare instances this is severe, causing an urgent clinical problem with pain and low blood pressure.) As the follicle caves in, the high levels of LH cause its follicle cells (or **granulosa cells**, as they tend to be called at about this time) to get plumper as they get better at producing progesterone instead of estrogen. The follicle turns into a new structure, the **corpus luteum**. (This is how the luteinizing hormone that brought it about gets its name.) To move the progesterone out of the follicle cells and into the circulation, the collapsed follicle is invaded by blood capillaries. As the corpus luteum matures into an efficient progesterone-producing structure, it accumulates fat, giving it a yellow color (hence the name corpus luteum, which is Latin for "yellow body").

Progesterone is the ovarian hormone that dominates the second half of the ovarian cycle, the **luteal phase**. Its levels in the blood (shown in Figure 3.2) reach a peak in the middle of the luteal phase, on about day 21. In the absence of a signal from an early pregnancy (through the pregnancy hormone **human chorionic gonadotropin**, or hCG), progesterone then falls, to again reach the low levels that characterize another follicular phase. The length of the luteal phase is normally between 11 and 16 days. If pregnancy occurs, the life of the corpus luteum is extended for several weeks through stimulation by hCG, until the placenta produces enough progesterone to take over responsibility for supporting the pregnancy.

The testes develop in male fetuses a week or two after the ovaries develop in female fetuses. Instead of follicles forming around oocytes, **tubules** form around the multiplying male germ cells, the spermatogonia. Unlike the ovaries' oogonia, the spermatogonia keep reproducing themselves for life. They are nurtured in the tubules by supporting cells, the **Sertoli cells**. The Sertoli cells in fetal life produce "anti-Müllerian hormone," which stops the male fetus from developing fallopian tubes, a uterus and a vagina.

Between the tubules are the "interstitial" cells, or **Leydig cells**, which make testosterone. In the fetus, enough of the mother's hCG (which stimulates Leydig cells to make testosterone in the same LH-like way it stimulates the mother's corpus luteum to make progesterone) gets into the developing testes for lots of testosterone to be produced. (It is not until puberty that the Leydig cells will become comparably active again.) Fetal testosterone has important effects on the developing brain (the brains of boys really are different from those of girls from this early time!), as well as on the internal sex glands and ducts. Externally, after conversion in the skin to **dihydrotestosterone** (DHT), fetal testosterone causes what would otherwise be the labia (which in girls lie on each side of the opening to the vagina) to first fuse together into a scrotum and then bring the urethra out to the tip of the phallus.

At puberty, as testosterone increases, a proportion of the spermatogonia in the tubules of the testes begins entering meiosis as **primary spermatocytes**; the first meiotic division then produces twice this number of **secondary spermatocytes**; the second meiotic division doubles the cells again, but now with just half the number of chromosomes in cells called **spermatids**. Thus spermatids contain the haploid number of chromosomes (23), and typically eight spermatids will have come from one diploid (46-chromosome) spermatogonium, all lying as a cluster of still-connected round-shaped cells, enveloped by the arms of a Sertoli cell. With nurture from the Sertoli cell, each spermatid will evolve into a **spermatozoon**.

## Meanwhile, Back in the Male

The testes (singular, **testis**) in boys and men also begin to function during fetal life, when the male sex hormone **testosterone** is responsible for the normal de-

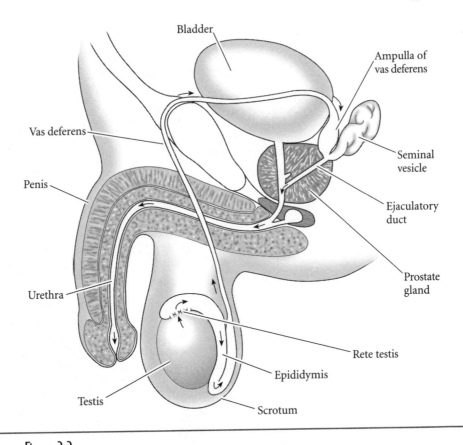

**Figure 3.3**   Male sex organs. On each side in a man, the testis, rete testis, epididymis and vas deferens transmit sperm cells (arrows) to the ampulla of the vas and the ejaculatory duct, located within the prostate gland, to await ejaculation. At ejaculation, secretions from the seminal vesicles and the prostate gland are added to the sperm cells to form the semen, which spurts out through the urethra.

velopment of the male sex glands and ducts, as shown in Figure 3.3. But mature sperm, like mature eggs, do not get made and released until puberty.

The **spermatozoon** is a long slender cell with chromosomes packed tightly into the sperm head and is equipped with a tail to propel it. The process by which the elongated spermatozoa are formed from the round precursor cells, with their loosely packed chromosomes in a conventional, round nucleus, is called **spermiogenesis**. A tubule of the testis at any place along its length or

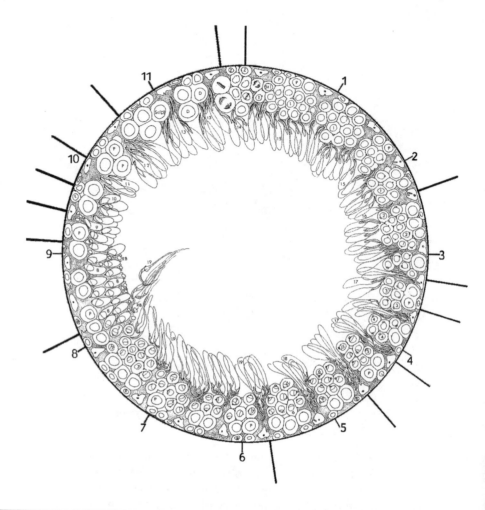

**Figure 3.4** Spermatogenic waves. Spermatogenesis is the process in mammals (in this case the rat) by which dividing spermatogonia in the tubules of the testis continuously produce sperm cells. The process is set out here as a clock, with maturation through four layers proceeding clockwise for four revolutions. In reality, one cut across a tubule will usually all be at the same stage (one sector or slice of the clock), and what is shown here going clockwise around the diagram would actually be occurring down the length of the tubule. The release of mature sperm in this way runs down the tubule, producing a spermatogenic wave—a perpetual moving harvest of mature sperm. Mature sperm leave one spot in the tubule of the rat every 14 days (thus, in the diagram it takes 14 days to move around the clock once), which means it takes 56 days for a newly formed spermatocyte to leave the tissue as a spermatozoon. In humans the "clock" (i.e. the spermatogenic wave) lasts 12 days.

## Sperm in the Epididymis

From the hundreds of tubules in the testis, the sperm cells are pushed into several very fine ducts, the **efferent ducts**, lying in a connector called the **rete testis**, to enter the epididymis (see Figure 3.3). The epididymis lies just next to the testis, in the scrotum, and is a single, long, coiled duct that would measure about six meters if uncoiled. It connects with the **vas deferens**, a tube that takes the sperm up out of the scrotum to meet the male accessory glands, the **seminal vesicles** and the **prostate gland**, just below the bladder. Here the semen is formed and stored, to be passed into the urethra at ejaculation.

The sperm cells in the rete testis and the upper epididymis are as unpurposeful as newborn ponies, staggering about in bewilderment, flicking their newfound tails about. Farther down the epididymis they will mature, but they will also be coated in special proteins that keep them subdued. As sperm come out of the epididymis and into the vas deferens (the long duct from the scrotum to the urethra), sperm will be mixed with the other components of **semen** (the fluid from the prostate and the seminal vesicles) and stored until ejaculation. The sperm should have good motility for up to a week or two, but the epididymal proteins are there to stop them from slipping into energy-expensive hyperactivity. Such hyperactive motility is what they will eventually need to force their way through the layers around an ovulated egg.

around its circumference will contain four generations of developing sperm cells. Pick any sector of the tubular clock stylized in Figure 3.4, and that sector will push out a new batch of sperm every 12 days, which means that it takes 48 days for a sperm cell to form. The sperm will spend yet another 14 days or more in the duct of the **epididymis** (see Figure 3.3) to mature before ejaculation sends it and millions of its fellows on their way. It is important to know this, because if a man has a severe illness, such as influenza, a single episode can disturb sperm production for more than two months.

At sexual intercourse, the sperm cells are ejaculated into the vagina, where the semen—the fluid holding the sperm and ejaculated by the man—comes into close contact with the mucus of the **cervix**. At ovulation the **cervical mucus** is receptive to the sperm, which can survive in it for several days or more, a steady stream being released upward through the uterus and out along the fallopian tubes.

# The Fallopian Tube, the Uterus and the Cervix

To understand what happens next, we turn now to the organs concerned—the fallopian tube, the uterus and the cervix.

## The Fallopian Tube

The fallopian tubes connect the cavity of the abdomen (the **peritoneal cavity**, in which the ovaries lie) with the cavity of the uterus (the **endometrial cavity**). The fallopian tubes in a woman thus link the abdominal cavity, by way of the uterine cavity, the cervix and the vagina, with the world outside the body. By conducting eggs—or ova—from the ovary ultimately to the outside, the fallopian tube earns its other name, the "oviduct."

Each fallopian tube (see Figure 3.5) is about 10 to 12 centimeters long and consists of an outer, wide, thin-walled part, the **ampulla**, close to the ovaries, leading to an inner, much narrower, more muscular part, the **isthmus**, close to the uterus. The isthmus connects to the narrowest part of all, the **interstitial segment**, which passes for one to two centimeters through the wall of the uterus to join the cavity of the uterus. The fallopian tube is lined by two types of cells: secretory cells, which produce mucus, glucose and other substances important for nourishing the egg and embryo, and ciliated cells, which bear tiny hairlike structures, the **cilia**, beating in the direction of the uterus and carrying the still-sticky cumulus mass down the ampulla soon after ovulation toward the junction between the ampulla and the isthmus.

It is at the fallopian tube's **ampullary-isthmic junction** that **fertilization** takes place. The fertilized egg stays at the ampullary-isthmic junction for two to three days before the tubal isthmus loses its dense secretions, and the muscle in its wall relaxes, enabling the early embryo, now rid of its cumulus cells, to reach the uterus. The hormone that causes these changes in the tube is progesterone.

## The Uterus

The uterus consists of a body (the uterine **fundus**) and a neck (the cervix), which joins it to the vagina. Its lining, called the **endometrium**, grows to be one centimeter in thickness, as seen on an ultrasound scan. The wall of the uterus, the **myometrium**, is muscular and about two centimeters thick. Outermost is a slippery layer similar to that which coats all the internal organs, the uterine **serosa.** As shown in Figure 3.5, the endometrial or uterine cavity is an upside-

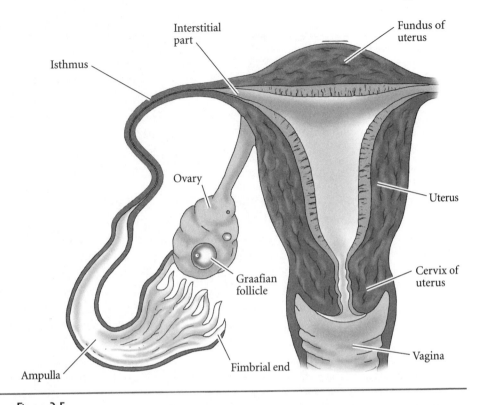

**Figure 3.5**   Internal female sex organs. The fallopian tubes connect the ovary on each side to the uterus (just one side is shown). The ovulating Graafian follicle releases the egg in its cumulus to the fimbrial end of the tube, from where it is carried quite quickly (half an hour) to the junction of the ampulla (which is wide) and the isthmus (which is narrow). Fertilization of the egg by sperm and cleavage of the pre-embryo occur at this ampullary-isthmic junction. Several days later, the developing pre-embryo is admitted to the uterus, where it will implant, about a week after fertilization.

down triangle in shape, with the tubes coming in on each side at the top; it is also flat, with the front and the back surfaces touching.

The endometrium grows under the influence of estrogen during the ovary's follicular phase; in the uterus we therefore call this the **proliferative phase**, and the uterus is lined then by "proliferative endometrium." During the ovary's luteal phase, progesterone causes the endometrium first to stop growing and then to make carbohydrate-rich secretions probably needed by an implanting embryo; in the uterus this is therefore the **secretory phase**, and the uterus is lined by "secretory endometrium."

The sequence of changes in the endometrium, particularly in the secretory phase, is ordered. The first noticeable change, two days after ovulation (or day 16 of a typical 28-day cycle), is for secretion to be visible in the endometrial gland cells under the nucleus ("subnuclear vacuolation"). By day 18 secretion fills the cells and appears within the glands themselves, and by day 21 there is a lot of watery-looking material in the **endometrial stroma** between the glands. Then, on day 24, the stromal cells get plumper, first around the spiral arteries of the endometrium, and then more generally, to the virtual point of confluence, which is a state called the **predecidual reaction** in a nonpregnant cycle and that can go on to a fully developed **decidual reaction** if pregnancy happens.

This sequence ticks like clockwork, to the point where a snapshot biopsy of the endometrium can tell a pathologist to within a day or two of how long it has been since ovulation occurred (or, more precisely, since exposure to progesterone began). If at the end of a cycle a well-developed predecidual reaction is seen on a biopsy, it can safely be inferred that the corpus luteum has produced enough progesterone, and for long enough, for pregnancy to have been possible, at least as far as the endometrium is concerned.

But, also like a clock, the endometrium will not tick backward. If the endometrium is too developed for an embryo, then bad luck, because it will not wait and the embryo cannot catch up. This could be one reason why **in vitro fertilization** (IVF) embryos sometimes have trouble implanting (which is discussed in Chapter 20). On the other hand, if the embryo is ahead of the endometrium, it *can* probably wait for the endometrium to catch up. Exploiting this difference is a current avenue for IVF research.

When estrogen levels, and especially progesterone levels, fall at the end of the ovarian cycle (see Figure 3.2), the endometrium breaks down and bleeds. This is the **menstrual phase**, during which FSH production in the pituitary gland rises to capture a new cohort of developing follicles, and a new follicular phase starts in the ovary.

## The Cervix

The cervix of the uterus does not show the same striking changes through the cycle as the endometrium, but it does have important responses. One of the jobs the cervix has is to keep sperm out if there is no egg present to be fertilized higher up. In the follicular phase, under the effect of estrogen, the cervix opens, and the mucus becomes greater in amount, wateriness, stretchability (**Spinn-barkheit**) and ferning (or forming a fernlike pattern when it is dried on a microscope slide) and, most important, in its receptiveness to and penetrability by sperm. If estrogen levels fall—or if progesterone is produced to counteract the effect of estrogen—these changes are all soon reversed and the mucus tightens up. Very soon into the luteal phase, therefore, the mucus in the cervix once more keeps sperm out.

# Conception

Of the millions of sperm deposited in the vagina during sex, perhaps fewer than 200 reach the fallopian tube. There may not be more than ten sperm in the ampulla at the time the egg is fertilized. We suspect that the tube does a lot to move the egg and the few sperm into close contact for fertilization to become probable, but we do not know how it does it. Fertilization needs to take place within about ten hours of ovulation for the embryo to develop normally, so it is best if the first sperm can get to the tube before the egg arrives.

Ejaculated sperm are motile, but they are inhibited from displaying their peak performance by a surface layer of protein molecules (see the box "Sperm in the Epididymis"); if the proteins were not there, the sperm would run out of steam too fast. The effect of taking off these brakes is to power up the sperm's swimming speed and to give the cell membrane over the sperm head the stickiness the sperm needs to cling to the egg's outermost membrane—in all, a process called **capacitation**. Sperm that are being stored in receptive mucus in the cervix are usually not yet in a capacitated state. Capacitation can happen naturally, by having the sperm swim up through the uterus and out along the tube, or it can be made to happen in the laboratory, by spinning and washing the sperm through a series of solutions.

# Fertilization

The ovulated egg has several layers that the capacitated sperm needs to power through, shown in Figures 3.6a and 3.7. First there is the jellylike cumulus, which the sperm likes to get its tail into (the beating sperm tail gets a better grip

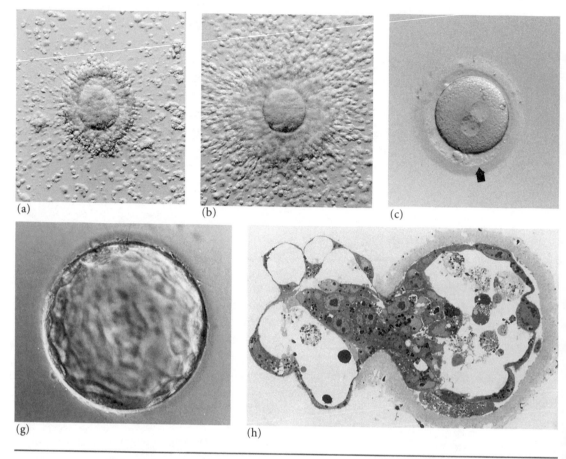

(a)  (b)  (c)

(g)  (h)

# Figure 3.6 Eggs and early embryos: (a) an immature egg derived from an immature follicle,

with the cumulus cells packed tightly around the egg; (b) a mature egg derived from a mature follicle, just before ovulation; the cumulus cells now have space between them, and the cumulus is said to be "expanded"; (c) a fertilized egg, or zygote, at 20 hours; there are two pronuclei, one female and one male; the arrow points to the zona pellucida (which is masked by cumulus cells in a and b); (d) a four-cell pre-embryo at 40 hours—the stage of the pre-embryo in special need of research; (e) a morula—a solid ball of about 16 cells; this is as far as the pre-embryo develops in the tube; (f) an early blastocyst; a fluid-filled cavity has formed, leaving a group of cells to one side (arrow) that are now destined to form the embryo itself; (g) an expanded blastocyst, poised to "hatch" through its now very thin stretched zona; the cells of the embryo are out of focus in the center; (h) a hatching blastocyst, escaping through a gap in the zona, seen in cross-section by electron microscopy. After hatching is complete, the blastocyst will attach to the lining of the uterus in preparation for implantation. If the blastocyst splits into two during the process of hatching, identical twins can result. (Photos a-g by Rosemary Cullinan, Sydney IVF. Photo h by Professor Alex Lopata, Melbourne.)

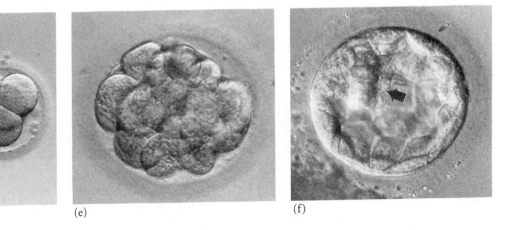

(d)                    (e)                              (f)

in the cumulus, propelling it forward more effectively). Second is a tough, glassy-looking membrane, the **zona pellucida** (Latin for "clear layer"), to which the sperm must successfully attach itself if it is to get through.

What happens next is complicated but important. The sperm cell up to this point has been wearing a crash helmet, the **acrosome**. Imagine pushing your fist into a soft balloon: the fist is the sperm head's nucleus (where its genetic material is packed densely into the 23 chromosomes); the balloon is the acrosome. The outside of the sperm head, provided the acrosome is intact (that is, the balloon has not popped), is specifically sticky for the zona pellucida—the way one side of Velcro is for its matching surface. The successful sperm binds tightly to the zona (see Figure 3.7). This causes the acrosome to break open, releasing, instead of air as a balloon would, a potent mixture of enzymes, which digest a path through the zona. These enzymes are helped by the capacitated sperm's forcefully beating tail, itself with a good grip in what is left of the cumulus. The process of the balloon bursting is called the **acrosome reaction**.

And so it is that the sperm, now bereft of its acrosome, finds itself next to the egg, within the **perivitelline space**; all it now needs to do is drift up to the "vitellus"—the egg itself. Now covering the acrosome-reacted sperm head is the inner layer of the acrosome, which, unlike the outer layers (now gone), is specifically sticky for the egg membrane. Contact is made and the trap is sprung (see again Figure 3.7).

Like nerve cells and muscle cells, the egg is electrically charged. The moment the sperm fuses with it an electrical signal causes several reactions inside the egg. Almost immediately (it takes about 15 seconds) the egg secretes what are called "cortical granules," which contain a mucus that fills the perivitelline space, smothering the egg membrane, and stopping any more sperm that might

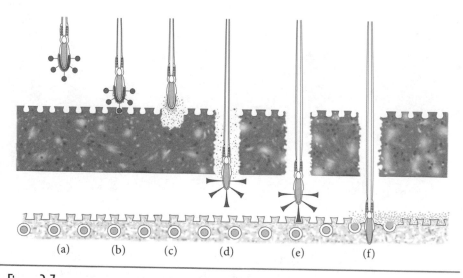

**Figure 3.7** Sperm attachment and fertilization of the egg: (a) the zona pellucida exhibits special binding sites complementary to those exhibited by the approaching, capacitated sperm cell; (b) binding between sperm cell and zona triggers the acrosome reaction in the sperm; (c) enzymes released from the acrosome digest a path through the zona; (d) the sperm cell, having penetrated the zona and entered the perivitelline space, has lost its plasma membrane and outer acrosomal membrane and now displays new binding sites complementary to those on the membrane of the egg; (e) binding of the sperm to the egg is followed by release of material from the egg's cortical granules into the perivitelline space; this released material will coat the egg to prevent further sperm from binding; (f) the sperm head, neck and part of the tail enter the egg to fertilize it.

be on their way in from attaching to the egg. If another sperm chances to reach the egg during this 15 seconds, more than one sperm will fertilize it and the embryo will be ruined by having at least 23 too many chromosomes—a process called **polyspermic fertilization**, or simply "polyspermy." At the same time, the egg finishes expelling its own extra chromosomes, reducing the number from 46 to 23, to match those of the sperm. Next, the machinery of the egg starts preparing it to become an embryo. In about 24 hours it will divide into two cells, then four cells, and so on.

The sperm head, now inside the egg, falls apart, revealing all as the egg strips it down to its chromosomes. This is no time for shyness! At no other point are the male's genes open to such scrutiny by his mate. Stripped bare, the egg fashions these male chromosomes to match its own; each set forms a watery blob

## Chromosomes and the Fate of Embryos

When the egg displays pronuclei it can be called a **zygote**, or even an **embryo**, although it is worth noting that traditionally trained embryologists would keep calling it an **ovum**, or egg, until well after implantation. Syngamy is soon followed by the first of a series of cell divisions called **cleavage**, which will result in a solid ball of cells, the **morula**, all kept together by the zona pellucida. A modern term for the ovum through these stages is **pre-embryo**, because all its cells are **totipotent**, each capable of producing, if isolated in appropriate circumstances, a whole new embryo.

Twins, incidentally, can come about in two ways. Either two eggs are ovulated and fertilized separately (nonidentical or **dizygotic twins**), or one egg is fertilized and at some stage, up to about the time of implantation, a group of cells splits off to form a separate embryo (identical or **monozygotic twins**). If the split happens late, monozygotic twins can share the same pregnancy sac and are called **mono-amniotic twins**. If such splitting off is incomplete there is the risk of Siamese (conjoined) twins.

Circumstances other than normal fertilization can result in cleavage. If the sperm head triggers the egg without managing to penetrate it, the essentially unfertilized but activated egg may start to develop but will display just one pronucleus;

sooner or later its development, called **parthenogenesis**, will be interrupted, probably well before implantation. If two sperm fertilize the egg, there will be three pronuclei, with 69 chromosomes (a **triploid** complement), and development will ultimately fail—but perhaps rather later, as a clinical miscarriage in which a partly formed fetus coexists with what is called a partial **hydatidiform mole**.

The female chromosomes are sometimes excluded completely. First, a single X-bearing (that is, female-determining) sperm can double itself in the egg, before undergoing syngamy. The result is a (46,XX) "complete" hydatidiform mole. If implantation occurs, there is no development of an embryo or fetus; instead, there is a grapelike bunch of swollen trophoblastic villi, which in a proportion of cases can become malignant. Second, two sperm can enter the egg and focus on each other, again ignoring the female chromosomes during syngamy—and resulting in a diploid product that can be 46,XX or 46,XY, but again completely paternal in origin. This is a less common form of complete hydatidiform mole. If both sperm engaging in male-male syngamy are Y-bearing (male-determining), or if a single Y sperm divides to attempt syngamy with itself, then the result (46,YY) is lethal straightaway and development stops.

within the substance of the egg (visible with the help of a microscope in Figure 3.6c)—the male and the female **pronuclei**. This is the first definite sign of fertilization for the watching scientist, and it is looked for in IVF laboratories between 16 and 20 hours after eggs are inseminated in vitro. The male and female pronuclei then join together so that the two sets of chromosomes can mingle and match, a process called **syngamy**. The chromosomes now number 46—the normal complement again. If the sperm had an X chromosome to pair with the egg's X chromosome, the resultant chromosome count, or **karyotype**, will be 46,XX (female); if the sperm had a Y chromosome, the resultant karyotype will be 46,XY (male). The fertilized egg then divides several times without increasing its overall size (see Figures 3.6d and 3.6e).

The developing embryo (or more accurately pre-embryo) enters the endometrial cavity three days after ovulation and fertilization. It is, or very soon will be, a **blastocyst**, a hollow ball of cells surrounding a cystlike cavity that will soon number a hundred or more cells (see Figure 3.6f ). As the blastocyst eases its way out of the now very thin and stretched zona pellucida (we do call it "hatching"), a few cells near its middle become dedicated to forming the embryo itself (see Figure 3.6h); the rest of the cells—by far the majority—constitute the **trophoblast** and will form the **placenta** and supporting membranes for the pregnancy. This is why many scientists like to refer to the stages so far as "pre-embryonic." The pre-embryo by now is already manufacturing that most "primitive" of the body's proteins, human chorionic gonadotropin (hCG), the signal that tells the corpus luteum to keep producing progesterone and that is, a little later, measurable in blood or urine (the usual basis for testing for pregnancy).

## Implantation

The blastocyst attaches to the endometrium on about day 21 of the menstrual cycle. It squeezes through the surface layer of the endometrium to lie within the endometrial stroma, the watery connecting substance between the endometrial glands, which is what we mean by **implantation**. Nutrition comes from secretions of the endometrial glands. The outer layer of the blastocyst, the trophoblast, is in touch with the mother's blood, so oxygen passes to the developing embryo. Sometimes as the blood first bathes the embryo (on about day 26 of the cycle), a small amount of blood leaks out of the uterus into the vagina, which is called **implantation bleeding**; if it occurs it is nearly always much lighter than a menstrual period. By day 28 a pregnancy test, set to measure hCG levels greater than 50 units in blood, will be positive.

The stroma of the endometrium reacts to the presence of the pregnancy and to the continued production of progesterone from the corpus luteum in the ovary by forming a thick, cell-filled layer called the **decidua** (because, like the leaves of a deciduous tree, it will, eight or nine months later, be shed from the uterus at delivery along with the placenta as part of the afterbirth). The modified stromal cells, now called decidual cells, produce at least two important hormones, relaxin, which helps stop the uterus from contracting prematurely, and **prolactin**, which in this location helps control the shifting of fluid into the **gestational sac**, the bag of fluid surrounding the embryo inside the pregnancy membranes.

# Early Pregnancy

By the time of the missed menstrual period, the embryo itself has begun to form, but it will be another week before its gestational sac becomes visible on ultrasound. It will be yet another few days before the detection of a beating heart can confirm the presence of an embryo (see Figure 3.8a ). A pregnancy sac can grow without an embryo in it (Figures 3.8b and 3.8d ) but is destined to miscarry.

When the embryo is 28 days old, it will typically be six weeks from the **last menstrual period** (LMP), and we say the woman is six weeks pregnant. Such an embryo will show a number of human features. The embryo's head and the head-end structures develop before the tail-end structures. While the face (and the brain) are just beginning to form, the most obvious structures are the heart and a balloonlike extension to the embryo's gut, the yolk sac. Both the heart and the yolk sac are easily seen at this stage on ultrasound (as shown in Figure 3.8a). The heart beats fast, about 140 beats per minute.

The embryo needs a big heart to move the earliest kind of fetal blood between the embryo's tissues and the ever-more-distant developing placenta (see Figure 3.8c ), where the "extra-embryonic" (outside-the-embryo) capillaries are located in the **chorionic villi**. These tongues of afterbirth tissue (or trophoblast) lap a lake of maternal blood just on the embryo's side of the decidua, through which pass the mother's spiral arteries. By eight weeks from the last period, the embryo has taken on enough recognizable features to be called a fetus.

The red blood cells of the fetus at this early stage are made in the yolk sac. (Later, the manufacture of red blood cells moves to the developing liver and finally to the bone marrow.) Fetal red cells contain a special hemoglobin,

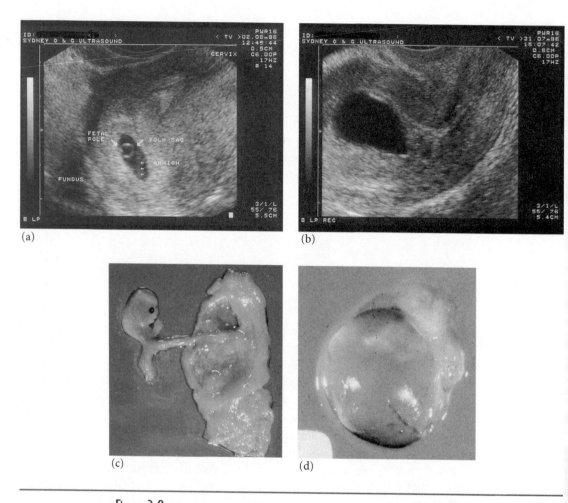

(a)　　(b)

(c)　　(d)

**Figure 3.8** Normal and abnormal pregnancy. An ultrasound view of pregnancy (a) less than six weeks from the last period shows the embryo, one quarter of a centimeter long, within the gestational sac. The beating heart is one of the most conspicuous, and important, features, but the fetus is dwarfed by its yolk sac; the gestational sac is surrounded by a bright decidual reaction. An ultrasound view of a six-week pregnancy that is destined to miscarry (b) shows an almost empty gestational sac surrounded by a poor decidual reaction. Miscarriage of an almost normally developed embryo and placenta (c), connected by the umbilical cord, shows the head and arms of the embryo have developed normally, but the tail end of the embryo has developed hardly at all. In such a situation, ultrasound may have recorded a beating heart prior to miscarriage. In a miscarriage of a blighted ovum (d), a gestational sac has formed, with membranes and placenta, but there has been no development of an embryo. Ultrasound examinations will not have disclosed a beating heart at any stage of the pregnancy. (Photos a and b by Dr. Jock Anderson, Sydney IVF. Photos c and d by Robert Jansen.)

## Trophoblast Stealth ...

Remember that half of the fetus's genetic endowment comes from the father, so the fetus is likely to differ from the mother in blood group, and almost certainly likely to differ significantly from the mother in its tissue groups. (Tissue groups or types, although more complicated to classify, are much like blood types, but are present on most of the body's cells; it is these tissue groups that doctors try to match for organ transplants.)

So why doesn't the fetus trigger an immune rejection reaction? The fetus uses a combination of passive and active measures to escape hostile immune attention. First, the fetus—and, way before it, the traveling sperm cell—is careful not to display its tissue groups on the surface of the trophoblast that faces the mother, where the immune system would see them. This is nature's non-radar-reflective stealth technology. Second, the early embryo produces a number of chemicals, possibly hCG itself, which in high concentrations numb the mother's immune system immediately around the embryo. Third, the lymphocytes (a type of white blood cell involved in immune recognition or sur-veillance) seem to assist. Lymphocytes are especially intrepid wanderers and snoopers and pass from mother to fetus and back again. These lymphocytes (by a process we completely fail to understand) will lead not to immune rejection of the fetus as foreign tissue but to an active "immune tolerance," by which the mother's immune system learns to accept her fetus as friendly.

### ... and Molecules We Never Forget

The primitive molecules produced by the fetus we have met so far include human chorionic gonadotropin (hCG) and alpha fetoprotein (AFP). They are produced so early that (especially for hCG) the body's cells do not forget how to make them. Thus, hCG and AFP are detectable in minute amounts throughout childhood and adult life. Occasionally, a cancer in adult life takes on the structure of trophoblast and produces lots of fully active hCG. Particularly rare tumors of the ovary mimic yolk-sac structures when looked at under the microscope; they are diagnosable in girls or young women by high levels of AFP in their blood.

called "fetal hemoglobin" (HbF), which binds oxygen more strongly than adult hemoglobin (HbA); thus, fetal hemoglobin is able to pull oxygen off maternal adult hemoglobin in the placenta. In the developing placenta, other nutrients are absorbed by the fetal circulation, while metabolic waste is passed over to the maternal circulation for excretion by the mother. In the yolk sac special **germ cells** have already been put aside; soon they move out into the developing ovaries and testes to form either eggs or sperm cells. Thus, the genetic line continues.

Fetal blood can give us useful glimpses of what is happening inside the gestational sac. Fetal blood has its own unique type of albumin—**alpha fetoprotein** (AFP). Fetal red cells, fetal hemoglobin and AFP, to a small extent, all leak across the chorionic villi of the placenta into the mother's blood, where they can be detected, measured or analyzed to give diagnostic information about the fetus. The chorionic villi of the trophoblast are diagnostically important more directly. This is the tissue we take samples of to look at the fetus's chromosomes in **chorionic villus sampling** (CVS). The chorionic villi also produce hormones, including "human chorionic somatomammotropin," which robs energy stores from the mother to benefit the fetus, and progesterone, which by about week eight of pregnancy takes over from the ovary's progesterone, allowing the mother's corpus luteum to be dispensed with.

The fetus, hopefully welcome, has thus positioned itself after a successful conception as snugly as any well-adapted parasite. But, like a more ordinary parasite, the fetus is biologically a friendly foreigner to its host.

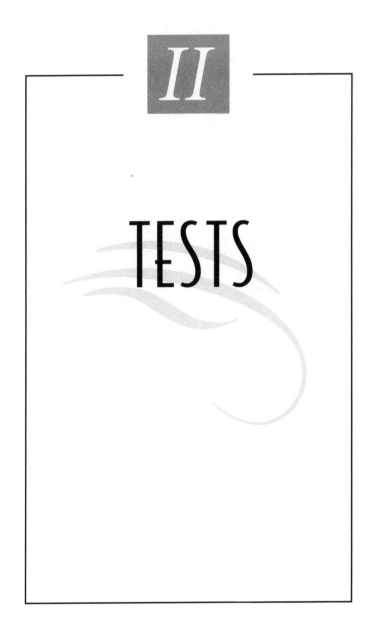

# II

# TESTS

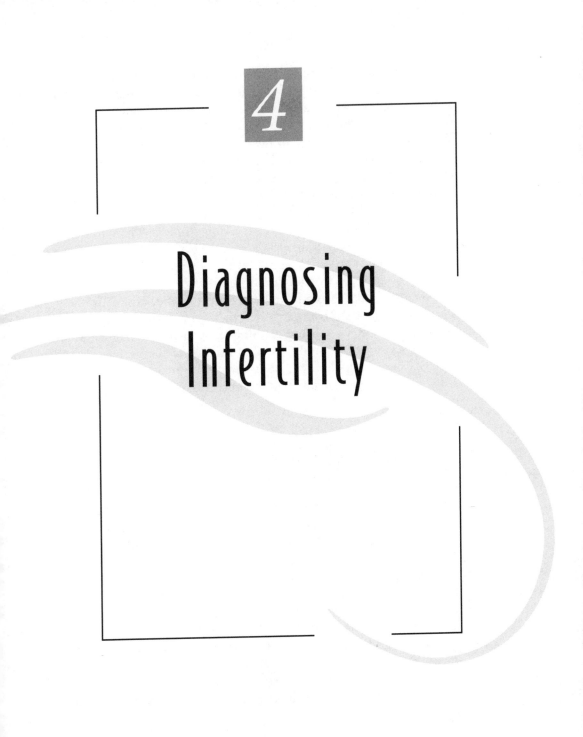

# 4

# Diagnosing
# Infertility

There are just four things that stop a woman from getting pregnant: too few normal **sperm** reaching the fallopian tube after intercourse; too few normal **eggs** leaving the ovaries; a **fallopian tube** blockage stopping egg from meeting sperm, and an **embryo**, because of a lack of oomph or too severe a barrier, unable to implant in the lining of the uterus, the endometrium.

The standard tests that distinguish these causes are a **sperm count**; a **post-coital test** (PCT); a measurement on about day 21 of the cycle of the **serum progesterone** (the amount of the hormone **progesterone** in the serum of the blood, which tells us if **ovulation** has occurred); and a test of tubal and endometrial function—either a **laparoscopy** (often with a **hysteroscopy**) or sometimes a **hysterosalpingogram** (HSG). These tests and others are explained in this chapter. With the exception of the laparoscopy and hysteroscopy, these tests can be arranged by your family physician.

We often make decisions about treatment on the basis of just these tests and the tests are thus done concurrently. If they are abnormal or equivocal, more detailed testing follows. Chapter 5 will discuss further testing if the preliminary tests appear to show an abnormality capable of preventing pregnancy completely. Chapter 6 looks at further testing if the preliminary tests are normal or if they show an abnormality that might still allow pregnancy to take place.

# Sperm Counts and Mucus Testing

A sperm count can be either the simplest or the most difficult of tests, depending on how cooperative a male partner is and, separately, how easy or hard it is for him to masturbate to provide the needed sample of semen (see the box "Doing What?"). The specimen also needs to be examined reasonably quickly, and generally during the ordinary working hours of the lab. He may need help from the female partner to overcome any of these difficulties.

Laboratories will stress the need for the specimen to be complete, that is, for none of the ejaculate to be lost. A Sydney sperm expert, Dr. John Tyler, has shown that under stress an ejaculate may be very unrepresentative, mainly because its volume will be low and sperm from the vas deferens may not be ejected into the semen effectively. An artificially low count can result, so a low sperm count always warrants that the test be repeated, under better circumstances, if there was stress during the first ejaculation.

Whether in a sterile container available from the laboratory or in a Silastic condom, the specimen should reach the lab within an hour or so. Keep it at or-

## Doing What?

"Yuckie poo!" is what I heard a man exclaim when one of my mentors in the 1970s detailed the need for a sperm count by collecting a semen sample—by masturbation into a clean, sterile, wide-open collecting jar after one, two or three days of no ejaculation. I thus had an insight into how overresponse to an indiscretion, presumably from the boy's parents, had caused a scar. Such social conditioning on the evils and perils of masturbation is fortunately very rare nowadays, notwithstanding the sin of Onan and its broad interpretation in some religions to mean that no semen be produced intentionally that does not enter a vagina. In Genesis, disobedient Onan was struck dead by God for spilling his semen onto the ground instead of into his brother's wife, after he had been told by his father Judah to get her pregnant on behalf of his dead brother. The religious systems that still insist on such biological and social folly are patriarchal to the extreme.

Still, not every male is experienced with masturbation. Producing a sample of semen on demand can be easier said than done, especially in an unfamiliar room and especially if there is not a total sense of privacy and security. Most modern assisted conception programs have well-designed, soundproof facilities, where the wife or female partner may also be present. Erotic literature helps some men, but not all. At Sydney IVF we make whisky, wine and beer available to help ease the tension.

An acceptable alternative to masturbation is to collect semen during sex using a special condom made of Silastic, which is a completely inert plastic. Ordinary condoms are usually toxic to sperm cells. Silastic condoms are thick and insensitive. One religiously correct version has a tiny opening in the tip to avoid (just!) the contraceptive sin of Onan.

How long do you need to wait after a prior ejaculation to have a sperm count done? Not long, but probably at least 24 hours. Do not wait more than four or five days, however, unless you are especially asked to; sperm movement, or **motility**, does not last forever in the male reproductive organs once the sperm have passed through the **epididymis**. Sometimes a very short interval is unavoidable, particularly when there is an unexpected shortfall in sperm cells at the time of an egg pickup procedure for assisted conception.

dinary room or body temperature to preserve the sperm's motility. Sometimes it is important for the sperm to be fresher than this, especially if the sperm count is known to be low and the sample is to be used for special diagnostic or therapeutic maneuvers. In such cases the semen is best collected at the IVF laboratory, which will have a special private area for doing so.

A normal sperm count will have an overall volume of at least one milliliter, a sperm density of more than 20 million sperm per milliliter, a motility of 50 percent or better (the percentage of sperm cells present that are moving, preferably purposefully) and a proportion of abnormal forms (odd-shaped heads, deformities of the midpiece and abnormalities of the tail) at less than about 50 percent (or, using the World Health Organization's so-called "strict criteria" for normal sperm appearance, there should be better than 14 percent of normal sperm forms). But these are mostly arbitrary figures. Some couples have no trouble getting pregnant with much lower sperm counts. Dr. Sherman Silber, a urologist and world leader in male infertility, has shown that almost no sperm count above a complete absence of sperm is so bad that pregnancy is impossible. Ultimately, it does just take one sperm to make it.

We can get a better idea of sperm function in practice by looking at sperm in the mucus of the cervix after sexual intercourse. This is the postcoital test (PCT) or Sims-Huhner (or just Huhner) test. Remember, however, that mucus in the cervix is only receptive to sperm during ovulation. To do a PCT at any other time is meaningless, because the normal result will be negative (a **negative test** shows no sperm or no motile sperm; a **positive test** shows more than five normally motile sperm per microscopic field of examination).

Indeed, it is so important to time the test correctly that at Sydney IVF we always measure **serum estradiol**, serum progesterone and **serum LH** when a PCT is done. Referring to Figure 3.2 (in Chapter 3), at ovulation the estradiol should be high, luteinizing hormone (LH) should be high, and progesterone should be low; if not, the test is being done too early or too late, or the ovulation is not strong enough for the PCT to be informative. The cervix and its mucus should also look receptive: (1) the cervix should be open; (2) the volume of mucus should be good (every woman will be different for both these parameters, but they will be consistent in one woman from ovulation to ovulation); (3) the mucus should be clear, watery and stretchy; and (4) the mucus should produce a complete ferning pattern when it is allowed to dry on a microscope slide. An **Insler score** (named after the infertility specialist who devised it) awards points from zero to three for each of these four parameters, the last two of which should really score three out of three.

If the PCT is positive, then we can forget about this aspect of getting pregnant. If the PCT is negative—and it was done during a good ovulation—then it gets complicated. Some infertile couples will go straight to **assisted conception** at this point (see Chapter 20) because of the practical difficulty there can be in sorting out the cause, or, second, because the treatment for whatever is found is often not successful. In fact, many couples will quite correctly opt for assisted conception whether the PCT is positive or negative, with the form of assistance decided by the sperm count (and whether or not there are antibodies to sperm present anywhere, which is discussed in Chapter 6).

What could be the causes of a negative PCT carried out during a normal ovulatory cycle on the day of ovulation? (I also discuss this in Chapter 6.) In practice, the complexities of timing the PCT, the indirectness of the limited information it provides and the probability of recourse to treatment such as IVF irrespective of its result mean that many physicians dispense with it in their infertility workup.

# Tests for Ovulation

Strictly, the only ways of being sure ovulation has taken place are by seeing the egg outside the ovary or by inferring it got out of the follicle because pregnancy occurred. Neither of these is usually very practical in investigating infertility. Generally, we rely on indirect evidence of ovulation, namely detecting the production of progesterone from the ovary after ovulation has taken place.

A single serum progesterone taken in the middle of the luteal phase may be all that is needed to be practically sure that ovulation is taking place; at that time

## Fake Ovulation

It is possible for a follicle to form a **corpus luteum** and make progesterone without the egg escaping from it. This is the **luteinized unruptured follicle** (LUF). It is detectable on careful ultrasound and hormone monitoring of ovulation. Instead of the follicle collapsing or apparently disappearing on serial ultrasound examinations of the ovary, it keeps getting bigger as progesterone production gets under way; typically, blood tests of progesterone start to go up while the follicle on ultrasound grows to 2.5 centimeters or more in diameter. The progesterone produced in that cycle may be less than in an ovulatory cycle; the length of the **luteal phase** may be less than the normal 11 to 16 days, and, of course, no egg is released to enable conception to take place. How often this happens normally is an open question. It is more common in **oligomenorrhea** and perhaps in **endometriosis**, both discussed in other parts of the book, and it may be part of what is sometimes called corpus luteum deficiency or **luteal phase defect**.

A good way of estimating the adequate length and degree of progesterone's action is through a **premenstrual endometrial biopsy**, which should show a **predecidual reaction** (see Chapter 3). These biopsies are often done as office procedures, with a thin endometrial biopsy curette that can be passed through an undilated cervix. But the procedure is painful, briefly. The chance of an early pregnancy being disturbed by taking the biopsy is small, but it can happen, so if a biopsy is planned, either as an isolated test or in conjunction with a laparoscopy, pregnancy should be avoided during the cycle when the test is performed. The advantage of a premenstrual biopsy for estimating the adequacy of progesterone production is that it looks directly at the accumulated effect of its action where it counts, in the endometrium. If the biopsy is normal, then whatever the blood levels of progesterone might have been during that cycle are not so important.

it should be more than 12 nanograms per milliliter (or more than 35 nanomoles per liter, depending on which units are reported by the lab). Preferably, there should also be some sign that the length of the luteal phase is at least 11 days, seen perhaps on the temperature chart and perhaps by remembering how many days separate clear symptoms of ovulation (such as ovulation pain or detecting the **LH surge** with a home-testing kit) and the start of the following period. In some situations more than one measurement will be useful in estimating the duration and extent of progesterone's rise.

The place of the sometimes irksome **basal body temperature** (BBT) chart in modern infertility treatment is still debated. There are clear cases when it is useful—and it is always cheap! I advocate it when ovulation itself is in doubt or under investigation and I am not monitoring the events of ovulation more exactly with blood tests and ultrasounds (see Chapter 10 for a discussion of induction of ovulation). A series of charts over several months can indicate when ovulation probably took place. This information can then be used to schedule having sex. Once the temperature is up, ovulation is over and done with for that cycle.

Where should the temperature be taken? Without a doubt a clearer pattern comes from measuring pelvic temperature by placing the thermometer in the vagina than if temperatures are taken in the mouth. But oral BBT charts can be revealing enough if taking the temperature in the vagina is awkward. (I know of no patients who prefer to use the thermometer in their rectum, so this now

## Why a Higher Temperature?

The rise in BBT with ovulation reflects the action progesterone has on the temperature regulating centers in the **hypothalamus** in the brain. Progesterone is an old molecule in nature, being found in fish, where it seems to have no special purpose except as a precursor for other hormones. In mammals, nature has employed progesterone as the hormone that sustains pregnancy. You may therefore presume that the evolution of progesterone's action on temperature was not just an accident—that it is an advantage for the embryo and then the fetus to be in a somewhat warmer internal environment than is the case before ovulation.

would seem old-fashioned.) Remember, too, that a thermometer for measuring the BBT, in order to be sensitive enough, should not have the wider range of clinical thermometers, which are designed to detect a fever. You can buy a basal body thermometer at any drugstore.

## Tests for Blockages

The most common place where a blockage keeps egg and sperm apart is in the fallopian tubes. There are two main ways that the tubes can be checked to see if they are open, or "patent" (called **tests for tubal patency**): by X-ray, or hysterosalpingogram, and by laparoscopy. Laparoscopy also enables endometriosis to be diagnosed, which gives it a special advantage (see Chapters 14 and 15 for more on endometriosis). Unfortunately, neither test provides all the information some situations demand, so at times it is wise to do both.

Laparoscopy is an operation, usually carried out under full, or general, anesthesia, in which a fiber-optic device (the laparoscope) about 1 centimeter in diameter is passed into the abdomen through a small cut in the navel (umbilicus). When investigating tubal blockages, a blue-colored dye is first instilled through the cervix into the cavity of the uterus. If everything is normal, the dye is then seen at laparoscopy to run from there out through the ends of the tubes. Laparoscopy takes about 20 minutes if it is done for diagnosis. Some conditions, such as endometriosis, may be able to be treated at once through the laparoscope.

## Minilaparoscopy—for a Minilook

Developments in finer laparoscopes, just a millimeter or two in diameter, are tempting gynecologists and patients into having this diagnostic operation using local anesthesia instead of general anesthesia. While exciting as a development for answering the simple question "Are the fallopian tubes free and patent?," I doubt that anything but the grossest endometriosis would be reliably detected. My personal preference is for diagnostic information to be as unequivocal as possible, and this means obtaining as good a view of the tubes and pelvic organs we can get. The minilaparoscope will not be replacing the conventional laparoscope in my practice any time soon.

Like all surgery, there are hazards, such as bleeding, infection or damage to an internal organ. The risk of these complications is low, usually less than one in a thousand, but can be higher in some conditions, such as when there has been extensive previous surgery.

A hysterosalpingogram (HSG) is an X-ray of the uterus and fallopian tubes. Some gynecologists carry out HSGs themselves, but nowadays most HSGs are performed by radiologists. Just about everyone who has had one says it hurts, but it is rarely practical to offer general anesthesia, mainly because the best X-ray machines are not portable enough to move into an operating room, where high standards of safety with anesthesia can be expected. The pain, somewhat like period pain, should not last longer than the time it takes for the X-rays to be taken. It is worth taking an analgesic two hours before and again about 20 minutes before the HSG is due to be done; whatever over-the-counter medication works for period pain will help.

The HSG proceeds with a vaginal examination carried out with a speculum (as when a Pap smear of the cervix is done). An instrument is fitted to the cervix by which some contrast medium (a liquid that is dense to X-rays and therefore visible) is slowly injected into the uterus and tubes. The test is judged normal if the medium passes out along the tubes, demonstrating no obstruction or significant irregularities, then into the abdomen, where it disperses among the intestines (see Figure 4.1).

There are two advantages that HSG has over laparoscopy. First, HSG shows the inside of the tubes in a way that cannot be inferred from looking at the outside of the tubes at laparoscopy; Figure 4.2 reveals an abnormal filigree pattern in the tube's lining that laparoscopy would miss. Second, when an oil-soluble contrast medium is used for HSG, Dr. Alan DeCherney at Yale University in the 1980s proved what gynecologists had long thought, that there are patients who go on to conceive after HSG who would not have otherwise become pregnant during this time. In other words, there is something about the oily HSG medium that improves fertility for about four months.

Infection is very rare after an HSG and the other tests of the fallopian tubes described in this section. If, however, there is already an infection present in the tubes, it will almost certainly be made worse. If there is a history of previous **salpingitis**, or if the doctor finds that the mucus in the cervix is yellow, then infection should be anticipated, a culture should be taken and antibiotics given before the test. Pain that persists or gets worse hours after the HSG should immediately prompt suspicion of infection and consideration of antibiotic treatment.

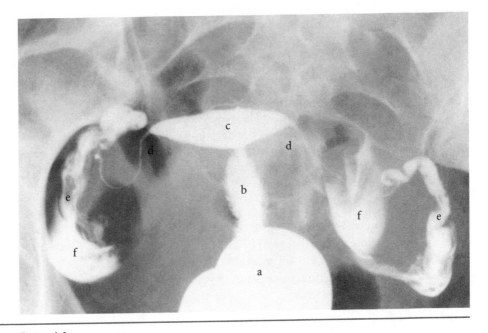

**Figure 4.1**   A normal hysterosalpingogram, or X-ray of the uterus and tubes. Appearing opaque (white) to X-rays are (a) the speculum in the vagina, (b) the cervix, (c) the triangular cavity of the uterus, (d) the narrow isthmus of the fallopian tube on each side, (e) the wider ampulla of the fallopian tubes, and (f) spill of the contrast dye out the end of the tube among the intestines.

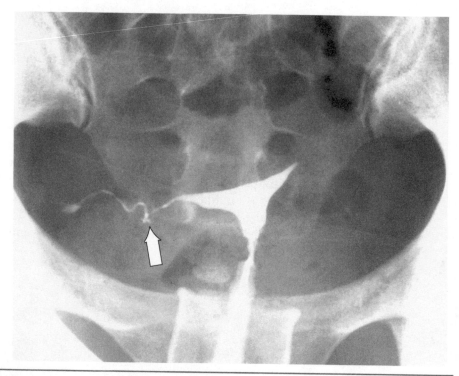

(a)

**Figure 4.2** An abnormal hysterosalpingogram taking place (a and b). The right tube (shown on the left side of the picture) reveals a filigree pattern developing in the isthmus of the tube, diagnostic of salpingitis isthmica nodosa (open arrows), and a dilated, smooth-outlined ampulla, characteristic of a hydrosalpinx (solid arrow). The opposite, left tube appears completely blocked.

Hysterosalpingography and laparoscopy complement each other in evaluation of tubal disease. Neither investigation is truly dispensable in planning a microsurgical approach to tubal blockage (see Chapter 12). A new investigation, **falloposcopy**, might end up replacing the HSG.

# Tests for Implantation

There are two sides to successful implantation of an embryo in the uterus—a competent embryo and a receptive and nutrient uterus.

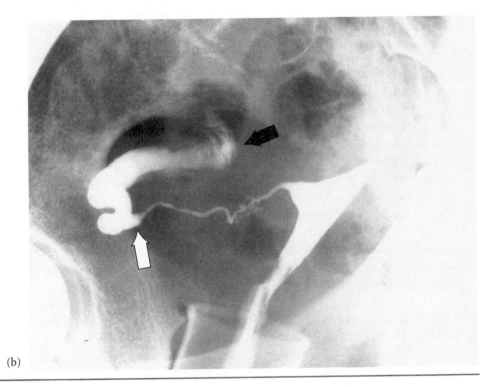

(b)

## Tests for the Embryo

The importance of the embryo's inner strength is shown by the ability it has to implant and, to some extent, to grow in many locations, some very abnormal and inhospitable, in the form of an **ectopic pregnancy** (discussed in Chapter 14). We need to remember, however, that the embryo developing in the fallopian tube or even in the ovary or abdomen often has its growth stunted. The embryo, or later the fetus, has formed itself abnormally. But this example from nature does demonstrate how an embryo that starts off vibrantly has much power to make its immediate environment provide it with what it needs.

We still have only very limited ways of testing for the health and viability of embryos **in vitro** (that is, in the laboratory) and virtually no ways of investigating embryos "in vivo" (that is, conceived and developing naturally in the fallopian tube). In vitro tests of embryo function are still firmly in the realm of embryo research (see the box "Properly Performing Embryos").

A modern way of carrying out an HSG is to pass a catheter into the opening of the tube into the endometrial cavity—a so-called **selective salpingogram**. Norman Gleicher, working in Chicago, has shown that a selective salpingogram, by increasing the pressure in the tube, may overcome a mild blockage in the tube's isthmus. Sometimes a catheter is passed through the blockage and the tube is opened. This is thus a second way that a salpingogram may be used to increase the chance of getting pregnant.

There are, however, disadvantages with hysterosalpingograms. The HSG is excellent at determining exactly where a tube is blocked, but if the tubes are open, it is not efficient at detecting adhesions on the outside of the tube, perhaps separating the tube from the ovary. I have already mentioned that endometriosis (often the main competing diagnosis) cannot usually be diagnosed without laparoscopy. I have also mentioned that the HSG is at best moderately uncomfortable and can at times be a painful experience. The fat-soluble medium can cause an inflammatory reaction in the abdomen in about 2 to 5 percent of people (this is rarely harmful, but it can be). The radiologist must also be careful that the fat-soluble medium does not enter blood vessels in substantial quantities, from where it might be transported to the lungs, causing breathlessness. A water-soluble medium is used by some radiologists because of its lesser tendency to cause reactions, but water-based mediums do not cause the improvement in fertility that results from oily HSGs.

## Tests for the Uterus

No single test tells us all we may need to know about the inside of the uterus. Having said that, however, the uterus is generally not as likely a place as the tubes for an abnormality. Abnormalities of the uterus can include uterine **fibroids**, **adenomyosis**, **intrauterine adhesions**, inflammation or infection of the endometrium (**endometritis**), **endometrial polyps** and **endometrial atrophy**. These conditions are described in Chapter 17. Occasionally an unsuspected but retained intrauterine device (IUD) causes apparent infertility.

The uterus can be inspected in several ways. Hysteroscopy is a fiber-optic examination of the uterine cavity by a hysteroscope, an instrument that looks like a short, thin laparoscope. It complements the HSG in revealing pathology that disturbs the shape of the endometrial cavity, especially adhesions (scar tissue between the front and the back surface of the cavity), fibroids projecting into the uterine cavity (**submucous fibroids**) and polyps. These can also show up on a HSG, although hysteroscopy is still needed to locate the pathology accurately and to deal with it. These conditions can thus often be treated during the diagnostic investigation, if it is carried out under anesthesia (often together with a laparoscopy); many gynecologists carry out hysteroscopy without anesthesia as an office procedure, using a thin hysteroscope that does not require the cervix to be dilated.

**Transvaginal ultrasound**, using a high-frequency probe, gives very clear images. Ultrasounds of the uterus done abdominally, through a usually uncomfortably full bladder, do not generally provide the detail needed for accurate diagnosis in the uterus. Transvaginal ultrasound allows the thickness and appearance of the endometrium to be followed through the menstrual cycle; it also allows polyps and endometritis to be suspected. Ultrasound also reveals changes in the **myometrium**, the muscle of the wall of the uterus; it is the best way of disclosing the position and size of uterine fibroids and may be the only way of suspecting adenomyosis (short of examining the whole uterus after a hysterectomy). A retained IUD is clearly seen by transvaginal ultrasound, even when it has lost its shadow, or opaqueness, to X-rays.

## Falloposcopy—A Fine View

Falloposcopy represents the present-day ultimate in exploring the inside of the body with fiber optics. Developed in Los Angeles by an Australian now in Adelaide, Professor John Kerin, falloposcopy uses a flexible scope less than a millimeter in diameter to image the lining of the tube. It enables adhesions to be seen within the tube that may not be detectable any other way. I have used it, for example, to show that a tube we had used twice without success in **gamete intrafallopian transfer** (GIFT) in fact was abnormal on the inside, when the other tube, although it had some adhesions around it, was normal on the inside; an HSG had not indicated an internal difference. When we switched sides for the GIFT procedure—just days after the falloposcopy—the woman conceived and had a healthy pregnancy in the uterus. It is clear that falloposcopy will add a new dimension to the information obtainable about the fallopian tube. It still remains to be seen if the images we get with it will replace the need for the HSG.

Available tests on preimplantational embryos presently include:

• Biopsies of cells for genetic analysis, developed by Dr. Alan Handyside and Professor Robert Winston and their colleagues at the Royal Postgraduate Medical School in Hammersmith, England. Remember that most embryos that miscarry do so because they have an incorrect number of **chromosomes**, usually revealed by a **karyotype**. But a karyotype is difficult to do on just one or two cells, so tests involving gene amplification using the **polymerase chain reaction** (PCR) were used instead in Handyside and Winston's series. Another, more reliable technique involves staining the cells with fluorescent chromosome markers, which show up as bright spots. This technique is called **fluorescent in situ hybridization** (FISH), so that seeing three colored spots for chromosome 21 (instead of two spots) means **Down's syndrome**, or **trisomy 21**. (Seeing two colored spots for the X chromosome means a female embryo.)

• Testing the inability of **follicle cells** to metabolize the adrenal gland hormone cortisol. Extra cortisol may be good for the egg just before it is ovulated, especially in stimulated cycles, and the test is for low levels of the enzyme 11ß-hydroxycortisol (which gets rid of cortisol) in cultured follicular cells. The people who discovered that only eggs from low-enzyme-level follicles in one series produced pregnancies have applied for a patent on this predictive test.

• Testing the integrity of the egg's (or embryo's) power supply, by sampling and

**Curettage** or **endometrial biopsy** reveals the tissue structure of the endometrium. We have considered this before in estimating normal ovulation, when this test is timed just before the date a period is expected. Biopsy can confirm the presence of endometritis, and this may be the only way this diagnosis is made; this is why it is usual, indeed almost invariable, for an endometrial biopsy to be done whenever there is the opportunity, such as during a laparoscopy.

In practice, we can assume that the uterus is doing its job properly for implantation if it is normal according to these conventional tests and if it is under the control of normal, ovulatory cycles from the ovary. It can be an advantage, at some stage of the investigations, to have a full curettage done, to ensure that the lining of the uterus is fresh.

## Properly Performing Embryos (concluded)

probing the **mitochondria** (see the box "How Eggs Get Their 'Use-By' Date: Mishaps in the Mitochondria" in Chapter 6). Genetic analysis of mitochondria is presently under development at Sydney IVF and elsewhere. It is a particularly promising method for assessing an egg or embryo's potential for growth, because accumulating injuries to an egg's mitochondria—especially its DNA—appear to lie at the heart of the way in which increasing age normally causes infertility well before menopause.

None of these tests is available yet for routine clinical work. Many IVF embryos that fail to implant can succumb simply because they are growing more slowly than the uterus is developing, so there is a mismatch. To a small extent we can tell how inherently healthy an embryo is by how quickly it is dividing, but there are many exceptions on each side. Some slowly growing embryos can, in a retarded uterus, do just fine; some fast-growing embryos may still not be normal. (The appearance of embryos most likely to be healthy is described in Chapter 20.)

One of the greatest challenges in embryo research today is to estimate in vitro the uptake of nutrients and the release of metabolic products of human embryos using microscopic measurements and to adapt this knowledge in order to develop embryo culture mediums that are at least as good for the embryo as the fallopian tube is for embryos in vivo. Active research programs are under way in the first of these areas in Great Britain.

## Your Road Map from Here

When you have had the tests described in this chapter, either an abnormality will be found, which means it is impossible to get pregnant without help (in which case read Chapter 5 and then whatever chapter is relevant to your diagnosis and its treatment), or there will be a more mild abnormality (or even no abnormality) found, which means pregnancy can still happen, but it has already taken too long (and perhaps time is getting short) and you would like to at least think about doing something (in which case read Chapter 6 and then the chapter on your diagnosis).

An endometrial biopsy timed for the end of the menstrual cycle, just before a period starts (a premenstrual endometrial biopsy), can reveal how normally the endometrium has responded to progesterone (see the box "Estimating Progesterone's Effectiveness" and Chapter 3). There should be, first, secretions in the glands (for nourishment) and, second, a predecidual reaction between the glands. For implantation to be successful, however, other things are needed. We think the endometrium needs to be capable of removing all the fluid from the uterine cavity (so that the front and back of the endometrium press onto the embryo). There is no routine test for this function, although researchers are looking with electron microscopes at the endometrial cells "drinking" the endometrial fluid by the process of pinocytosis, by which the cell takes small, membrane-bound "gulps" of fluid into its interior. The biopsy is usually normal however, and, as explained earlier, the common difficulty for IVF embryos is that endometrial development is happening too quickly rather than too slowly. Electron microscopy can also reveal what are called "tight junctions" between the surface cells of the endometrium, perhaps sometimes too tight to allow the embryo to squeeze past and to implant.

### D&Cs May Come Back into Fashion

When my colleagues and I were medical students, just about the only thing a family doctor could do—or did do—for infertility was a **dilation and curettage** (D&C), in which the lining of the uterus is scraped away and thereby forced to grow again. As students we could not see the logic for it, and because family doctors were not very adept at protecting their ideas against newly taught medical students, this (to us) rather drastic and senseless maneuver fell into disuse. Now, however, we are looking at it again. We suspect that after repeated menstrual cycles the surface lining of the endometrium is not necessarily shed or replenished from scratch; it may be that it accumulates too many tight junctions, binding individual cells together and ultimately resisting the implanting embryo. We are currently doing a study to see if curettage helps women get pregnant naturally or with assisted conception.

# When Natural Conception Is Not Possible

Once the basic tests described in Chapter 4 have been done, we know whether there are one or more obvious causes for not getting pregnant. This chapter covers the situations in which these tests show that pregnancy is, or seems to be, impossible the way things stand, that there is something wrong that no amount of time will overcome. Something has to be done—and usually can be—or there will definitely be no baby.

**Complete infertility**, sometimes called **sterility**, can be the case for these reasons: the **sperm count** shows an absence of sperm; **ovulation** is not taking place at all (this may have been suspected because there are no menstrual periods), or there is complete obstruction of both **fallopian tubes**. Let us consider these circumstances in turn and see how best to move forward.

# No Sperm Present

Very uncommonly, a sperm sample obtained for a sperm count under great stress can show a virtual exclusion of sperm, and, rarely, there just might have been a mix-up at the lab. Put simply, test results showing an absence of sperm, **azoospermia**, should mean examining a second specimen, just to be sure.

Confirming azoospermia is an upsetting event that can make a man feel isolated, bereft and withdrawn, often with transient **impotence** and an understandable loss of self-esteem. His partner may feel anger, guilt, and a wish to make reparations, often switching between these seemingly contradictory emotions but at times feeling them all at once. Sooner or later both will think about donor sperm and sperm banks (see Chapter 21). Using donated sperm will usually appeal sooner to the woman, but it is rarely a straightforward decision for either partner. Modern technology—the hope that emerging microsurgical or **in vitro fertilization** (IVF) techniques might work—has made it even less straightforward.

The two reasons azoospermia comes about are a blockage on each side between the **testes** and the **seminal vesicles**, usually in the **epididymis** or the **vas deferens**, and an absence of production of mature sperm in the tubules of the two testes, known as "maturation arrest." These conditions are discussed in greater detail in Chapter 9. Theoretically, and sometimes in practice, a blockage can be overcome, but it is rare for treatment to work if no mature sperm are being produced. It is therefore important to make the distinction.

The simplest way to find out if a blockage might be the cause for azoospermia is to measure **follicle stimulating hormone** (FSH) in the blood by a **serum**

FSH. (See the box "Follicle Stimulating Hormone in Men" in Chapter 9 for an explanation of this hormone's relevance.) For a complete picture, a **serum LH**, a **serum testosterone** and a **serum prolactin**, plus perhaps a **serum sperm antibodies** (also discussed in Chapter 9) should also be done. If the FSH level is increased, then there is irreversible damage to the tubules and no treatment is available. If the FSH is normal, then the cause might be an obstruction. A detailed review by a urologist skilled in infertility microsurgery in men is called for, including a **biopsy** of the testes to confirm that sperm production is in fact normal and that an obstruction must therefore be present (see Chapter 9). If the FSH is low, and especially if measurements of **luteinizing hormone** (LH) and testosterone are also low, then it can mean a loss of the pituitary gland's drive to the testes. Detailed review by a specialist endocrinologist or andrologist is then warranted, because the situation is potentially treatable with hormone injections.

Once an obstruction to sperm passage is confirmed, there are two ways in which pregnancy can be made possible—through **microsurgery** to excise the blocked part and join the two ends to overcome the obstruction permanently or through **microsurgical epididymal sperm aspiration**, from the epididymis or rete testis (the ducts between testis and epididymis) for assisted conception using IVF, usually with **sperm microinjection** (see Chapter 20).

When IVF is used to overcome infertility from an absence of sperm (see Chapters 9 and 20), it involves more physical involvement for the woman than assisted insemination with donor sperm. On the other hand, it will be the sperm of the man that the woman has chosen as a spouse or partner that will get her pregnant, not that of a stranger. Different couples will value the two sides to this equation differently. It is usual for the couple themselves to differ in their opinions; time, and a great deal of understanding, is needed to keep the relationship on an even keel. It helps most couples to be tactful but open about their thoughts, and skilled counselors (see Chapter 24) can help.

# No Ovulation

In contrast to an absence of sperm release, an absence of ovulation, or **anovulation**, is much less often due to a serious, untreatable abnormality. Chapter 4 explains how anovulation is diagnosed. To distinguish the different conditions that can be responsible, we measure serum FSH, LH, prolactin and testosterone, and usually what is called a **free androgen index**, which reflects biologically available testosterone, a more sensitive indicator of excess.

One of the causes of anovulation is **hypothalamic anovulation**, a relative or absolute lack of FSH produced by the pituitary gland to drive the ovaries' follicles, usually based on a lack of **gonadotropin-releasing hormone** (GnRH) drive of the pituitary gland from the **hypothalamus** (with the result that the serum FSH and serum LH will be normal to low). Other causes of anovulation include **hyperprolactinemia**, an increase in the production of prolactin by the pituitary gland (the serum prolactin is high), and the **polycystic ovary syndrome**, in which the pituitary hormone FSH is relatively normal or low, LH is usually high and testosterone production from the ovary can be increased (so serum FSH is normal to low, serum LH is normal to high, serum testosterone is normal to high and the free androgen index is increased).

In each of these conditions ovulation can be induced. Tablets of **clomiphene** will stimulate FSH production in at least some instances of hypothalamic anovulation and the polycystic ovary syndrome. Tablets of **bromocriptine** will treat hyperprolactinemia. Injections of **human menopausal gonadotropin** (hMG) or **recombinant follicle stimulating hormone** (rFSH) will work in any of these conditions, and **intravenous pulsatile GnRH** is extremely effective for hypothalamic anovulation. The individual conditions and these treatments are described further in Chapter 10.

It is only when there are no responsive follicles in the ovaries—that is, there is **primary ovarian failure** (meaning that the ovarian failure is not secondary to a problem mediated by the pituitary gland)—that ovulation cannot be induced with hormones or drugs. This diagnosis is pointed to by FSH levels that are high, particularly if high levels of serum FSH have been shown on more than one occasion. It means that the pituitary gland is trying to overcome—to compensate for—an absence of responsive follicles in the ovaries, which is just what happens naturally at menopause, when FSH levels in blood also get very high. A diagnosis of primary ovarian failure will be the case in 5 to 10 percent of patients under the age of 40 investigated for absent periods and absent ovulation. A symptom that might make the physician or woman suspect primary ovarian failure is the occurrence of menopause-like symptoms, including hot flashes. This condition and the place of a **biopsy of the ovary** are discussed further in Chapter 10.

Ovarian failure is as disappointing and devastating a diagnosis as sperm failure. It means that pregnancy can only be achieved by receiving a donated egg or embryo—programs that are more complicated to arrange than sperm donation programs. (Egg and embryo donation are discussed further in Chapter 22.)

# Blocked Tubes

When tubal blockages are detected at **laparoscopy** or with a **hysterosalpin-gogram** (HSG), as described in Chapter 4, whichever of these two tests that has not been done yet is usually performed to confirm tubal blockage. Why does tubal blockage need confirmation? There is a small chance that apparently blocked tubes at HSG are the result of spasm—painful contractions of the uterus that block the tubes where they pass through the wall of the uterus. In this case a **hysteroscopy** and laparoscopy can clarify the situation. Alternatively, at laparoscopy, performed under general anesthesia, there may have been technical difficulties injecting the blue dye that is used for testing patency of the tubes through the cervix, thus not getting enough pressure for it to pass down both tubes. Sometimes plugs of secretion may block the narrow isthmus of the tubes and may not have been overcome by enough pressure. A **selective salpin-gogram** may clarify these equivocal situations, and **falloposcopy** may also provide relevant information (see Chapter 4). A hysteroscopy is useful to show the anatomy of the points at which the tubes enter the cavity of the uterus.

Sometimes a very localized blockage close to the uterus can be overcome by passing a fine catheter through the blockage with the help of an X-ray or

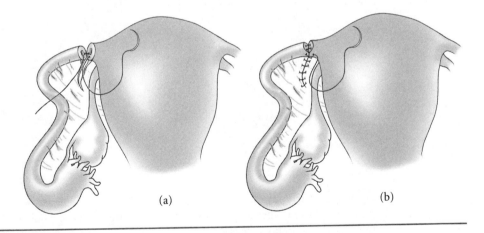

(a)                                        (b)

**Figure 5.1** Microsurgery of the fallopian tubes: reversal of sterilization by tubal anastomosis: (a) the two freshly cut ends of the tube are being joined by the first of six fine sutures to the inner, muscular layer of the tube, just outside the tube's endosalpinx; (b) the muscular layer has been joined, and the outer layer of the tube (the serosa) is being closed.

ultrasound examination (discussed in Chapter 13). If tubal blockage is confirmed and is not overcome by the diagnostic maneuver itself, the choice in treatment lies between **microsurgery** to the tubes and **assisted conception** with IVF. Generally a blockage of the narrow **isthmus** of the tube, close to the uterus, can be overcome by resecting it and rejoining the tube using careful microsurgical methods (see Figure 5.1 and Chapter 13). With more widespread blockages, there can be a better chance of pregnancy with one cycle of IVF (see Chapter 20 and Appendix B) than there is with a year of attempting pregnancy after microsurgery (shown in Figure 5.2).

Whereas any of the conditions described in this chapter will mean that, at least without treatment, there is sterility—unequivocal infertility that no amount of time will overcome—there are similar but less complete situations that leave a chance of getting pregnant naturally. Because knowing what to do is then much less clear, we devote a separate chapter to them.

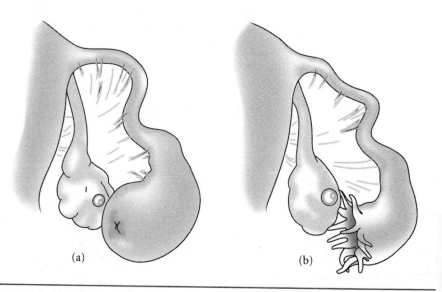

(a)                                                        (b)

**Figure 5.2**  Microsurgery of the fallopian tubes: salpingostomy: (a) a hydrosalpinx, in which the tube is blocked at its outer end and, as a result, is distended with fluid; (b) the tube has been opened microsurgically with "radial" incisions that follow the line of the folds in the endosalpinx.

# When Natural Conception Is Possible but Not Happening

If your infertility tests show that there are one or more minor abnormalities that may or may not explain your not getting pregnant, you are in a different, and in some ways more frustrating, position than if the tests show a complete barrier to pregnancy (the subject of Chapter 5). We sometimes call this condition **relative infertility**, or if all the tests are completely normal, the condition is called **unexplained infertility**. Management of each of these two situations has a lot in common.

In this chapter we will look at several more investigations needed to fully evaluate infertility. We will also start to get a handle on assessing the importance of what we might call partial problems—the various diagnoses that can be made (most of which have their own chapters on treatment in Part Three of this book) and what to do when these partial problems occur together—or when there does not seem to be any abnormality at all.

# Causes of Relative Infertility

A number of abnormalities can be found from the basic tests described in Chapter 4, abnormalities that cause a delay in getting pregnant but that might still enable pregnancy if enough time is available to keep giving pregnancy a chance.

## Oligospermia

As distinct from azoospermia (discussed in Chapter 5), a **sperm count** may show **oligospermia**, a reduction in the number of sperm, usually associated with reduced sperm motility (the kicking motion the sperm are seen to have under the microscope) and with an increase in the percentage of the sperm cells that have abnormal shapes. It is not hard to understand how this decreases the chance of getting pregnant in a particular month. The lower the actual number of motile, normal-looking sperm in the ejaculate, the lower the chance is of pregnancy happening quickly. How to investigate and what to do about low sperm counts is discussed in Chapter 9.

## Ovulation Disorders

Disorders of **ovulation**, or infrequent ovulation, will ordinarily produce **oligomenorrhea** (or infrequent periods). The causes are the same as those for **anovulation** (not ovulating; see Chapters 5 and 10). There are then several problems with getting pregnant.

First, less frequent ovulation itself means fewer opportunities to get pregnant over a period of time. Second, the **follicle** can open but the egg may not be released, remaining in the ovary in the **corpus luteum** (the **luteinized unruptured follicle**, discussed in the Box "Fake Ovulation" in Chapter 4). Third, the development of the egg may not coincide with ovulation, so the egg can be released but may not be able to be fertilized or may not be fertilized normally, making a **miscarriage** more likely. Fourth, ovulation can be followed by too short a **luteal phase** to enable successful implantation of the embryo, even if the egg has been fertilized normally (a **luteal phase defect**).

## Age

A man's fertility decreases with age but not in any way that is not reflected in the sperm count. Creeping age is also, of course, known to decrease the frequency with which men and women have sex. But it is also clear now that it is the age of the woman that is the critical factor in determining age-related fertility. When a woman is about ten years from the time menopause will happen, she will be getting low on high-energy eggs that are capable of producing a successful pregnancy. Because we cannot forecast when menopause will take place for a particular woman, we cannot know when this decrease in fertility will happen.

We do know, however, that the average age at which Western women go through menopause is 50 or 51, with a normal range from age 40 to 55. This means that fertility falls fairly suddenly at an average age of about 38 to 40, with the range at which this fall in fertility *can* occur being about 35 to 45. The only sign that this is taking place may be a shortening of the menstrual cycle (although this may not be the only reason menstrual cycles get shorter). The only test presently available to establish whether this decrease to fertility is under way is an indirect one, namely a **serum FSH** done during a period. A high serum FSH result is abnormal, because it means the pituitary gland is encountering resistance in the ovaries at the beginning of a new cycle and is trying to

## How Eggs Get Their "Use-by" Date: Mishaps in the Mitochondria

Every cell in the body, including egg cells and sperm cells, needs to be powered by a source of energy. The structures responsible for producing this energy are minute organelles inside the cell called mitochondria. Under an electron microscope a mitochondrion looks like a bacterium (and that is what we think the mitochondrion evolved from billions of years ago). Every cell in the body contains hundreds of mitochondria, each busy burning up sugar molecules with oxygen to release carbon dioxide as well as usable energy (in the form of high-energy phosphate compounds that are shifted around in the cell to where their energy is needed for some critical action).

What makes these mitochondria fascinating is that each one has its own bit of genetic material—their own bit of DNA, just like bacteria have their own DNA. This is the only place outside the cell's **nucleus** (where the **chromosomes** are) that DNA is found. Mitochondrial DNA (mtDNA) is different from nuclear, or chromosomal, DNA in a number of ways. First, instead of a single strand in each chromosome (producing two of each gene, one maternal and one paternal), mtDNA is a circular molecule, present in thousands of copies per cell. Second, mutations (mistakes in the sequence contained in the DNA) are more frequent,

and repair of the genetic code does not take place, so that as cells get older they gradually accumulate more and more mitochondria that do not work properly. Third, all of the mitochondria in your body came from the mitochondria in the egg when you were conceived—none came from the mitochondria in the sperm cell that fertilized the egg. Thus, mtDNA is a form of inheritance you get entirely from your mother.

So why do eggs all get produced before birth (see Chapter 3)? Why do new sperm cells keep forming, even into a man's old age? Consider that every time a cell divides, the mitochondria have had to divide much more often, and every time a mitochondrion divides, the DNA divides first. And each time DNA divides there is probably an opportunity for a mistake in the genetic code (a mutation), and an accumulation of mistakes or mutations, in the long run, is called "genetic drift." Therefore, if egg cells kept dividing through life, the older a woman is, the more genetic drift there will be in the offspring—almost certainly beyond what nature is prepared to tolerate. (This seems to be such an important principle that it probably holds true for every vertebrate species of the animal kingdom; in all animal studies, all the eggs are produced before the animal becomes fertile.)

compensate with the production of more follicle stimulating hormone. Nevertheless, serum FSH levels at the beginning of the cycle can vary from one cycle to the next.

At Sydney IVF we are looking at judging the stage of this age-related decline in female fertility by examining the **mitochondria**, those quintessentially age-governed little structures inside cells responsible for providing a cell's energy and potential for development. We are looking specifically at **mitochondrial DNA** (mtDNA), especially in the follicle cells and in the eggs themselves.

Genetic integrity for *sperm* mitochondria? Forget it. Sperm mitochondria have a different job— providing the energy the sperm cell needs to swim to the egg. **Capacitation** of sperm (when they swim fastest to get through the egg's **cumulus** and **zona pellucida**) probably represents the firing of the sperm's afterburners, deriving each last ounce of energy from the mitochondria before the successful sperm enters the egg, delivers its chromosomes and tosses aside the depleted, exhausted, oxidized mitochondria that got it there. These defunct mitochondria would probably be the last thing you would choose to deliver genetically true mtDNA to the embryo.

But in none of the body's tissues do mitochondria, and the integrity of their DNA, last forever. Aging of mitochondria in muscles, for example, accounts for the fact that no amount of training in middle age keeps your muscles as efficient as they were during your youth. Aging of mitochondria in heart muscle starts later, during your forties. Aging of mitochondria in the cortex of the brain, on the other hand, does not happen much until age 70. When does it happen in eggs? Several studies are beginning to show that it occurs in the late thirties and early forties—just the time that we know miscarriages are more common and just the time that otherwise unexplainable infertility becomes prevalent.

## Peritubal Adhesions

When there is an **adhesion** or scar tissue around the **fallopian tube**, separating the tube from all of the surface of the ovary or limiting the movement of the tube's **fimbrial end** to "touch and feel" the ovary's surface at ovulation, the chance of pregnancy is also reduced, although this depends on the location and the extent of the adhesions. The worse these are, the lower the chance of pregnancy happening quickly. The subject of peritubal adhesions is discussed in Chapters 12 and 13.

## Only One Tube Open

Because ovulation happens from just one ovary at a time, a woman who has ha*
one tube removed or has one tube blocked and the other open will on averag*
take twice as long to get pregnant. Ovulation is slightly more likely to move al*
ternately from one ovary to the other in successive months, but this is not a firm
rule, and sometimes it is only the one ovary that ovulates consecutively fo*
months on end, especially if part of the other ovary has been removed. I*
younger women with otherwise normal fertility it might not matter at all, i*
terms of getting pregnant, but in older women (who have less time to spend)*
or if there are other reasons for not getting pregnant easily, doubling the tim*
needed to conceive does matter.

## Endometriosis

**Endometriosis** is a common condition that seems to diminish fertility by lim*
iting the life of sperm in the fallopian tube. Other effects of endometriosis o*
ovulation, or at least on egg pickup by the tube, and on the early embryo, or **pre***
**embryo**, may also be important. The harm seems to come from a chemical ef*
fect, and one not related to where the endometriosis is located among the pelvi*
organs. It is only in the most severe instances that there is scarring that result*
in a blockage of the tubes. In most cases it seems to be that the more severe th*
endometriosis—especially if it is causing other symptoms—the longer it wil*
take to get pregnant, but there are many exceptions and some women with ap*
parently significant endometriosis get pregnant quickly, particularly if th*
sperm count is excellent. (Chapters 15 and 16 are devoted to detailed discussions of endometriosis.)

## Abnormalities of the Cervix: The "Cervical Factor"

Sperm are intrepid, and if menstrual blood can get out through the cervix, then
sperm ought to be able to get in. Nonetheless, it cannot help matters if the mucus in the cervix (**cervical mucus**) is inflamed due to infection (**cervicitis**) or i*
the cervix is scarred from previous surgery, such as a major cone biopsy.
Modern methods of treating an abnormal Pap smear for "cervical dysplasia"
(also known as "cervical intraepithelial neoplasia" or CIN) or a papilloma-virus
infection with cautery, cryotherapy (freezing) or laser are very unlikely to have
a harmful effect on sperm getting through the cervix. By removing abnormal

tissue in the canal of the cervix, these therapeutic maneuvers may actually improve sperm transit.

The effects of an abnormality of the cervix show up on a **postcoital test** (PCT) and an **in vitro penetration test**, which investigate sperm and mucus function in the laboratory. The in vitro penetration test we favor at Sydney IVF is the **Kremer test**, named after the Belgian scientist who devised it. The Kremer test is a four-way test done with the woman's mucus, her partner's (fresh) semen, a standard sample of normal mucus and an apparently normal semen specimen. The possible outcomes and their interpretation are given in Table 6.1.

What could be the causes of a negative PCT carried out during a normal ovulatory cycle on the day of ovulation? First, the cervix may be resistant to estrogen due to previous surgery, in which case the quantity of mucus can suffer. Second, the cervix may be infected or inflamed, in which case the quality of the mucus sometimes (but by no means always) suffers; it then has a yellow color instead of being clear. But there may be no apparent cause at all, with the mucus looking perfectly normal; in this case there may be poor sperm function or there may be antibodies to sperm present (called **sperm antibodies**), either in the mucus or in the semen. Before antibodies are looked for, the mucus itself needs to be examined carefully.

Further testing involves interactions between cervical mucus and semen in the laboratory, and is again so dependent on the normal estrogen exposure of the cervix that it is best not to leave matters to chance. We give estrogen tablets from day two of the menstrual period (75 micrograms of ethinylestradiol per day works fine), both to produce standard estrogen conditions for the mucus

**Table 6.1** Sperm-Mucus Interaction Testing and Its Interpretation

Penetration of sperm into the mucus is simply referred to as "good," "bad," or "fair," but in practice the results are not always clear-cut.

| Husband/Wife | Husband/Donor | Donor/Wife | Donor/Donor | Interpretation |
|---|---|---|---|---|
| good | good | good | good | normal |
| bad | bad | good | good | sperm problem |
| bad | good | bad | good | mucus problem |
| bad | fair | fair | good | sperm and mucus problem |

(obtained after about 8 to 10 days exposure to the estrogens) and to stop natural ovulation—and the possibility of unwelcome progesterone that comes with it—from spoiling the test. If the mucus still is not good on this dosage of estrogen, we sometimes double it for a few more days.

## Sperm Antibodies

Sperm antibodies occur when for some reason the man or the woman has an immune response against sperm cells. This potentially limits the sperms' movement and their ability to get to the egg. Not all sperm antibodies are important. The antibodies can be directed at any of three parts of the sperm: the head, the middle or the tail. Those directed at the tail are most likely to stop movement but all antibodies will slow sperm movement to some extent. The antibodies can be "agglutinating" (and make sperm stick together in clumps) or "immobilizing" (which are less common but more serious). The antibodies are looked for

### Sperm Antibodies: Chickens and Eggs

In women it is not unusual for low levels of sperm agglutinating antibodies to develop after a number of years of infertility. This is not likely to be anything other than a physiological response to sperm unaccompanied by the immune tolerance brought on by a pregnancy and is not in itself medically important. In men, sperm antibodies, both agglutinating and immobilizing, virtually always develop after a **vasectomy**, and they usually persist after **vasectomy reversal**. The longer the interval between vasectomy and reversal, the more likely it is that sperm function will be permanently disrupted by sperm antibodies.

Why some women develop the more serious sperm immobilizing antibodies is quite unknown. It is possible, but not certain, that anal intercourse makes production of sperm antibodies more likely. Certainly it is not the only reason sperm antibodies can form. It is also plausible—although I stress that the hypothesis is completely untested—that sperm antibodies might form from intercourse during menstruation. In both situations there is the possibility of sperm escaping the normal reproductive tract to make direct contact with immunologically competent tissues, similar situations that might predispose to transmission of **HIV,** the **AIDS** virus.

in both partners' blood serum (**serum sperm antibodies**), in the semen (**semen sperm antibodies**) and in the mucus (**cervical mucus sperm antibodies**). There is generally no need to look for them if the PCT is normal, except that if serum is to be used for assisted conception it needs to be shown that it is free of antibodies.

## Abnormalities of the Uterus

Abnormalities of the uterus do not often cause trouble in getting pregnant; they are more likely to cause miscarriage once the pregnancy is under way (see Chapters 7 and 8). The more severe forms of these abnormalities, however, will also delay or prevent conception. The most common uterine cause of infertility is the presence of a **fibroid** or a **polyp** that distorts the cavity of the uterus (the **endometrial cavity**). The bigger the fibroid or polyp, or the more of the cavity it occupies, the lower the chance of successful implantation. Other causes of relative infertility in the uterus include inflammation (**endometritis**) and **intra-uterine adhesions** (adhesions affecting the uterine cavity). These problems in the uterus are discussed in detail in Chapter 17.

# How Much Does It Matter ?

As we saw in Chapter 1, just one of these abnormalities on its own, if mild, will not necessarily *stop* someone from having children, even if it takes longer than normal to get pregnant, but the effects are multiplied if there is more than one abnormality. For example, if oligospermia decreases to 20 percent of normal the chance of getting pregnant in a particular month, and if endometriosis is also present, which alone would also diminish the chances to 20 percent of normal, then the overall decrease in the chance of pregnancy in one month is 20 percent of 20 percent, or 4 percent! Straightaway there is likely to be a real problem—real infertility (see the box "Mild Problems Seem to Go Together").

With more than two of these partial abnormalities, each, say, diminishing fertility to 20 percent per month, but all multiplying together, we can get to the situation where pregnancy is no more likely than it is among couples using effective contraception! This effect is explained in Appendix I, although we should understand that in practice we have no sure way of knowing how much a particular diagnosed abnormality or combination of abnormalities is actually

Often a single mild abnormality will not reach your awareness or that of your physician. Pregnancy might occur a few months later; you may have been concerned transiently, but then pregnancy happens and all is well. The same thing may happen the next time. After this, contraception instead of conception becomes the priority for you both. No single diagnosis will have been made. For example there will have been no (single) diagnosis of mild endometriosis, no diagnosis of a lowish sperm count, no diagnosis of a mild or intermittent ovulation disorder (perhaps just being in your late thirties), no diagnosis of some mild adhesions from an ovarian cystectomy and so on. But if two of these mild conditions had been present together it may well have been a different story. Because the effects are multiplied, it becomes a lot more likely

that you will have had tests done (see Appendix I for the arithmetic). In this way, when we do tests for infertility, we physicians paradoxically more often see mild conditions in combination than we see them in isolation.

### The Worse the Problem, the Better the Treatment

The more severe any one cause of infertility described in this chapter is discovered to be, the more likely it is that it will be the reason—the only reason—why you are not getting pregnant. And, if it can be treated effectively, without the treatment itself causing any new problems, the more likely it is that treating it will lead to your getting pregnant reasonably quickly. Put simply, the worse the problem, provided it can be fixed, the bigger the difference the treatment will make to your fertility.

diminishing the monthly chance of conceiving, except by estimating how long, so far, getting pregnant or not getting pregnant has taken.

## Treating Relative Infertility

The options for treating these partial or mild conditions are to do nothing and just wait; to try and correct separately each problem that is discovered; or to skirt around all the problems at once with an appropriate form of **assisted con-**

**ception**. When is it best to do nothing? How do we judge what role a particular set of apparently mild or incomplete barriers to fertility are actually playing?

We saw earlier how several mild conditions can multiply to create a major problem. But how do we assess how such a theory translates into practice? The best way to judge their effect is to look at how long it has taken to get pregnant so far (or how long it took to conceive a previous pregnancy) and to compare this with how long you have to conceive before you are too old or before you think it is taking an unjustifiably long time. The longer it has taken so far, the less the chance per month of conceiving (an effect explained in more detail in Appendix A). Remember, however, that pregnancy can happen any time by luck. Just because a couple achieved pregnancy quickly the first time they tried—and it was only when the second pregnancy took too long and tests were done that revealed the presence of diagnosable problems—does not mean that those problems were not there all along. The problems are not, in such a situation, necessarily new.

The second option, correcting each of the separate minor abnormalities found, can be a difficult one. It is always the job of a physician to try to return abnormal to normal. The art and science of medicine is most effective, however, when what is being treated is a long way away from what is normal. An operation for a ruptured appendix, for example, is life saving—it is a highly efficacious thing to do. Bringing a blood sugar level back to normal with insulin in someone in a diabetic coma is equally obviously effective. But removing the appendix in a patient with vague pain or laboriously keeping a blood sugar level at 100 percent of normal instead of 110 percent of normal is much less likely to make a big difference. Remember that any form of medicine or surgery risks making the situation worse instead of better, by introducing new, treatment-related abnormalities to replace the abnormalities being treated. In short, the more minor and the more numerous the abnormalities, the less likely it is that treating them will have a net beneficial effect.

These considerations make the third option, assisted conception, more attractive, especially if you consider that endometriosis usually has no harmful effect on getting pregnant with **gamete intrafallopian transfer** (GIFT) or **in vitro fertilization** (IVF); that GIFT and IVF readily compensate for moderate degrees of oligospermia; that provided one tube is normal internally, then GIFT or IVF can make use of it; and that the cervix becomes irrelevant to getting pregnant with GIFT and IVF.

Not everyone will decide at this point to pursue pregnancy. It is your choice—one taken together with your partner, in full knowledge of all the options and what these options involve. Perhaps read the specific chapters in Part Three that relate to your diagnosis (or diagnoses).

# Unexplained Infertility

If the tests show no abnormality then it is doubtful that you will be reassured. If you are not getting pregnant when you want to, it is often harder to come to terms with being told, "Everything's normal," than it is when one or another reason is found. The temptation—at least for some people—is to say that it is psychological or that medical science is stupidly missing some exotic diagnosis that, if it were known, could be treated simply. Both these conclusions are usually wrong, as I explained in Chapter 1. So do not listen to people who tell you it is *in* your mind. It's *on* your mind, for sure, but that is not why you are not getting pregnant.

As far as exotic reasons for not getting pregnant are concerned—causes of infertility that are somehow out of reach—they do sometimes occur but they seem to be rare. Chapter 3 made it clear that it is part of being human that pregnancies should not happen too frequently. Unexplained infertility is actually normal, even if not very desirable as we move from the twentieth to the twenty-first century. Relatively simple kinds of assisted conception such as GIFT work well; they would not work if there was something exotic stopping pregnancy.

Our experience with IVF over the past 15 years has shown us that, if anything, it is usually a subtle difficulty with the sperm that stops women under about 38 years of age from getting pregnant, whereas after 38 (although sometimes before) it is more and more likely to be a subtle problem with the eggs. This shows up during GIFT and IVF cycles by there being fewer follicles and eggs than expected when the ovaries are stimulated. Exceptions to this rule, however, are common enough. Take your reading further with Chapters 19 and 20.

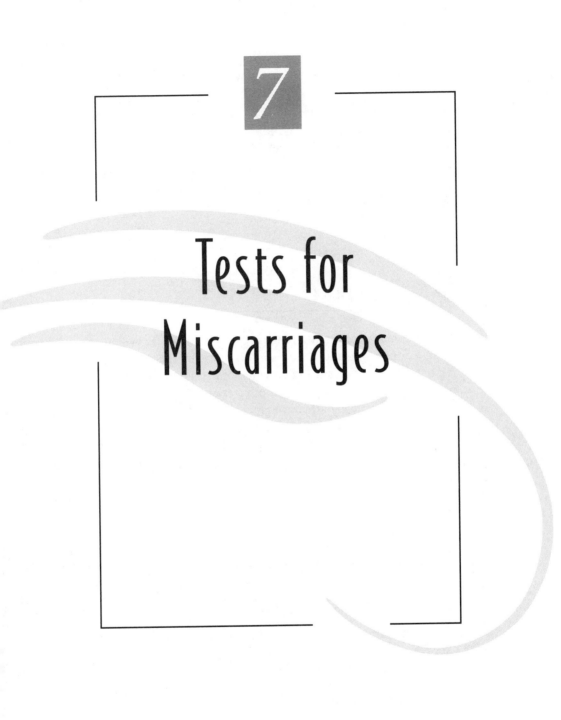

# 7

# Tests for Miscarriages

For most women most of the time, a miscarriage in isolation is sensibly regarded as just bad luck. Generally, a miscarriage is more likely than not to mean that the body's reproductive system is working, that next time, and without specific intervention, a normal, healthy pregnancy and a baby will most often result. But a miscarriage that is followed by a second one, and then perhaps a third, or a miscarriage that occurs after a long period of infertility, is another matter. Rather than being reassuring, such a miscarriage is a sign—or a reminder—that all is not well and tests should be done. Let us start by considering the forms a miscarriage can take, and then how common miscarriages are in nature.

## Are You Miscarrying ?

The first indications that a pregnancy is not doing as well as it should consist usually of bleeding and then cramps. Eventually there may be an uncanny feeling of wellness—the nausea of pregnancy disappears, the nipples lose their soreness. None of these symptoms is an invariable harbinger of doom. They usually lead to tests, typically a **transvaginal ultrasound**, perhaps with a **serum hCG** (depending on the stage of the pregnancy), that will decide if all is well or not. Interpreting these tests depends on the stage of pregnancy. Miscarriages differ in the form they take, depending on the stage of pregnancy at which they occur.

## Menstrual Miscarriages

One could use the term **menstrual miscarriage** for a pregnancy that is so brief that it does not significantly delay the period. There are no symptoms of pregnancy. Even with a delay of a few days, and with perhaps more period pain or more premenstrual tension than normal, it is not possible, without doing a blood pregnancy test, to distinguish a menstrual miscarriage from a delayed period. (Remember that these symptoms—exaggerations of normal—are also likely when a period is late and the lining of the uterus, the **endometrium**, is thicker because of a prolonged **follicular phase** and a late **ovulation**.) An ultrasound examination will not reveal a pregnancy sac. Some gynecologists call such a miscarriage a "biochemical pregnancy," because the only hard evidence for pregnancy comes from a biochemical test (the pregnancy test, or level of serum hCG).

## Subclinical Miscarriage

A **subclinical miscarriage** is the miscarriage of an early pregnancy that delays the period a week or two and that can result in the appearance of a small **gestational sac** on transvaginal ultrasound, but when the miscarriage takes place it is like a delayed period, although it can be heavier and longer. No **curettage** of the cavity of the uterus is necessary. Not all gynecologists consider this to be a separate category of miscarriage, so it is also sometimes called a biochemical pregnancy.

## Clinical Miscarriage

The best recognized type of miscarriage can be called a "clinical miscarriage," to set it apart from the other miscarriages. In this case, a transvaginal ultrasound will reveal a gestational sac, and there may be symptoms of pregnancy. A fetal heart can develop and be seen on ultrasound, but it can be late in appearing (more than six weeks after the last menstrual period, or, more accurately, longer than four weeks from conception), and when the embryo does not grow, the fetal heart slows and then stops. When miscarriage takes place, with bleeding and then pain, it is common to have a curettage of the uterus to make sure the uterus has emptied and that infection and bleeding do not complicate matters. If there is no serious bleeding or if a transvaginal ultrasound shows that miscarriage has been complete, then curettage is not necessary.

Before the days of ultrasound, we used to distinguish a **threatened miscarriage** (bleeding, generally without pain, and a cervix that remained closed) from an **inevitable miscarriage** (with painful contractions accompanying bleeding and the cervix then dilating). Nowadays, a miscarriage will be regarded as inevitable if the gestational sac on ultrasound is smaller than it should be and when the fetal heart is absent or is slow, at a time when the heart should be visible and beating faster than about 120 beats per minute. In cases of doubtful dates, a second ultrasound is carried out a week or two later. The symptoms of miscarriage can sometimes be confused with the symptoms of an **ectopic pregnancy** (discussed in Chapter 14); the ultrasound is useful in making this distinction.

A physician will be particularly interested in what parts of the pregnancy form before miscarriage takes place. The earlier the damage to the pregnancy, the less developed the embryo or fetus will be, so that with many conceptuses (or the "products of conception") that have abnormal **chromosomes**, there is no embryo at all, just **trophoblast** (placenta) and membranes. If embryonic structures are present, it is the head-end of the embryo and the heart that develop first; the tail may be very deficient. The further the pregnancy has progressed, the more complete the development will have been of the embryo or fetus. It is unusual for a normal, completely formed embryo to be lost in the first three months of pregnancy.

Just how complete the development of the pregnancy is at the time of miscarriage can also be judged by having a pathologist examine the miscarriage tissue, either after it has been expelled from the uterus spontaneously (the natural process of miscarriage) or after the tissue has been proactively removed from the uterus by **vacuum curettage**.

The other useful test to do on miscarriage tissue (before it has been placed in a fixative solution for the pathologist) is to send some trophoblast tissue for culture to permit a **karyotype**, or analysis of the chromosomes. If a karyotype is done on incompletely formed miscarriage tissue, in more than 60 percent of cases the chromosome constitution will be abnormal. Vice versa, an abnormal chromosome constitution in the embryo means that, with a few exceptions, a miscarriage will have been inevitable. If the chromosomal constitution is normal, on the other hand, there must be another explanation for the miscarriage. With repeated miscarriages, therefore, or when a miscarriage looks inevitable after a period of infertility, a karyotype of the miscarriage tissue is an important test to determine the problem. I discuss this in more detail further on.

## Missed Miscarriage or Missed Abortion

A pregnancy where there is no embryo growing normally may persist into the second three months (the second **trimester**) of pregnancy, especially if **progesterone** treatment has been used to try to salvage the pregnancy but only succeeds in delaying the natural process of miscarriage. (Such treatment with progesterone or a **progestogen** is almost always futile.) A true **missed abortion**, as this is known, is not a good thing, because the tissue of the miscarriage hardens and can be very difficult to curette from the cavity of the uterus, risking damage to the endometrium in the form of **intrauterine adhesions** (discussed in Chapter 17).

## Midtrimester Miscarriages

Should a normally formed fetus miscarry, usually in the middle three months of pregnancy (the second or midtrimester), then the essential distinction for the cause of the miscarriage a gynecologist will want to make is the one between **cervical incompetence** and **premature labor**. The pattern of the events is different, and the treatment of the two conditions is very different, so careful recall of the order of events is important.

With cervical incompetence a normally formed fetus can be lost after about 14 weeks of pregnancy due to softening, shortening and then opening of the cervix. Such an "incompetent" cervix allows the membranes of the pregnancy to bulge through. Symptoms can be minimal until it is too late, consisting just of backache and an increase in wetness or discharge from the vagina. There may be no symptoms at all before the membranes (the waters) break, a rush of fluid occurs and the fetus is expelled into the vagina with minimal bleeding and pain. The placenta will usually follow and bleeding is then common.

Premature labor (or "immature" labor, if the fetus is still well short of viability), in the absence of cervical incompetence, is said to happen when the process is like labor, with the onset of painful, episodic contractions of the uterus and bleeding before the waters break. The fetus and placenta are then expelled. With such a pattern the common causes are an infection (sometimes, ironically, associated with the presence of a stitch in the cervix, or a cervical ligature, used to treat cervical incompetence) and abnormalities of the uterus. Sadly, it is still not always possible to find a treatable cause even in repeated cases, and then a variety of antibiotics, medications and hospitalization may be called for to try to keep the pregnancy in place until it can be expected that the newborn will be viable. I discuss this treatment further in Chapter 8.

# How Usual Are Miscarriages?

Table 7.1 shows the average chance of a pregnancy ending in miscarriage according to the age of the woman. (The male partner's age has very little if any effect.) There is a steady rise with age from the early twenties (when it is about 13 percent for clinically obvious miscarriages) and substantial increase in risk after the late thirties (when it is about 20 to 25 percent for clinical miscarriages). After about age 42, more than half of pregnancies will miscarry.

It was once thought that it was the aging uterus that caused miscarriages to be more common in older women, but clinical studies with donated eggs and embryos from younger women show that this is not the case. Instead, the aging process affects the eggs (see Chapter 6, especially the box "How Eggs Get Their 'Use-by' Date: Mishaps in the Mitochondria," and Chapter 23), leading to

| Table 7.1 | Effect of a Woman's Age on the Risk of Having a Miscarriage |
|---|---|
| *Age of Woman* | *Average Chance of Miscarrying* |
| younger than 20 years | 12% |
| 20 to 24 years | 13% |
| 25 to 29 years | 14% |
| 30 to 34 years | 16% |
| 35 to 39 years | 19% |
| 40 to 42 years | 25% |
| 43 years and older | 50% |

Based predominantly on data from Dorothy Warburton and Clarke Fraser

chromosomal or mitochondrial embryopathy, which I discuss further on. As a result, many women in their forties, and some even in their fifties and sixties, have recently conceived and successfully undergone pregnancy with eggs from much younger women.

## Recurrent Miscarriage

Just as getting pregnant is a matter of chance, so is a miscarriage. It is uncommon for every pregnancy to miscarry, although in some women it does seem to happen this way. Gynecology textbooks say that repeated miscarriages should be investigated if a woman has had three or more miscarriages in a row, a condition called **habitual abortion** (or, more gently, **recurrent miscarriage**). This is an old-fashioned perspective.

It was 1982 before it was generally known that there is an increased chance of miscarrying with just about every cause of **relative infertility** (discussed in Chapter 6) and with most treatments for infertility. If a miscarriage takes place with a background of infertility, it can help—by getting a total view of the reasons behind the disability—to investigate even one miscarriage by sampling the miscarriage tissue and performing a karyotype. If the karyotype is normal, then the chances are that the miscarriage was caused by whatever is causing the infertility.

Whether the karyotype of a miscarriage is normal or not, we can find a cause for about two-thirds of couples who have had three or more miscarriages;

about half of these couples will have a successful pregnancy as a result of treatment. There is probably no medical condition that produces a longer list of appropriate tests than those that investigate recurrent miscarriages, although the good news may be that most of them can be done with one sample of blood. A gynecologist, however, will probably be selective, and exactly which tests are most likely to be helpful will depend on the circumstances.

I will approach the relevant tests according to a consideration of the possible causes of miscarriage. I should say right off that these different categories are not well known outside this book, and your gynecologist might or might not consider or categorize the causes of miscarriages this way. It is a sensible approach, however, and explaining miscarriages this way works.

# Causes of Miscarriages

We consider here the causes of miscarriages in the following four groups: **chromosomal embryopathy**, in which a genetic error at **conception** dooms the embryo; **preimplantational embryopathy**, in which the genetic makeup of the pre-embryo is normal but there is a harmful event that cripples the embryo before it has a chance to implant properly; **postimplantational embryopathy**, in which the implanted embryo is interfered with and then fails to develop further, and "fetal loss," where a normal embryo or fetus is expelled from the uterus. Repeated or recurrent miscarriages may run true to type or they may be mixed or be interspersed with live births. We use the term **mixed reproductive loss** when pregnancies are lost at very different stages of pregnancy.

## Chromosomal Embryopathy

The condition described as chromosomal embryopathy produces miscarriages in which the embryo does not develop properly because of a genetic error present from conception. (The embryo is pathological, hence the word "embryopathy.") If the chromosomes are abnormally endowed at conception, then there will often be little or no chance of the pregnancy coming to term as a baby, especially if there are, for example, 69 chromosomes instead of the normal number of 46 chromosomes, a state known as **triploidy** (see Figure 7.1b). There are exceptions, however, and a proportion of the **trisomies**, or one extra chromosome, such as **Down's syndrome**, or **trisomy 21** (see Figure 7.1c), and

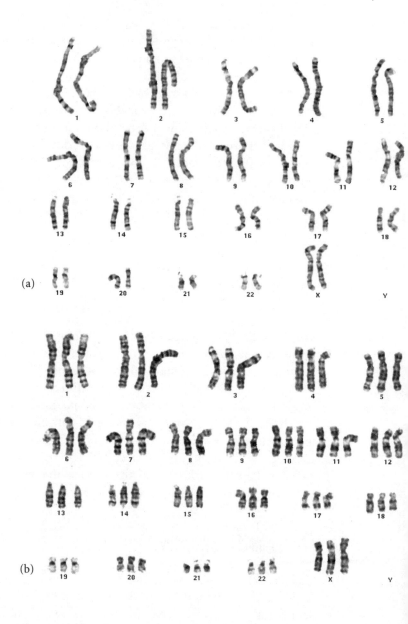

(a)

(b)

**Figure 7.1** Karyotypes. In a normal karyotype (a) there are 46 chromosomes; the presence of two X chromosomes here indicates a female. In triploidy (b) there are three of every chromosome and miscarriage is inevitable. With trisomy 21 (c) there are 47 chromosomes, with three of chromosome 21 (arrow), indicative of Down's syndrome; the presence of an X and a Y chromosome here indicates a male. If there is a balanced translocation (d), a part of a chromosome is

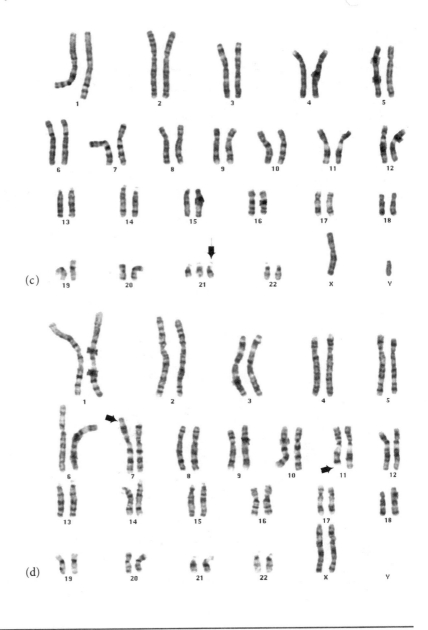

(c)

(d)

moved (here from the long arm of chromosome 11) to a different chromosome (here on the short arm of chromosome 7 (arrows)); the fetus (or person) will be normal, but, at least theoretically, half of this woman's eggs when fertilized will carry too much or too little chromosomal material, resulting in implantation failure, miscarriage or a birth defect. (Karyotypes performed and photographed by Dr. Cynthia Roberts, Sydney IVF.)

**Table 7.2**    Karyotypes of Miscarriages in First Three Months of Pregnancy

More than 60 percent of such miscarriages have abnormal chromosomes. The table gives the breakdown among the chromosome abnormalities.

| Abnormality | Explanation | Relative Frequency |
|---|---|---|
| *Aneuploidies* | | |
| Monosomy (particularly 45,X) | One chromosome not enough (i.e., 45 chromosomes) | 16% |
| Trisomy (especially trisomy 16) | One chromosome too many (i.e., 47 chromosomes) | 54% |
| *Polyploidies* | | |
| Triploidy | Three times the haploid number (i.e., 69 chromosomes) | 20% |
| Tetraploidy | Four times the haploid number (i.e., 92 chromosomes) | 6% |
| *Unbalanced Translocations* | | |
| Unbalanced translocation | Too much of part of a chromosome | 4% (at least) |

Adapted from figures published in 1975 by J. G. Boué and A. Boué and colleagues in France

especially the trisomies of the sex chromosomes (X and Y chromosomes), can survive through to birth. The frequent abnormal karyotypes that cause miscarriages are listed in Table 7.2.

How is a karyotype done? Answer: with difficulty and a lot of work (see the box "Karyotyping Step by Step"). We begin by getting some living tissue from the conception, in the form of **chorionic villi** in early pregnancy, **amniotic fluid** cells later in pregnancy or from either the **placenta** or the fetus's skin in the case of an immature delivery. This tissue is then set up in a tissue culture, so that the cells continue to multiply in the laboratory. After this, the chromosomes are

In a culture, as in the body, cells divide by **mitosis**. Once the tissue culture for performing the karyotype is under way, mitosis is stopped in its tracks by adding a drug called colchicine to part of the culture. This freezes mitosis at a stage of cell division called **metaphase**, when the chromosomes are separate and can be photographed. They are then either literally cut out from the photograph with scissors and pasted up in order or now more often by the help of a high-definition computer screen, so that each chromosome pair is displayed in sequence to check for completeness. This is done for typically 20 or so metaphases—an enormous amount of work.

Normal karyotypes are indicated this way: a normal female karyotype is 46,XX (to indicate 23 chromosome pairs, of which one pair comprises the sex chromosomes and the other 22 pairs are **autosomes**, or nonsex chromosomes); a normal male karyotype is 46,XY.

We have already encountered the term **triploid**, which means three times the haploid number of chromosomes (see Chapter 3), and usually comes about if two sperm fertilize an egg. The general term for the gain or loss of a single chromosome is **aneuploidy**. The most common aneuploid chromosome complements are the trisomies, where there is an extra chromosome because of incorrect movement of the chromosomes during **meiosis** into the egg or the sperm, for example, trisomy 21 (Down's syndrome), in which an extra chromosome 21 gets into egg or sperm and therefore into the embryo, and trisomies of the sex chromosomes (**Klinefelter's syndrome** = 47,XXY, **triple-X syndrome** = 47,XXX and **extra-Y-chromosome syndrome** = 47,XYY), in which the embryo is endowed with an extra sex chromosome. The loss of one of a chromosome pair, a "monosomy," is not compatible with even early embryo development, unless the chromosome lost is a Y chromosome, namely **Turner's syndrome** (45,X), although even then a majority end as miscarriages, with just a small proportion surviving as babies.

photographed through a microscope while the cells are dividing. Even with the help of a computer one extremely highly trained technician (a cytogeneticist) will be able to do just ten or so karyotypes per week. The karyotype is therefore a rather expensive test.

Unfortunately, however, by the time a miscarriage is expelled, the trophoblast tissue may have degenerated too much for the cells to survive in tissue culture for karyotyping. If finding a reason for a particular miscarriage is

Balanced translocations do not produce abnormal embryos with quite the frequency you would expect by chance. The reason must be either because there is preferential selection of normal eggs or sperm cells somewhere along the line or, more likely (we believe), because **syngamy** fails more often than is usual and the embryo's development is stopped before the pregnancy is revealed. On the other hand, there may be a balanced reciprocal translocation, the "reciprocal" referring to the fact that two different chromosomes have swapped pieces, which

gives a much, much greater chance of the fertilized egg having an abnormal amount of chromosome material, for two reasons. First, there is not just one chromosome that risks being unbalanced but two (with a third possibility that both end up unbalanced). Second, a translocated bit of chromosome can be so small that it does not ever segregate properly, rattling about chaotically, and ends up just about anywhere by random chance and disrupts the picture further. The miscarriage rate with a balanced reciprocal translocation can therefore get rather close to 100 percent.

important enough, a physician might recommend a curettage or a **chorion villus sampling** (CVS) as soon as practicable after a transvaginal ultrasound shows no surviving embryo.

Whether miscarriage tissue has been available for karyotyping or not, recurrent miscarriages in the first trimester should mean that the couple should have *their* karyotype checked to exclude a **balanced translocation**, in which a piece of one chromosome has been translocated to another position. This does no harm to the person concerned, because there is no gain or loss of chromosomal material, but when the chromosome pairs split up and move into eggs or sperm (discussed in Chapter 3), there will be a shortage of genes for one egg or sperm and an excess of genes for its sister egg or brother sperm. Other eggs and sperm can be normal, the ones that receive the normal member of the pair. (For more on balanced translocations of the chromosomes, see the box "Unbalancing Translocations.")

## Embryopathy Before Implantation

It is nature's way that injuries sustained by an embryo or pre-embryo are "all or nothing." Either the injury will be mortal, ending in miscarriage days or a week or two later, or it will be shrugged off by the exuberance embryos show in grow-ing. Such injuries, endowed prior to conception or occurring between the time of conception and implantation, which thus result in what we call preimplanta-tional embryopathies, include undue aging or other nonchromosomal abnor-malities of egg and sperm leading up to conception. These abnormalities may affect the egg's **mitochondria**; nutritional support for the pre-embryo, as hap-pens with disease of the **fallopian tube** and, to some extent, fertilization and de-velopment in vitro (IVF), and a noxious external event, such as a high fever or an alcoholic binge (it probably needs to be a real bender).

Apart from tubal disease (see Chapters 4 and 12), these injuries to the early embryo are generally not likely to be repeated and no special tests are useful. Note, however, that if an episode such as a fever occurs and the pregnancy con-tinues, then the chance of a birth defect is just barely different from the gener-ally expected incidence of birth abnormalities. Most people, in other words, will not choose to have an abortion just because such an event has taken place.

## Embryopathy After Implantation

The possible reasons for an embryo or fetus to sustain injury after implantation are many. In general, the later in fetal life such an injury occurs, the more likely it will reveal itself as an abnormality at birth instead of as a miscarriage. The de-veloping pregnancy needs a quickly expanding blood supply through the wall of the uterus to the placenta. The blood supply to the fetus may become insuffi-cient if implantation is on a **uterine septum** (a wall partly dividing the uterus in two—see Chapter 18), if implantation is over a uterine **fibroid**, or if growth of the placenta is constrained by intrauterine adhesions or **endometrial atro-phy**. These causes are best looked for with a **hysterosalpingogram**, a transvagi-nal ultrasound of the uterus and a hysteroscopy (see Chapter 4).

Not enough progesterone early in pregnancy will result in miscarriage if, for example, the **corpus luteum** (the progesterone-producing tissue that the recently ovulated **follicle** develops into) is mistakenly removed for being cystic or painful before the placenta has taken responsibility for producing proges-terone. Whether or not an early progesterone deficiency is truly a cause of mis-carriages is doubtful, but remember that a **luteal phase defect** usually comes about because the follicle that preceded it was less than optimal, implying that the egg may have been compromised from the start (a cause, therefore, of preimplantational embryopathy). A **premenstrual biopsy** is reassuring if it is normal (see Chapter 4), because it indicates that progesterone production has been normal.

An overactive thyroid gland can cause miscarriages, perhaps because it increases the rate of metabolism in the body and progesterone is disposed of too quickly. **Thyroid function tests** comprise assays in blood of **thyroxine** and **thyroid stimulating hormone** (TSH). The miscarriage shown in Figure 3.8c in Chapter 3 resulted from an overactive thyroid gland; the embryo is almost normal for its stage of development.

Textbooks list diabetes as a cause of miscarriage, and women with recurrent miscarriages have in the past undergone formal tests to exclude diabetes. This is unnecessary. Diabetes causes miscarriages only when it needs insulin for treatment and it is in poor control. The diagnosis for these people will have been made already. If in doubt, it is simple to test for sugar in the blood with a **plasma glucose** level.

Any severe upset to the mother's health or metabolism can affect the fetus, but these upsets will generally already be very obvious. Failure of the kidneys, causing uremia, is one example and is checked with a **serum urea and creatinine**. One of the more subtle but rare metabolic causes of miscarriage is Wilson's disease, in which there are high levels of copper in the serum (measured as **serum copper**), but is usually in association with abnormal tests of liver function (and with a yellow ring visible within the iris of the eye).

Remember that from an immunological point of view the fetus is a foreigner. The mother's immune system must learn to tolerate the fetus. If her immune system goes wrong, the mother can reject the fetus—first by making antibodies and immune cells and then through miscarriage. A good deal is known about these events, although more is still to be learned.

There is one blood-group antibody, or agglutinin, that causes recurrent miscarriages in families that have it: the rare anti-TjA antibody. It and other agglutinins are looked for with a **blood group and antibody screen**.

Patients with the disorder known as systemic lupus erythematosus (SLE) form antibodies against their own tissues. People without this disease may also have antibodies against some of their own tissues detectable in the blood, often with no indication of disease. The antibody, or the group of antibodies, most likely to cause miscarriages is known in several different guises as the "lupus anticoagulant" or "lupus inhibitor" (it slightly inhibits blood coagulation) and as antiphospholipid antibody or anticardiolipin antibody. The tests we order to see if such antibodies can be implicated are the **lupus anticoagulant** and the **serum anticardiolipin antibody**, which are important tests, because treatment is available with aspirin, heparin and such corticosteroid drugs as prednisone. Blood levels of **antinuclear antibody** (ANA, or sometimes ANF for "antinuclear factor") are often increased in women with recurrent miscarriages and in patients with SLE, but unless there are other antibodies there in very high levels, it will

## A Little Rejection?

An ingenious theory was devised in the 1980s to account for the apparent benefit of immunization of the wife with white blood cells from the husband. Not all the facts fit, but for the moment at least, let's not have that stand in the way of a good story.

It was proposed that if a man and woman happen to share many of their blood and tissue groups (the groups that matter, for example, when choosing kidney transplant recipients), then the pregnant woman will not recognize the fetus as being different early enough to mount what is called immune tolerance. By the time the minor immune differences are picked up by the mother's immune system, it is too late and the immune response is one of rejection. By sensitizing her to her partner's tissue groups—through inoculation with white blood cells—it is meant to sharpen her immune surveillance so that in a future pregnancy a response will take place more quickly, allowing tolerance to develop and enabling the fetus to survive without rejection. Attractive though the story is, unfortunately no one has ever been able to show a breaking down of the normal immune barriers of pregnancy as a cause for miscarriage. If it happens, it does so without the overwhelming inflammation one sees, for example, in the rejection of a transplanted skin graft or kidney.

Recently, Dr. Maria Teresa Illeni and her colleagues from Milan, Italy, published perhaps the best study so far on immunotherapy for recurrent miscarriages. Forty-four women with at least three straight miscarriages—all unexplained— entered the study and were either treated or not treated according to (figuratively speaking) the toss of a coin. Of the 22 women immunized, 16 became pregnant, and 16 of them (or 27 percent) miscarried. Of the 22 women who were not immunized, 14 became pregnant (the difference between 16 and 14 is small and almost certainly explainable by chance), among whom there were just two miscarriages! Based on these results, we can now safely say that treating recurrent miscarriages with white blood cell inoculations no longer has a justifiable basis. Incidentally, you may notice from Dr. Illeni's study that considering the whole group of 44 women with recurrent miscarriages, 30 became pregnant again, among whom just 8 miscarried, but 22 were successful in having babies. Thus, don't lose hope too quickly.

be unclear whether ANA is the cause or the result of the miscarriages or whether it is completely unrelated.

One of the most tantalizing hints about possible immunological causes for recurrent miscarriages has come from the discovery that a proportion of women can be treated by being immunized to their partner's (or to a stranger's) white blood cells. A number of studies have shown that the beneficial effect is stronger than if the woman's own white blood cells are used for the inoculation. The way it works is unknown, but in order to have a chance of working, there should not be any of the antibodies described in the previous paragraph. There is, unfortunately, no specific test that forecasts whether this rather complex treatment will work. How it might or might not work is described in the box "A Little Rejection?"

# Fetal Loss

The distinction between embryopathy arising after implantation and the loss of a completely normal fetus is not always clear in medical practice, but it helps to understand the things that can go wrong to an otherwise normally developing fetus and what tests can be done. The most common structural failure of the uterus to contain the pregnancy is a prematurely opening, or dilating, of the cervix, called **cervical incompetence**. It requires careful and repeated vaginal examinations during pregnancy to exclude it as an imminent cause of miscarriage. Sometimes a shortened, possibly incompetent, cervix is seen on transvaginal ultrasound of a pregnancy. Treatment of an incompetent cervix involves placing a ligature or suture in the cervix (a **cervical ligature**; also discussed in Chapter 8), usually at about 12 weeks gestation so that the suture will not get in the way of an unrelated early miscarriage, for example from a chromosomal cause.

If left untreated, miscarriages due to cervical incompetence tend to occur earlier and earlier (although never before about 14 weeks). Cervical incompetence may be more common among infertility patients because of the number of procedures that have been done through the cervix that may have weakened it. Most gynecologists will be on the lookout for cervical incompetence in patients who have spent years trying to get pregnant; even if the chance (or risk) is low, the penalty for missing the diagnosis while it is still treatable (the hazard) is severe.

Although placing a suture or ligature in the cervix for an incompetent cervix is usually not a difficult operation, there is a risk that if the prior miscarriages were more of the immature labor variety than true cervical incompetence, the irritating presence of the suture in the cervix will make the situation worse instead of better. This is why a rather definite diagnosis of cervical incompetence should be made before a decision is reached to place a suture.

Abnormal constraint on the growing gestation can lead to miscarriage. Miscarriages can thus result from abnormalities of the shape of the uterus, abnormalities that can either result from disease of the uterus (Chapter 17) or have been present from birth (Chapter 18). Miscarriages due to a wall dividing the cavity of the uterus in two (a **uterine septum**) and miscarriages due to a fibroid, or benign tumor of the uterus, encroaching into the cavity (a **submucous fibroid**) typically happen in the first three months, perhaps, but not always, after a fetal heart has been detected (and are therefore of the postimplantational embryopathy kind). Miscarriages that are due to other birth abnormalities of the uterus, such as a **bicornuate uterus** or a **unicornuate uterus** (see Chapter 18), are typically of the premature labor and "fetal loss" variety. Sometimes the run of miscarriages with these sort of abnormal uteruses occur later and later into the pregnancy each time, and a viable pregnancy can be anticipated without special treatment being necessary. These abnormalities are looked for before pregnancy with a hysterosalpingogram or by hysteroscopy. Treatment may be directed at the underlying abnormality (see Chapters 17 and 18) or at inhibiting contractions of the uterus that would expel the fetus (see Chapter 8).

Constraint on the growing pregnancy can also come about if the gestation happens to implant in the outer angle of the uterine cavity, very close to where the fallopian tube enters it, namely an **angular pregnancy**. If they do not miscarry early, angular pregnancies often settle into the cavity proper of the uterus as they grow and cause comparatively little further trouble, except perhaps for an increase in the likelihood of experiencing retention of the placenta after the baby is born. (I discuss the diagnosis of angular pregnancy in relation to ectopic pregnancy in Chapter 14.)

An infection of the fetus leading to miscarriage can happen in three ways: the infection can have been there from the start, within the endometrial cavity, in the form of **endometritis**; it can ascend through the cervix when the pregnancy is already established; or it can get to the fetus by way of the bloodstream, through the placenta. The most obvious infective or inflammatory cause of miscarriage is when pregnancy occurs despite the use of an IUD. Miscarriage is more common if the IUD is left in place than if it is removed as soon as pregnancy is confirmed and before the IUD's tail disappears into the uterus. If the IUD is left in place, not all pregnancies miscarry (most will not), but those that do can do so at any stage of gestation. Endometritis or another infective cause before conception can result in miscarriages in the same way, irritating the fetal membranes and causing premature contractions of the uterus.

Once the pregnancy membranes have sealed off the uterine cavity, it is much less common for infective organisms to gain entry. If the membranes rupture prematurely, however, infection is sooner or later inevitable, followed by expulsion of the fetus.

The most prominent organisms that regularly reach a fetus by the blood stream, through the placenta, include certain viruses, such as rubella, the German measles virus, the attenuated rubella virus used for immunization, cytomegalovirus, herpes zoster, the chicken pox virus, herpes simplex, and, although not considered to be a cause of miscarriages, **HIV**, which causes congenital **AIDS**. Certain bacteria (tuberculosis, syphilis, brucellosis) and certain parasites (malaria, toxoplasmosis) also cross the placenta to infect the fetus.

Because infections are typically followed by immunity, it is rare for any of these infections to cause miscarriages repeatedly. Syphilis is an exception. Latent syphilis causes no symptoms but is nonetheless **chronic** and active, so a **serological test for syphilis** is a traditional and still standard blood test done in pregnancy and should especially be done for recurrent miscarriages that take place in the second trimester.

Some of these infections do cause birth defects (rubella and syphilis being among the best known, even though the diseases are rare nowadays). If the infections are suspected clinically, then prior exposure (and probable immunity) can be determined by measuring IgG antibodies in the blood, whereas a recent infection causes a distinguishable transient rise of IgM antibodies in the blood.

How the information of a recent infection is acted on at the time of pregnancy depends on a number of things—the stage of the pregnancy, the likely involvement of the fetus, the circumstances of the conception and the risk, not just of transmission of the organism to the fetus, but also of the likely severity of fetal damage.

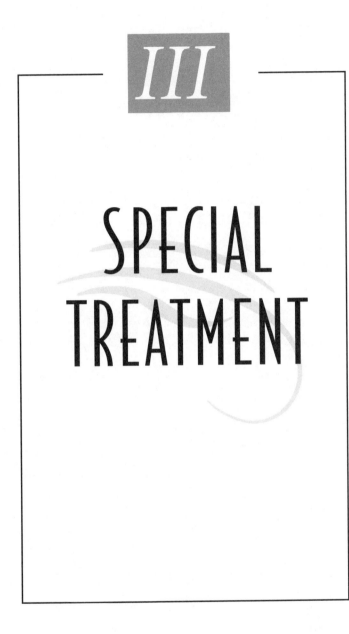

# III

# SPECIAL TREATMENT

# 8

# Treatment for Miscarriages

There is always the chance that a pregnancy will miscarry. As I say in Chapter 7, a miscarriage soon after a couple start putting their fertility to the test is sensibly regarded as just bad luck; it is reasonable to expect that the next pregnancy will be normal. A miscarriage after years of infertility, however, may not mean that cure is around the corner, and when one miscarriage follows another, and then there is another, a search for treatment becomes urgent.

# Treatment During Pregnancy

Can we stop a particular miscarriage? The very great majority of early miscarriages are predestined from conception or soon after. By the time a miscarriage threatens, especially in the first trimester, the die is well and truly cast, and nothing—including hormone injections—will make a difference in the outcome. An occasional exception is the detection of the **lupus anticoagulant**.

The presence of the lupus anticoagulant or the presence of significant **anticardiolipin antibodies** (described in Chapter 7) is managed by encouraging the circulation through the placenta, or afterbirth, using aspirin (in a similar way that aspirin is used in men to reduce the risk of heart attacks), heparin (an anticoagulant drug that can be given by subcutaneous injection), and the class of immunosuppressant drugs called corticosteroids (the cortisone-like pharmaceuticals, such as prednisone, prednisolone and dexamethasone). These treatments are rather specific for this particular cause of miscarriages, and in the majority of miscarriages they will not influence the outcome.

In the second trimester, early diagnosis of **cervical incompetence**, by timely examinations of the cervix in women at risk of it (including previously infertile women who have had procedures done that may simultaneously have weakened the cervix—see Chapter 23), can lead to urgent placement of a cervical ligature—a stitch in time. More often, unfortunately, symptoms of abnormal discharge from the vagina and back pain herald an imminent disaster.

Sometimes the contractions of the uterus in the **premature labor** kind of miscarriage can be treated early and vigorously enough to make a difference in the outcome. The drugs used include progesterone-like drugs (**progestogens**), such as 17-hydroxyprogesterone caproate, given as twice-weekly injections of Delalutin (United States) or Proluton Depot (Australia, United Kingdom); antiprostaglandin drugs, such as aspirin, mefenamic acid (Ponstel in the United States, Ponstan in the United Kingdom), indomethacin (Indocid) and chlorpromazine (Largactil); and inhibitors of uterine muscle contractions such as albuterol (Ventolin). Some of these drugs have important side effects. Because an underlying infection is not uncommon, treatment with an antibiotic also might be sensible. Generally, however, once the symptoms and signs of a miscarriage become apparent, it is for the subsequent pregnancy that we can hope to make a difference.

# Treatment Between Pregnancies

A possible cause for recurrent miscarriages will be found about half the time, although there is usually some lingering doubt whether the apparent cause diagnosed will turn out to be the actual cause of the miscarriages. Keep in mind also that few causes of miscarriage operate all the time, and, on the other hand, correcting a diagnosed cause does not necessarily protect against a miscarriage of a different, incidental cause, such as an isolated instance of **chromosomal embryopathy** or an unanticipated case of cervical incompetence.

## Treatment of the Uterus

An abnormality of the uterus can sometimes be fixed surgically. A **uterine septum** can be treated by dividing the septum during a **hysteroscopy** (see Chapter 18). A **bicornuate uterus** causes miscarriages less often; a corrective operation involves a laparotomy and plastic surgery to the uterus (a **metroplasty**—see Chapter 18). A **submucous fibroid** can often be treated by resecting it during a hysteroscopy, whereas more extensive fibroids extending through the wall of the uterus need more extensive surgery, involving **laparotomy** (opening of the abdomen) and excising the fibroids (**myomectomy**—see Chapter 17). **Intrauterine adhesions** can be difficult to treat, even with repeated hysteroscopies, but it is worth persisting with until a good cavity of the uterus results (see Chapter 17).

## Treatment of the Embryo

Nothing can be done about abnormalities of the chromosomes found by doing a karyotype on the prospective mother and father, but if either partner, for example, carries a **balanced translocation**, there should be a measure of reassurance that not every pregnancy will have unbalanced chromosomes and be

In a proportion of cases, a series of miscarriages will simply be a confluence of bad luck. You can estimate that if a woman has a 10 percent chance of miscarriage in her first pregnancy, she will have a 10 percent chance of miscarrying a second pregnancy and a 1 percent (10 percent of 10 percent) chance of miscarrying the first two pregnancies. The chance of miscarrying the first three, just through bad luck, will be 0.1 percent, or one in a thousand (rare, but it has to happen to someone!). The same calculations for a 40-year-old would give a chance of two miscarriages in a row as 4 percent and three in a row about 1 percent.

In real life the chance of a sequence of miscarriages taking place is higher, because there are real and persistent causes of miscarriages added to those caused simply by the way the odds fall. Truly **empirical studies** (studies based on observation, on empirically derived facts) show that the risk after one or more miscarriages can get high, but it is almost never 100 percent.

I can now get you to appreciate why there is so much quackery and witchcraft in the "treatment" of recurrent miscarriage, even those treatments published in otherwise distinguished medical journals. There are two main reasons. The first reason is the phenomenon that statisticians call "regression to the mean," or "a tendency for things to move toward the average as experience accumulates." If, for example, you take 100 couples who have had three successive miscarriages, do tests, find nothing especially wrong, treat them with a special potion derived from a cockscomb boiled up during a full moon and finally encourage the 100 couples to conceive again, perhaps half will miscarry a fourth time, but the other half will have a baby. You might be tempted to attribute your success to the magic potion—and use **statistics** to prove that the miscarriage rate that has fallen from 100 percent (in the first three pregnancies) to 50 percent (in the fourth) is **statistically significant**, but all that has happened is that the couples were selected *because* they had 100 percent miscarriages (ignoring those who had fewer miscarriages and who broke the sequence through chance before reaching the number three) and then behaved in the expected, average way.

The second basis for errors dates from 1938, when the statistician P. Malpas, writing in the *Journal of Obstetrics and Gynaecology of the British Empire*, drew up a table of the likelihood of one miscarriage following the next, based on debatable assumptions of "chance causes" and "100 percent recurrent causes." An American, N. J. Eastman, revised the assumptions in 1956 but reached similar conclusions. They ended up with the following calculations, based respectively on their various assumptions and on an 18 percent first-pregnancy risk of miscarriage (Malpas) and on a 10 percent risk (Eastman):

| Calculated Risk of Miscarriage After: | Malpas | Eastman |
|---|---|---|
| 1 previous miscarriage | 22% | 13% |
| 2 previous miscarriages | 38% | 37% |
| 3 previous miscarriages | 73% | 84% |

For many years, study after study showed that just about any kind of treatment would reduce the risk of a further miscarriage quite markedly from these grim predictions. Among the more notorious of the drugs for which this claim was made was DES (diethylstilbestrol), later held responsible for frequent birth abnormalities of the vagina, cervix, uterus and fallopian tubes in the babies who did not miscarry. The same statistical and Malpasian fallacies dog the naturopaths, herbalists and hypnotists (and so on) who today claim to cure repeated miscarriages.

In 1961 Dorothy Warburton and Clarke Fraser, from the Montreal Children's Hospital, demolished the fallacies in Malpas and Eastman's reasoning, namely that there is (or was at that time) no evidence that there is an appreciable group of women who throughout their lives have an indelible, 100 percent recurrent cause for miscarrying every pregnancy. Instead, they correctly predicted that "the gestational process depends on such a complex interaction between maternal and foetal factors, both genetic and environmental, that it must be susceptible to a very large number of agents."

In 1964 and again in 1979, Warburton actually studied miscarriage histories in women who had at least one baby. She showed with her colleagues that while the risk of miscarriage does rise appreciably after every further miscarriage, the risk in fact is nowhere near as high as Malpas and Eastman had predicted in theory. Still, through the bias she introduced by studying only fertile women (evidenced by at least one baby), Warburton's estimates might be a little low. The hardest studies to do are those that, instead of looking back at reproductive histories (retrospective studies), start by ascertaining couples before they get pregnant and then follow them up to see what happens (prospective studies).

Malcolm Macnaughton, from Aberdeen, Scotland, was the first to do such a study. Warburton and Macnaughton's findings are set out below and serve as the best guides we have to the true chance of miscarrying a further pregnancy after one or more previous miscarriages:

| Calculated Risk of Miscarriage After: | Warburton | Macnaughton |
|---|---|---|
| 1 previous miscarriage | 23% | 20% |
| 2 previous miscarriages | 28% | 44% |
| 3 previous miscarriages | 33% | 58% |

These are guides for you, the reader, and for me, the explainer, but even these data are not reliable enough for scientific studies of treatments. What investigators should try to do is divide couples randomly into two groups, avoiding other variables like age and occupation from causing bias, then treat one group with the new potion or remedy and not treat the other group (the **control group**). We can all then be convinced if there is a difference in outcome between the two groups.

Such controlled trials are difficult to mount and to pursue (and of course they must have the approval of an **institutional review board**), but they *have* to be done to overcome quackery. They may seem unfair, in that half the couples do not get the supposed benefit being tested, but in practice you would be surprised how often the people in the control group end up doing better than people in the specifically treated group. Such properly controlled trials have *not* shown that, for example, progestogens or injections of **human chorionic gonadotropin** (hCG) are effective for preventing miscarriage.

doomed. Fortitude is needed, however, to press on with successive pregnancie to the point where, by chance, one either is genetically normal or has balance chromosomes and survives. Should a pregnancy continue, the question in evitably arises whether to look at the chromosomes of the fetus. The procedure for this, **chorionic villus sampling** (CVS) and **amniocentesis**, themselves carr a small risk of causing miscarriage. There is no easy answer. Genetic counsel ing—and your intuition and perhaps that of your doctor—may help.

Unfortunately, there may be a genetic cause for the occasional long and un remitting sequence of miscarriages for which no chromosomal cause is other wise obvious. There are two possibilities. First, we believe but cannot yet show that when there have been five, six or more miscarriages, the sequence ma mean a coming together in the two partners of one or more lethal recessiv genes—genes of which two are needed for the gene to be expressed and are o no importance to either bearer alone or, with a majority of most other partners, are devastating when doubled up in the particular partnership. Alternatively, and just as hard to demonstrate, a new dominant mutation might have occurred in either partner that cripples development of all embryos carrying the gene. In these cases, however, not more than 50 percent of the pregnancies would be expected to be affected. Logically, the use of donated sperm, eggs or embryos (see Chapter 21) ought to overcome such a disability, but no systematic appraisals of these forms of help have been done for recurrent miscarriages.

Second, there could be an abnormality of the egg's **mitochondria** (the little powerhouses that generate any cell's energy), either through a mutation or set of mutations occurring in the prospective mother's cells when she herself was just an embryo and before her ovaries became populated by the eggs carrying the mutant **mitochondrial DNA** (mtDNA) or accumulated among the older eggs as the mother reaches her late thirties and her forties (as discussed in Chapter 6 and the box "How Eggs Get Their 'Use-by' Date: Mishaps in the Mitochondria"). This circumstance, if we could only be certain of the diagnosis for a particular woman's miscarriages, might lend itself to treatment with donated eggs (see Chapter 21) or (at the risk of being overly fanciful) even to a transfusion of mitochondria from a younger egg to the older fertilized egg in vitro as part of an in vitro fertilization program.

## "Empirical Treatment"

If no cause for miscarriage is found or if miscarriages persist after a diagnosed "cause" has been treated, there is much difference of opinion over what to do next. The range of possibilities—called "empirical treatment" by some physicians—includes herbal remedies, acupuncture, hormone tablets or injections and immunization with your partner's white blood cells (see the box "A Little Rejection" in Chapter 7). Few of these have been properly tested for effectiveness and those that *have* been tested have generally been found to be wanting. (See the box "Malpas's Mistake" for reasons why there has been such a plethora of treatments for pregnancies after recurrent miscarriages—treatments that go in and out of vogue.)

I am not out to persecute herbalists, naturopaths, acupuncturists and faith healers. They fill a need, especially when the attention they pay to patients comes with understanding and compassion, and they often seem to have more time than busy family doctors or specialists. It is just that they—like some gynecologists in the past—have not put their remedies to the test of a properly controlled trial.

## Supplements of Folic Acid

There is some evidence to suggest that taking extra folic acid may help prevent miscarriages. At Sydney IVF we recommend this as a routine. One 5-milligram tablet a day is enough. You can buy folic acid without a prescription, but eating plenty of fresh vegetables probably does the same thing.

We know that some cases of major abnormalities of the brain and spinal cord (neural tube defects such as anencephaly and spina bifida) can come about because of a deficiency of folic acid in the diet and can be prevented by taking folic acid at the time of conception. This is the main reason why we recommend all women on our assisted conception programs take folic acid during the program. We also know that women who have had a baby with such a neural defect are much more likely than other women to also have had a miscarriage. It is therefore possible that at least one kind of miscarriage actually represents an even grosser failure of development of the embryo than spina bifida or anencephaly and could result from the same deficiency. Because deficiency of folic acid remains common in our society and because taking folic acid supplements does no harm and is cheap, it is reasonable to recommend it to all women attempting to get pregnant, including women who have had one or more miscarriages.

## Infertility and Miscarriages

Often the same reproductive disorder that causes infertility lies behind miscarriage when conception has, by chance, taken place. Medically, there is no sharp distinction between not conceiving and conceiving and miscarrying. Managing the infertility properly can put an end to such miscarriages and lead instead to a healthy baby. The miscarriages common in infertility situations usually occur early, including those due to high concentrations of abnormal sperm (for treatment, see Chapter 9), disorders of ovulation (see Chapter 10), disease of the fallopian tubes (see Chapter 12) and, possibly, endometriosis (see Chapter 16). The best treatment in these situations is to make an accurate diagnosis and then carry out specific treatment, ensuring the best possible start to the pregnancy. Such treatment can include formal assisted conception (see Chapter 20).

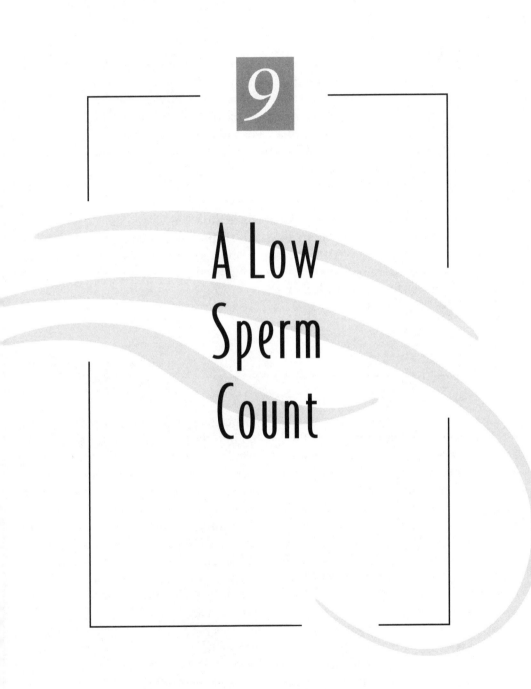

# 9

# A Low Sperm Count

Millions of sperm cells are ejaculated, but only one is needed to make it to the egg. That is the way it needs to be in order to get pregnant naturally. It would be nice to know why this is so, but, to put it succinctly, we still do not. This chapter will look at three main aspects of male-related infertility—a complete absence of sperm (**azoospermia**), a decrease in sperm (**oligospermia**) and inhibition of sperm by immune reactions to sperm (**sperm antibodies**)—and how to overcome these problems.

Treatment of male infertility can be directed at the man (which, few though the possibilities are, I describe in this chapter) or it can be directed at the woman, in the form of **assisted conception** (see Chapter 20). The one form of assisted conception I describe in this chapter is **assisted insemination** using the husband's sperm (AIH). The use of donated sperm for assisted insemination, or **donor insemination** (DI)—the ultimate fallback for overcoming male infertility—is discussed in Chapter 21.

## Sperm Terms

It is useful to understand a few special terms correctly. **Semen** refers to the fluid emitted at ejaculation with male orgasm. The sperm cells account for only about 1 percent of the volume of the semen, so there is absolutely no way of knowing whether sperm are present in the semen unless a microscope is used to examine either the semen after a specimen is collected (essentially a **sperm count**) or the mucus of the cervix after sexual intercourse (a **postcoital test**).

An inability to reach orgasm and thus to ejaculate is called **impotence** and usually manifests also as an inability to obtain, or to sustain, erection of the penis with sexual excitement. In some diseases that affect nerves, including some cases of diabetes, ejaculation can occur backward, up into the urine lying in the bladder, instead of out the tip of the penis; this is called **retrograde ejaculation**. **Aspermia** means that there is *no* ejaculate with orgasm, usually indicating malfunction of the glands that provide the seminal fluid, the **prostate** and the **seminal vesicles**.

When we perform a sperm count (see Chapter 4 for details), the result will be one of three: it is normal; one or more parameters are below normal (loosely called oligospermia, or "not enough normal sperm"); or no sperm are present at all (azoospermia). Even an apparently normal sperm count, however, does not always rule out a male contribution to infertility.

# No Sperm

We learned in Chapter 5 that there are two reasons why sperm can be missing from the semen: a failure of sperm production and release in the male sex organs, the **testes**; and an obstruction in the male genital ducts that lead on each side from the testis to the penis, including the **epididymis** and the **vas deferens**. The way to be sure what is happening is to carry out a **testicular biopsy** (taking a small piece of tissue from the testis for a pathologist to examine) and measure **serum follicle stimulating hormone** (serum FSH).

## No Sperm Production

Sperm cells are nurtured to maturity in the tubules of the testis (the **testicular tubules**). These tubules are lined by **Sertoli cells**, which envelop the immature sperm cells, providing them with the nutrition they need to develop. Although complete absence of sperm cells is rare, it does happen with, for example, errors of the **chromosomes**, such as with **Klinefelter's syndrome**. The diagnosis "Sertoli-cell-only syndrome" is confirmed by a biopsy of the testis, although there is no need for this test if a **karyotype** shows the abnormality of Klinefelter's, namely 47,XXY—an extra X chromosome.

A more common problem in the tubules is when sperm cells are present, but their numbers are reduced and those that are there do not complete their development into mature sperm. The serum FSH can be increased, although a

## "Follicle" Stimulating Hormone in Men?

**Follicle stimulating hormone** (FSH) is the hormone women make to stimulate **follicles** in the ovary (see Chapter 3), but men have it too. In women, the follicle cells nurture the developing egg. In men, the Sertoli cells nurture the sperm, and the same hormone, FSH, is needed. Just as the serum FSH goes up in women when there are few or no eggs left in the ovaries, in men the serum FSH goes up when mature sperm are not being produced in the testis. A high serum FSH in the absence of sperm in the ejaculate means that there is testicular damage and that the problem is thus not likely to be a blockage (or, if a blockage is present, that it is not the only problem).

In about one in 200 cases of male infertility, the testes are inactive because of a deficiency of FSH and **luteinizing hormone** (LH) from the pituitary gland, just as this deficiency can cause **anovulation** in women (see Chapter 10). As well as inhibiting the maturing of sperm, such a deficiency causes the other main tissue in the testes, the **Leydig cells**, which produce the male sex hormone **testosterone**, to also be inactive, which means the male sex characters are stopped from forming or from being maintained. If the deficiency is present from birth or from childhood, puberty fails to happen normally; if the deficiency is acquired after puberty, there will be less of a need for shaving and, gradually, impotence or loss of sexual desire will follow. The abnormality is diagnosed by finding low levels of serum FSH, **serum LH** and **serum testosterone**.

A deficiency of FSH and LH in men, as in women, can in turn be because of a deficiency of **gonadotropin releasing hormone** (GnRH), produced by the **hypothalamus** to drive the pituitary gland, as described in Chapter 3. In some cases of FSH and LH deficiency present from birth there can be a faulty sense of smell (a physiological function also dependent on the hypothalamus), an association known as **Kallmann's syndrome**, which can occur in either sex.

Deficiency of FSH might also be the result of disease of the pituitary gland itself, but this is even rarer. A prolactin-producing tumor in men, also much less common than such tumors are in women, generally produces profound impotence as the sperm count falls. The diagnosis is made by finding a high **serum prolactin**, after which special tests for imaging the pituitary gland need to be carried out.

Although rare, these causes of azoospermia are important because they can be treated, using the same preparations of FSH and LH that are used in women for ovulation induction, namely **human menopausal gonadotropin** (hMG, such as **Humegon** and **Pergonal**) and **human chorionic gonadotropin** (hCG, such as **Pregnyl** and **Profasi**). Treatment is prolonged, however, and needs to be carried out over many months before a response is seen. In between attempts at pregnancy, treatment with injections of testosterone is enough for normal sexual function.

late-stage arrest in the development of the sperm may show a normal serum FSH. A testicular biopsy is needed to define the diagnosis. Why some men have such a "maturation arrest" has been under active investigation for a number of years. The causes in general seem to be the same as many of those that result in less complete sperm-forming problems (see the section "Oligospermia"). If there is a genetic cause for lowish sperm counts (see Chapter 2 and below), then random, unfortunate combination of the genes responsible for limiting sperm counts might produce azoospermia.

Both maturation arrest and Sertoli-cell-only syndrome can also be the result of radiation treatment or drug treatment (chemotherapy) for cancer. Environmental factors more often produce oligospermia and are discussed further on. A shortage of follicle stimulating hormone, the testicles' driving hormone in the **pituitary gland** (and a common cause of absent **ovulation** in women), is rare.

## Sperm Obstructions

Obstructions lying between the testis and the urethra, which carries semen down the penis at ejaculation, can be **congenital** (present before birth) or can be acquired later, most commonly through infection, especially gonorrhea, which by causing epididymitis (inflammation of the epididymis) can obstruct the epididymis. Congenital forms of epididymal and vas deferens obstruction can arise in a number of situations, including exposure as a fetus to diethylstilbestrol (DES), which was taken by many women in the 1950s and 1960s in an attempt to stop miscarriage and also caused genital abnormalities in women (see Chapter 18). Another situation that has been known to give rise to congenital obstruction, or to obstruction occurring in infancy, is an association with chronic bronchitis and sinusitis, known as "Young's syndrome," which was probably related to a poisonous effect of mercury used in teething powders and, since mercury was removed in 1960, is now more rare. A third cause of congenital obstruction arises if the man has the genes for **cystic fibrosis** (a severe congenital disease of the lungs); all male sufferers have an absence of the vas deferens on each side, called **congenital absence of the vasa deferentia** (CAVD).

## Absent or Retrograde Ejaculation

Absent ejaculation or retrograde (backward-directed) ejaculation can occur after spinal cord injury (paraplegia) and after surgery to the bladder or prostate, as well as with diabetes. The diagnosis of retrograde ejaculation is made by finding sperm in a sample of urine passed after orgasm in sexual intercourse or masturbation. With absent ejaculation, sperm for use with assisted conception, including assisted insemination, can be obtained by electroejaculation (whereby an electrical stimulus applied under anesthesia using a special probe is passed

## Nature's Orneriness

Why would nature allow inherited causes to gain ground when nature's aim in evolution, on the face of it, ought to be to maximize reproductive fitness? I discuss this paradox in Chapter 2, where I show that there are advantages to the species generally for reproduction to be limited. This limiting of fertility is more important as couples get older, when they still enjoy (often *require*) sexual intercourse for their continued bonding, but they have children who need looking after. These children must not have their mother worn out through the repeated bearing of more children while they depend on her, or there will be the risk that without a mother none will survive to achieve adolescence and independence. Remember that it is not until children are grown and themselves conceive that you can truly say that you have successfully reproduced—that you have left your genetic legacy.

Thus, nature will favor *some* genes that decrease fertility. Nature pays little attention to personal suffering, however, and the reality is that some people or couples will by chance be overdosed with infertility genes, either individually (with severe oligospermia) or in combination with their partner, when mild oligospermia complicates, for example, mild endometriosis (see Chapter 15). The purpose of the profession of medicine here, as in every other field in which there are physicians and nurses, is to ease the suffering caused by nature's shortcomings or excesses.

through the anus into the region of the prostate gland). With retrograde ejaculation, sperm cells can be recovered from the urine, "washed," concentrated and then used for assisted insemination or for **in vitro fertilization** (IVF). If this is to be done, the urine should first be deacidified (rendered alkaline) in the man, by his swallowing a tablespoon of baking soda dissolved in a small glass of water on three occasions over the 24 hours before obtaining the specimen.

# Oligospermia

A low sperm count is like greatness: some are born with it, others have it thrust upon them.

# Inherited Oligospermia

Many cases of low sperm counts are caused by inherited factors. In a paper published in the *British Medical Journal* in 1994, Professor Richard Lilford and colleagues showed that 17 of 148 men who attended either of two infertility clinics in Leeds had brothers who had also sought help for infertility, an incidence of more than 11 percent. On the other hand, of 169 men who were questioned while their wives were having babies or who were requesting sterilization by **vasectomy**, none had a brother infertile from oligospermia. Careful analysis pointed to the likelihood that 60 percent of infertility in men was inherited by a recessive mode of inheritance, meaning that two abnormal genes are needed to inherit the oligospermia.

The types of genes that may be involved are those that code for the hormone receptor for the main male hormone, testosterone. Testosterone's action in the sperm-forming tubules of the testis is needed for sperm to develop to maturity. A number of genes could be involved. Although we do not know much about these genes, we do know that the genes for decreased fertility in men are not the same as the genes for decreased fertility in women.

Another prominent congenital cause of oligospermia is incomplete descent of one or both testes into the scrotum. This condition is called **cryptorchidism**

## Hidden Testes: Truly Hidden or Just Hiding?

Normal testes in young boys do not spend all their time in the scrotum, so the diagnosis of undescended testes can be tricky. The reason is that the tissues that lead down to the testis in the scrotum include a muscle that can contract, as a reflex from anxiousness or from cold, and pull the testis up out of the scrotum. This is the so-called "retractile testis," which needs no treatment and thus needs to be distinguished from a truly cryptorchid testis.

Experienced physicians sometimes advise a boy's parents to gently feel for the testes in the scrotum (with appropriate explanation to the boy) while he is relaxed in the bath; if they are both in the scrotum, all is well. Likewise, if both testes have been noted to be present in the scrotum at birth, before the retractile reflex has developed, then all will be well. Not all normal testes are in the scrotum by birth, however, especially if birth has been premature. Careful examination over the few months after birth will usually confirm their normal arrival in the scrotum.

(from the Greek for "hidden testicle"). The testis may lie anywhere from high in the abdomen, within the wall of the abdomen in the area of the groin, down to the soft tissues around the top of the scrotum. The higher the location, the higher the risk these testicles have of developing cancer. Diagnosis in early boyhood is important, because there is evidence that the sooner the situation is corrected by an operation (called an **orchidopexy**), the better for the later production of sperm. The diagnosis in young boys can be difficult.

## Environmentally Caused Oligospermia

If the genetics of oligospermia is still a little obscure, environmental causes of low sperm counts are even less understood. Sperm experts still do not agree that the average sperm count in men in Western societies has fallen in the last generation or two, although the evidence that this has been happening is getting stronger. In particular, there seems little doubt that the incidence of more serious problems with men's testicles is increasing, such as a failure of one or both testes to descend into the scrotum and, even more serious, cancer of the testis, which can be associated with very low sperm production.

What could the mechanisms be? An early favorite among clinicians has been the ambient temperature in which testes find themselves. It is well known that the normal temperature in the scrotum is several degrees lower than it is in the abdomen. The testes of many mammals seem to need this lower temperature to work properly, and many scientists (me included) have shown that bringing the testes back into the abdomen of rats by an operation causes the Sertoli cells to malfunction within 24 hours! Thus, it is wise to avoid hot baths and saunas if there is any question about the sperm count. Hot showers are not a problem, because there is enough evaporation over the scrotum while standing under the shower to keep the testes from heating up too much. Whether tight underwear is a culprit remains to be proven.

One treatable cause of oligospermia is a **varicocele**, a varicose vein inside the scrotum, usually on the left side, which may allow blood at too high a body temperature or blood containing too much carbon dioxide or other substances to spill backward from the abdomen into the scrotum. Varicoceles can be felt in the upper part of the scrotum, typically by noting more tissues between the fingers on the left side than can be felt on the right; the examining physician may feel an impulse upon the man coughing, which sends a spurt of blood backward. The diagnosis of varicocele can be confirmed by an **ultrasound** of the scrotum. The treatment involves removing the abnormal vein or, better, tying it off higher in the body, up in the wall of the abdomen. (It means a day or two of discomfort, no worse than the discomfort a woman undergoes with a **laparoscopy**.) The problem with treating varicoceles, however, is that not all detectable varicoceles are actually doing much harm, and treatment is uncommonly followed by much improvement.

The sperm count is susceptible to environmental poisons, occupational toxins and drugs used for medical purposes. Smoking is probably the most avoidable of environmental noxious substances. Harmful oxidation of sperm is typical in any situation where the sperm count is reduced environmentally and smoking can only make this worse. So-called recreational drugs are also harmful, including marijuana. Alcohol in moderation probably does not affect the sperm count; wine, which contains many natural antioxidants, could possibly turn out to be beneficial—in moderate amounts. Exposure to industrial pollutants at work can be harmful; these include the constituents of printing inks and adhesives, as well as paint pigments containing the metals lead, cadmium and mercury.

Unfortunately, little is known about which medical drugs are liable to depress the sperm count. Many of the common drugs for high blood pressure and peptic ulcers can lower the sperm count, although not for everyone who takes them. Sulfasalazine, used to treat colitis, is known to reduce the sperm count (sometimes to azoospermia), as do anabolic steroids, which are misused for body building. Chemotherapy drugs used for treating cancer can affect any tissue where cells are being made quickly, including the tubules of the testes; the effects such drugs have on the manufacture of sperm is often permanent.

The substances polluting the environment are even less understood in this regard. Dioxin, an infamous component of the defoliant known as Agent Orange, used for removing vegetation in the Vietnam War, has been implicated in oligospermia, as it has in the causation of endometriosis (see Chapter 15). The pesticides DDT, dibromochloropropane, chlordecone and ethylenedibromide, among others, have also been blamed. A group of researchers from Aarhus University in Denmark recently had the opportunity to examine sperm counts from members of the Danish Organic Farmers Association, and these farmers had significantly better sperm counts than comparable men who did not so fastidiously avoid using potentially polluting chemicals.

Infections of the male reproductive organs can be harmful either by causing an obstruction (discussed earlier) or by harming the sperm directly. A history of a discharge that stains the underclothes, of painful urination or of unusual tenderness of the scrotal organs are all reasons to have a consultation with a urologist, with a view to treatment with antibiotics. A particularly serious infection is one caused by the mumps virus, especially if mumps is contracted during adolescence and is associated with pain (hence inflammation) of the

Human sperm counts seem to be more susceptible to harm than many animal sperm counts, but studies on animals in the wild may be particularly useful in identifying harmful pollutants in the environment. Dr. L. J. Guillette from the Department of Zoology at the University of Florida in Gainesville, in an address to the Fourteenth World Congress of Gynecology and Obstetrics held in Montreal in 1994, argued convincingly that human agricultural and industrial by-products and toxins are very widespread, even in environments we might think are pristine. Measurable amounts of DDT, for example, are found even in the polar regions.

Dangerous man-made contaminants share three special features, as well as being human in origin: they evaporate easily, they are very poorly soluble in water but soluble in fat and they are not able to be metabolized or destroyed. They therefore disperse widely and get trapped in the fat stores of plants and animals, working their way thoroughly through the ecosystem. Because of their persistence, organisms feeding on each other cause these substances to accumulate and be magnified as they get worked up in the food web.

Top-level predators, and this includes human consumers, can thus carry body burdens of contaminants at levels a million or more times greater than the environmental background level. The resulting reproductive disorders that have been found among wildlife, according to Dr. Guillette, include reduced fertility, reduced ability to hatch (among birds), reduced viability of offspring, reduced hormone activity and altered adult sexual behavior.

### ... and from Beef Cattle

The detrimental effects of substances such as DDT, dioxin and polychlorinated biphenyls (PCBs) may be because they and their metabolites can act as **estrogens** and as antiandrogens. To add insult to this injury, synthetic estrogens active by mouth, such as diethylstilbestrol (DES), were used widely for many years to increase the weight of beef in the livestock industry, before being banned in the 1980s. Professor Niels Skakkebaek of the University Department of Growth and Reproduction in Copenhagen has been a leader in drawing attention to what more and more of us are convinced is a major decline through the second half of the twentieth century in human sperm counts, the increase in cryptorchidism and the increase in cancer of the testis. He, too, believes that estrogens and antiandrogens accumulating in the environment may be to blame.

testes. Permanent damage to the testes is likely. Mumps in childhood, well before the process of puberty starts, rarely affects the testes.

The testes can come to harm from injury to the scrotum. Torsion of the testis, or twisting on its blood supply, can also cause substantial damage, although torsion is not very likely to affect both testes. Pain in the scrotum, spontaneously or after injury, is always a reason to seek medical help quickly.

# Immune Reactions to Sperm: Antisperm Antibodies

The sperm-forming tubules in the testicles and the ducts that carry the sperm to the exterior are physically isolated from the body's immune system. Should the barrier between the bloodstream and the male's reproductive tissues be breached, however, the immune system is likely to form antibodies to the sperm cells. As we noted in Chapter 6, these antibodies can be formed to the head of the sperm, to its midpiece (its waist) or to its tail. The antibodies may be agglutinating, causing the sperm to stick to each other and thus not be able to swim properly, or they may be directly immobilizing, causing the sperm cell to die. More insidiously, they may just coat the sperm, producing no visible result but blocking the sperm from attaching to the egg. All these antibodies can be revealed by those **sperm antibody tests** that are carried out using **immunobeads**.

The most common cause for sperm antibodies forming in men is the sterilizing operation, vasectomy. At the cut end of the vas deferens on the side of the testis (where, therefore, the sperm are obstructed), an irritation is set up, with inflammation and, inevitably, an immune reaction against the accumulating sperm, with production of sperm antibodies. Worse, at least for men who later want the sterilization to be reversed, the immune reaction persists, permanently compromising sperm numbers and sperm motility, even when the vasectomy reversal procedure itself—the new plumbing—is a success. Sperm antibodies are also likely to form when the epididymis or the vas gets blocked from infection. On the other hand, they do not often form when these ducts have been blocked from birth. The reason for this discrepancy is not known.

Women can also develop sperm antibodies. Sperm are highly penetrative, routinely reaching the abdomen after sexual intercourse. The surprise perhaps is that antibodies do not form much more often than they do (see the box "Sperm in Women and Sperm in Men"). A moderate level of sperm agglutinating antibodies is not uncommon in women after many years of infertility.

## Sperm in Women and Sperm in Men

The body is no zoological fortress; if it were, there would be no need for virologists, bacteriologists and parasitologists. Sperm in the body are intrepid—and rather long lasting. Sperm heads engulfed by **macrophages** (the body's scavenging cells that ultimately dispose of foreign material) last in recognizable form for a week or more. Inseminated mice, for example, can reveal that genetic material from sperm cells ends up not just in the abdomen and the lymph glands but eventually in far-off tissues such as the heart (although not, I should say, as identifiable sperm cells).

Nature probably has a purpose in a woman getting to know her partner's genetic material firsthand before pregnancy. Studies show that there are fewer complications in pregnancies that start after a suitable conditioning period of exposure to sperm. Professor Ian Craft, an IVF gynecologist in London, has found that a woman who conceives by receiving donated embryos, and thus has no prior exposure to the relevant male's genetic material before she is pregnant, runs a higher risk of experiencing pregnancy-related high blood pressure than women who conceive naturally.

In addition to sperm cells, semen contains white blood cells that can colonize the recipient, particularly if intercourse takes place in a way that causes abrasion or trauma. This is the way that the **AIDS** virus, **HIV**, is transmitted. At vaginal sexual intercourse, male to female transmission of AIDS is twice as likely to happen as female to male transmission. The risk may be higher with anal intercourse, as is, possibly, the risk of developing antibodies to sperm, when sperm gain access to tissues in ways the reproductive system has not necessarily evolved to cope with.

Curiously, sperm antibodies, if found in one partner, are more likely to also be present in the other partner. Sperm antibodies have also been found among women who have never had sexual intercourse. The reason for the production of sperm antibodies in these situations is thought to be the coincidental resemblance some viruses or other infections may have to the surface molecules on sperm cells, an immune phenomenon called "cross-reactivity." Because such an infection is reasonably likely to affect each of the partners, the common occurrence of antibodies that just happen to also react against sperm is explained, as is the occasional development of sperm antibodies among virgins.

The reason why some men without blockages form sperm antibodies and why some women form serious levels of sperm antibodies that account for infertility is still obscure. Treatment is unsatisfactory, short of assisted conception involving IVF (see Chapter 20). Immunosuppressive drugs, including the adrenal-like steroids cortisone, prednisone and prednisolone, are sometimes claimed to be effective, but when given in adequate amounts for long enough there is a small chance of a serious penalty—a crippling complication of the hip joint, called **aseptic necrosis of the femoral head** (literally, noninfective tissue death of the top end of the thigh bone). Even a small risk of such a serious hazard keeps most physicians and most potential patients away from more than a short course of treatment, usually closely related to an assisted conception maneuver.

# Treatment of Male-Factor Infertility

In reproductive medicine it is not difficult to cause outrage among some more extreme feminists, such as a group called FINRRAGE (Feminist International Network of Resistance to Reproductive and Genetic Engineering). Eating at their souls, it seems, is the biological reality that it is women who conceive children and in whom, through reproductive medicine, the proof of successful pregnancy needs to be achieved. Their gripe is the absence of available effective treatment for the great majority of men with low sperm counts, our efforts instead being directed at the woman, where with assisted conception we get by with smaller and smaller numbers of normal, even immature, sperm. These methods of treatment, which involve fertilization of a woman's egg or eggs in vitro, have been a generally successful approach (and are discussed from a medical perspective in Chapter 20 and from a more social perspective in Chapter 24).

Dr. Renate Klein, in the late 1980s and early 1990s a research fellow at the Department of Women's Studies at Deakin University, Victoria, maintains that too often the woman in this situation is coerced into accepting such intrusive treatments to gain "his" child, instead of being given an evenhanded choice. This choice includes the option of donor insemination, or assisted insemination using the semen of a normal man who donates semen for the purpose (see Chapter 21). There is also the option of not having children at all.

How couples react to male infertility and how they then relate to each other is as variable as the affected couples. Discussion of this personal side I leave to other chapters. Our purpose here is to keep to the biological and medical facts as we presently understand them.

## The Few Treatments That Work in Men

The fact is that, with rare exceptions, the only effective options for treating men with oligospermia consist of surgical treatment of varicocele in some men and paying general attention to not smoking and avoiding the more obvious workplace pollutants. Drugs such as **clomiphene** (used to induce ovulation in women; see Chapter 10) have not been shown to be effective in men and they are expensive. Antioxidant vitamins, such as vitamins A, C and E may or may not be helpful, but most people are not short of them or of other antioxidants found in the diet. The sperm count in any case is not likely to be more than marginally improved. For most men with low sperm counts, orders of magnitude of improvement (tenfold, a hundredfold, a thousandfold) are needed to make a material difference to their wives' conceiving easily.

Azoospermia is amenable to corrective treatment in men only when it is the result of a localized blockage of the epididymis or if the vas deferens is amenable to microsurgical repair. Remember that a diagnosis of blockage is usually made by a urologist carefully feeling the structures in the scrotum; it is confirmed by finding a normal serum FSH and perhaps by showing normal sperm-forming tubules in the testis with a testicular biopsy. (The ducts are too fine to allow an X-ray to be done without risking a blockage resulting from the test itself.) The surgery needed is highly specialized—do not let just any urologist attempt it. The success of such microsurgery depends on the skill of the microsurgeon, the location of the blockage (reversal of male sterilization by vasectomy, a **vasovasostomy**, is usually the most straightforward) and the degree of problem caused by lingering sperm antibodies.

Beyond these forms of treatment, we have to move to the person in whom pregnancy is to happen, namely the woman. In this chapter we look only at assisted insemination using the husband's semen (AIH) and, to prepare for the more substantial interventions that involve the woman (and which are described in Chapter 20), we consider the rapid progress that has been made in recovering sperm cells for IVF from men with very few or no sperm in the ejaculate.

# Assisted Insemination with Husband's Semen (AIH)

When impregnation through sexual intercourse fails to secure pregnancy it can be due, for example, to sexual impotence, very low semen volumes, retrograde ejaculation, severe **hypospadias** or an obstruction in the woman in the region of the **cervix**. In these circumstances, AIH can be carried out with good effect. AIH is the simplest and the oldest of the reproductive technologies.

Is there value in using AIH for couples whose infertility is due just to oligospermia? Is it any better than similarly timed, natural sexual intercourse (see Chapter 19)? Many of us have long doubted that it is, especially with mere insemination of the ejaculate into the cervix. If, however, the sperm is prepared by washing it as if for use with **gamete intrafallopian transfer** (GIFT) or in vitro fertilization (IVF) by separating it from the semen's other components and resuspending the sperm in a special salt solution, then inseminating not into the mucus of the cervix but up through the cervix into the uterus itself—**intrauterine insemination** (IUI)—can have some benefit, although the benefit is limited.

In a study performed at the Free University Hospital in Amsterdam, Holland, and published in 1990, Dr. Antonio Martinez and colleagues randomly allocated women with either unexplained infertility or infertility associated only with oligospermia to one of four treatments: timed sexual intercourse; timed IUI; timed sexual intercourse after the woman had taken clomiphene (which induces ovulation, perhaps of more than one follicle, but at the price of some negative effects on mucus in the cervix and on the lining of the uterus—see Chapter 10); and timed IUI after clomiphene. The incidences of pregnancy were, respectively, none of 34 cycles of timed sex alone, three of 32 cycles (9.4 percent) of IUI, one of 31 cycles (3.2 percent) of clomiphene plus sex, and five of 35 cycles (14.3 percent) of clomiphene plus IUI. They concluded that there was significant value in intrauterine insemination compared with sexual intercourse, but not much, if any, additional benefit came from using clomiphene, despite a significant increase in the number of eggs obtained with its use.

## Intrauterine Insemination and Superovulation

The benefit of ovulating multiple eggs (**superovulation**) in association with IU is demonstrated much better by using follicle stimulating hormone (FSH) instead of clomiphene. FSH avoids the negative effects clomiphene has on the uterus, and it has become a popular form of assisting conception with IUI whether there is oligospermia or unexplained infertility. It also produces more ovulating eggs than clomiphene. The arithmetic to justify it is straightforward. If few sperm cells are reaching the fallopian tubes, the presence of two eggs at the site of fertilization will double the chance of pregnancy; four eggs will just about quadruple it and so on. The hazard that comes with the use of FSH is the one of higher-order multiple pregnancy—triplets, quadruplets, quintuplets and beyond—possibly then managed by **fetal reduction**, which has its own ethical and moral dangers. Comparing the risk of not getting pregnant with IUI and superovulation with the hazard of multiple pregnancy should the treatment prove too effective is not straightforward.

## Risks and Hazards

For an intelligent assessment of the risks and benefits of multiple ovulation induction—as is the case so often with evaluating choices in treating infertility—we need to distinguish **risk** from **hazard**. Strictly speaking, the risk of a high-multiple pregnancy with intrauterine insemination and superovulation (multiple ovulation induction) is low—there is a low chance of it happening. But if it does happen it is a very serious hazard and the penalty is considerable. The hazard is such that one should accept it only if it has a very, very low chance of eventuating. The difference between a risk and a hazard is that *risk* is a probability you can put a number on, and a *hazard* is an all-or-nothing event—it happens or it does not.

For example, whether you sail a 12-foot or 40-foot boat across the Atlantic Ocean from the Florida Keys to Bermuda, one *hazard* is the same (namely, drowning), but, other things being equal, the *risk* or *chance* of drowning is much greater with the smaller boat. For another example of the distinction, the risk of getting caught shoplifting might be small, but the hazard, the penalty if you are caught, is prohibitive. In practice it is often not so easy to balance the risk of not getting pregnant with the hazards introduced by modern infertility treatment, such as high-multiple pregnancy. Read more about the compromises in Chapter 20.

In those parts of the world where IUI is still used with superovulation (chiefly North America and Asia), I believe that its popularity will decrease with time. There is now such concern about the long-term health effects of repeated multiple ovulation in women, particularly the eventual risk of cancer of the ovary (see Chapter 11), that there will be more and more emphasis on taking the utmost advantage of every such ovarian stimulation, using GIFT and IVF. Studies in 1989 in California showed that AIH after treatment with FSH gave a pregnancy rate of 6.7 percent per cycle, compared with 32.9 percent per cycle using GIFT. The Amsterdam doctors I referred to achieved pregnancies with IUI only if more than 2 million washed, normal, motile sperm were available for insemination into the uterus, and this is not achievable for many men with oligospermia. With GIFT, good results are possible with just 100,000 such sperm. I would conclude from this that the usefulness of AIH, with or without stimulation of the ovaries, is very limited for couples with significant oligospermia.

## Cancer Insurance

AIH is the traditional way by which sperm banked by men who are to receive sterilizing treatment for cancer is used to try and secure pregnancy. Nowadays, as with oligospermia generally, the amount of sperm stored and available is so limited that it is usually kept for IVF.

# Where There's Sperm There's Hope ...

Never say never. In medicine, as in life, we learn not to be too surprised by the unexpected. Provided there is not a complete absence of sperm—azoospermia—pregnancy can and does sometimes happen. It really does ultimately take just one sperm to make it (and, despite the cynics, it's usually not the milkman's). Experienced infertility physicians have seen pregnancies ensue with sperm counts of fewer than one million and despite dismaying levels of sperm antibodies. Whatever assistance and whatever intrusions couples endure to get around the problem of low sperm counts, they should try not to lose sight of this ever-present possibility. Chapter 19 takes my advice on this further.

## AIH Ethics: When to Offer It and When (Perhaps) Not

The failure to offer sperm banking to a man in 1981 when he was about to receive cancer treatment that would lead to azoospermia was in 1991 the subject of legal action for damages in Great Britain. The action was not successful, but now that sperm banking is more generally available, a future legal action based on such an omission might well succeed, according to Diana Brahams, a London trial attorney who writes for *The Lancet.*

Notwithstanding Onan's sin (the sin of masturbation), AIH is mostly untroubled ethically, but there are three exceptions: when it is accompanied by stimulating the ovaries to achieve multiple ovulation and thus hazarding triplets, quadruplets or beyond; when the semen comes from a prisoner, separated from his wife or previous partner by the command of society; and when the semen is to be used posthumously, after the death of the sperm provider.

If most sperm in the world are produced to be lost, it is especially true for all of a prisoner's sperm. I have read in books that jails can stink of semen. While prisons are for punishment, so a man's reproductive destiny (or that of a woman, unless she is already pregnant) will be locked up with the prisoner. The occasional requests we get at our own donor insemination program in Sydney for help in obtaining, stor-

ing and using semen from a prisoner have quickly become lost in confused motives on the part of the prisoner and his wife or friend, in the unwillingness of administrators to cooperate and risk setting a prece-dent and in the general helplessness that afflicts prison inmates and their dependents. The Virginia Supreme Court in 1993 denied the appeals of two prisoners under sentences of death who wanted to freeze their sperm in an attempt to preserve "their bloodline"; at least one man's girlfriend had agreed to be named as the legal recipient of the sperm. The men's pleas were reportedly described by Virginia's governor as "brazen" and "appalling," while the court characterized them as "frivolous." Rejecting all arguments, the court ruled that it was not an unconstitutionally cruel or unusual punishment to execute the men without first freezing their sperm for possible future use.

In 1984 Dame Mary Warnock, an Oxford professor of philosophy, gave her name to a celebrated report produced by a committee she had chaired. The Warnock Report was in very many ways a sensible acceptance of the then recent and profound developments that had occurred in reproductive technology. But without justification, in my view, Warnock sought to stop the use of sperm by a woman after the death of her husband. Under the U.K.

## AIH Ethics (concluded)

Human Fertilisation and Embryology Act of 1990, the male whose sperm is used successfully after his death is not to be treated as the father of the child. The "expected psychological complications for the child and the mother" were the grounds given for this infringement of the reproductive and social autonomy of women who have once chosen a mate.

Warnock did not explain why and how these problems (if they truly are problems) might come to be the primary concern of people other than the woman herself, the woman who is, with her other children, really the only person who has a personal stake in the issue. A similar case in France was decided in favor of the woman after public opinion forced the release of her husband's sperm from the National Sperm Bank after his death. The woman's perspective in such circumstances is crucial; it is enough here to say that she should have a large part in making the final decision on the matter and should be unhampered in her right to decline.

Sperm banking and embryo banking (see Chapter 20) are increasingly available to young adults faced with treatment likely to lead inadvertently to sterility. On the face of it, they are assuming that they will survive the treatment and that they will wish later to reproduce, like any normal person. Consciously or subconsciously, however, they want to preserve their genetic potential in case they die. Many dying patients take comfort from having children, because it means that it is not strictly the end of the road biologically; on the other hand, among the reasons for the anguish adolescents have in facing death is that their procreative instincts have not been fulfilled. I have observed that young adults faced with death often have a considerable and urgent wish to have children.

This does not give society an obligation to use reproductive technology to achieve offspring for every person, young or not, faced with death (or to try and satisfy the wishes of their understandably distressed parents), but if the reason a husband leaves stored sperm behind after death is to secure descendants, then his saying so in his will should, in my opinion, be respected, if his surviving wife wants it that way. In New South Wales, the Law Reform Commission has sympathetically and sensibly recommended that the deceased husband should be recognized as the father provided that the woman is his widow and is unmarried at the time of insemination and the birth, but that the child should have a right to the father's inheritance only if this is specifically provided for in his will.

# ... and There's Now Hope Even with No Sperm

Meanwhile, there is no doubt that overcoming the effects of extremely low and even zero sperm counts is the area where huge progress is being made with IVF Chapter 20 describes the microscopic insertion of sperm directly into the egg

## From Father to Son

Can the genes for oligospermia be passed on? Yes, in some instances. Men born with blockages of the epididymis or an absent vas deferens can be carrying one or more genes for cystic fibrosis, a severe disease of the lungs in children who inherit the gene for it from both parents. A screening test is wise for men with such a blockage, and if it is detected, the wife should be screened for the gene before a decision is made to get pregnant.

Men with extreme oligospermia, whose wives can now conceive with their sperm using IVF with sperm microinjection techniques instead of from donated sperm (see Chapter 21), may carry a chromosomal abnormality that could be transmitted to the offspring. We sometimes screen such men with a karyotype before proceeding. It can also be prudent for the pregnant woman to have a karyotype done on the fetus, either using **chorionic villus sampling** (CVS) or **amniocentesis** to obtain fetal cells. In either case, the couple needs to understand that if an inherited condition has caused the sperm count problem (and this may be

more common than we might think), this condition may well be passed on to the child conceived this way.

There is no evidence so far of an increase in birth defects with sperm microinjection generally or with ICSI in particular. With one kind of exception, karyotypes of the pregnancies after ICSI are turning out to be normal much more often than we expected. The exception is that there appears to be a significant increase in the risk of a baby with an **aneuploidy** for an X or a Y chromosome: karyotypes such as 45,X (**Turner's syndrome**), 47,XXY (Klinefelter's syndrome), 47,XXX (**triple-X syndrome**) and 47,XYY (**extra-Y-chromosome syndrome**) can be expected with a risk of perhaps one or two per 100 births, which is several times more than expected among natural conceptions. Whether this represents an increased risk for the families involved (most of whom have pregnancies naturally too few and far between to be able to estimate the risk they would run with natural conception) remains to be seen.

More and more, these sperm are being obtained directly from the testis or from the ducts leading out of the testis, before they risk damage from oxidation and before they are exposed to sperm antibodies in the epididymis and the vas deferens.

Since 1993 sperm have regularly been obtained from men with an obstruction to sperm production present in the epididymis or vas deferens, whether from birth or acquired from an infection or from a vasectomy for sterilization. The procedure is called **microsurgical epididymal sperm aspiration** (MESA). The recovered sperm can be used straight away for IVF (generally by direct insertion into eggs; see Chapter 20) or frozen for use later. Since 1995 immature sperm cells have been removed directly from the testis in men who produce too few sperm cells for there to be any in the ejaculate. This breakthrough for couples with azoospermia caused by maturation arrest is called **testicular sperm extraction** (TESE).

For the millions of ejaculated sperm nature needs to have one egg fertilized, we are now able to help to the extent that one egg and just a single recovered normal sperm can mean an embryo more than half the time. With several eggs and several sperm there are now almost always normal embryos to be transferred. But see the box "From Father to Son" for a word of caution.

Let us conclude this chapter on low sperm counts by asking a question. Will a technical fix for low sperm counts suffice? Surely not. If the evidence pointing to a global decline in human sperm numbers over the last generation or two turns out to be correct, some biologists predict that by the year 2050 we could see the collapse of traditional means of getting pregnant. Even today, for couples who can afford the sophisticated assistance described in the last parts of this chapter, we have seen that there are the hazards of transmitting male reproductive deficiencies to male offspring (at least in those cases that have an hereditary basis). As there might be for endometriosis in women (see Chapters 15 and 16), confirmation of environmentally induced oligospermia would mean that there is an increasingly obvious need to do a better job of identifying environmental toxins that we can do something about.

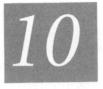

# Not Ovulating

Menstruation, or bleeding from the lining of the uterus (the **endometrium** is usually brought on by a fall in hormone support from the ovary for the linin The timing of menstruation is determined by the cyclical activity (or otherwise of the ovaries. If a woman is not ovulating—a condition called **anovulation** her menstrual cycle will be disturbed or lost.

## Symptoms of Anovulation

The most common menstrual sequel to anovulation is absent periods (**ameno rhea**), but sometimes there is enough estrogen being produced to cause irregu

| Table 10.1 | Patterns and Causes of Abnormal Menstruation Including Disturbances of Ovulation | |
|---|---|---|
| *Technical Name* | *Meaning* | *Reasons* |
| Amenorrhea | absent periods | (1) anovulation<br>(2) absent uterus,[1] obstruction in uterus or intrauterine adhesions[1] |
| Oligomenorrhea | infrequent periods | (1) infrequent ovulation<br>(2) anovulation with varying estrogen levels |
| Irregular dysfunctional intrauterine bleeding (DUB) | irregular heavy periods | (1) anovulation with varying estrogen levels |
| Regular DUB | regular heavy periods | (1) pathology of the uterus[1]<br>(2) bleeding tendency |
| Hypomenorrhea | regular light periods | (1) intrauterine adhesions[1]<br>(2) oral contraceptive pill, clomiphen<br>(3) normal aging |
| Intermenstrual bleeding or premenstrual spotting | bleeding between or just before periods | (1) pathology of the uterus[1]<br>(2) pathology of the cervix<br>(3) endometriosis[2] |

[1] See Chapter 15
[2] See Chapter 13

## Hormones Behind Periods and Periods Behind Obstructions

Regular menstrual bleeding depends on a regular rise and fall in hormones from the ovary, the details of which are in Chapter 3. Briefly, this is generally achieved only by formation of **follicles**, which secrete the ovary's first hormone, estrogen (specifically estradiol), followed by ovulation and then production by the **corpus luteum** of progesterone, the ovary's second hormone. Because it takes an average of about two weeks for a follicle to grow to the point of ovulation (the **follicular phase**), and because the corpus luteum lasts about two weeks (the **luteal phase**), the ordinary menstrual cycle lasts about four weeks (with a normal range that varies between 24 days and 35 days). Shorter or longer cycles are chiefly brought about by variation of the follicular phase; the luteal phase is rather constant.

**Estrogen** and **progesterone** sequentially build up and then transform the lining of the uterus, the endometrium. The follicular phase in the ovary, during which only estrogen is released, is the **proliferative phase** in the endometrium (meaning that the endometrium proliferates, or grows, getting thicker and thicker). The luteal phase in the ovary, when progesterone is produced, is the **secretory phase** in the endometrium, as proliferation stops and the endometrium transforms its energies from growth to differentiation, accumulating secretion to benefit an implanting embryo. If there is no ovulation—if there is no progesterone or exposure to a **progestogen**—the endometrium can keep proliferating, getting thicker and thicker, and become "hyperplastic," a condition called **endometrial hyperplasia**.

In the absence of ovulation (and in the absence of progesterone or a progestogen), the endometrium can bleed from just the loss of estrogen support. A mild up and down exposure to estrogen can be enough to cause serious bleeding when

lar bleeding (anovulatory periods, or **anovulatory dysfunctional uterine bleeding**). Anovulation is the main cause of amenorrhea, but not the only one. Table 10.1 lists the main disturbances of the menstrual cycle, their association with ovulation or anovulation and what can cause the disturbed menstrual patterns.

What are anovulatory periods like? Anovulatory menstrual periods, produced by fluctuating levels of estrogen alone, usually but not always occur irregularly; they may be completely painless and they vary a lot in length and amount from one period to the next. In contrast, normal ovulatory menstruation, produced by falling levels of progesterone, is more regular and predictable, is usually accompanied by at least mild period pain on the first day and is about the same in duration and heaviness from one period to the next.

the endometrium is thick. Unlike a normal menstrual period at the end of progesterone (or progestogen) exposure, such an anovulatory period does not cause the whole endometrium to shed. The bleeding often occurs from patches of the endometrium, and sooner or later it starts growing again and building up further. We call this anovulatory dysfunctional uterine bleeding. There is a fine hormonal line between amenorrhea and anovulatory dysfunctional uterine bleeding. The hormone disturbance underlying them can be virtually the same.

There will also be amenorrhea if there is no uterus (see Chapter 18) or if the endometrium in the uterus has been destroyed or replaced with **intrauterine adhesions** (Chapter 17).

**Cryptomenorrhea**, or "hidden menstruation," is apparent amenorrhea, resulting from an obstruction to menstrua-

tion, such as an incompletely formed vagina or a low **transverse vaginal septum** (see Chapter 18). Whereas amenorrhea itself is usually harmless and painless, cryptomenorrhea is cyclically painful and can cause pathology, including endometriosis, while it is unrelieved.

**Primary amenorrhea** is when there have been no periods in a woman's life. The most common causes, beyond a simple delay from perhaps insufficient weight, are **primary ovarian failure** (puberty fails as well) and congenital absence of the uterus and vagina (breast and pubic hair development are normal; see Chapter 18). **Secondary amenorrhea** is when the periods have stopped after having been present; its most common causes are **hypothalamic anovulation, hyperprolactinemia, polycystic ovary syndrome** and early **menopause** (all discussed in this chapter), and intrauterine adhesions (discussed in Chapter 17).

# Causes of Anovulation

There are a number of causes of amenorrhea due to anovulation, some of which may also present with anovulatory bleeding. The tests for these are described in Chapter 5, including **serum FSH, serum LH, serum prolactin, serum testosterone** and the **free androgen index**. If there are infrequent periods, or **oligomenorrhea**, then these tests are best done during the time of the period. In this chapter we look further into the biology of what has gone wrong.

## Hypothalamic Anovulation (HA)

Hypothalamic anovulation, sometimes referred to as **simple hypothalamic amenorrhea**, results from stress or weight loss, especially a weight reduction to below the teenage weight when the first period, or **menarche**, took place. Stress or weight loss reduces the brain's drive to the **pituitary gland**, which in turn reduces that gland's drive of the ovaries, stopping proper development of the follicles and causing ovulation to stop. The extreme weight loss of **anorexia nervosa** produces a doubly profound suppression of ovulation and periods because of the combined effect of weight loss and psychological stress.

Extreme exercise is capable of inhibiting ovulation whether weight loss occurs or not. Dr. P. T. Ellison, a Harvard anthropologist, has shown that energy expenditure—exercise associated with ballet dancing is a good example—is more likely to cause periods to stop than weight loss alone. The same happens

### The Body Mass Index, the Stars and Monsieur Quetelet

There is a normal range for the relationship between a person's weight and height, called the **body mass index** (BMI), which gives a rough estimate of how much spare tissue there is in the body, especially fat, which the female body needs to have in reserve for pregnancy to be safe. Nature thus postpones menarche until this range is reached. The BMI, sometimes called the **Quetelet index**, equals the weight (expressed in kilograms) divided by the square of the height (expressed in meters) and is normally in the range 20 to 25. Nature shuts off the periods and ovulation if body fat falls out of this range.

A woman's reproductive fortunes might or might not be held in the power of the constellations through astrology. But why in the nineteenth century a real stargazer gave the matter of varying body fat his careful philosophical attention is a puzzle. Lambert Adolphe Jacques Quetelet (1796–1874), a Brussels mathematician and astronomer, made up the rule that an adult's body weight should be as many kilograms as that adult's length in centimeters exceeds 100. Nowadays we overlook his arithmetic and instead confer his name on the BMI, which he did not invent.

Obesity, with a BMI greater than 25 or 30, also may stop periods, but unless there is a tendency toward the **polycystic ovary syndrome** (see discussion further on), it is better to be a bit overweight than underweight for optimum fertility.

The common pathway through which the brain affects the way the pituitary gland controls the ovaries (and the testes in men) is by releasing a burst or pulse of **gonadotropin-releasing hormone** (GnRH) every 60 to 90 minutes (explained in Chapter 3). In chronic hypothalamic anovulation levels of GnRH are low, which can result from changes in the balance between neurotransmitters, substances that mediate impulses across nerve junctions in the brain, particularly, in this case, the hypothalamus. Such imbalances might include insufficient levels of norepinephrine (noradrenaline), which is what mediates

amenorrhea both with weight-loss and endorphin-releasing exercise, and thus also lies behind the effects of such opiates as heroin in those addicted to it; excess serotonin, as in anorexia nervosa; and a deficiency of dopamine in hyperprolactinemic amenorrhea, in which the raised levels of prolactin depress GnRH.

On the other hand, either an excess of GnRH or an exaggeration of GnRH action in the pituitary in the polycystic ovary syndrome causes the pituitary to produce luteinizing hormone (LH) at the expense of follicle stimulating hormone (FSH), again producing anovulation.

with long distance running, especially if it causes "highs," a sensation due to the production in the brain of **endorphins**, natural, opium-like substances that confer a feeling of well-being. Illicit use of synthetic opiates such as heroin does the same thing more dangerously; amenorrhea of this kind is common among drug addicts.

By "simple" hypothalamic amenorrhea, we therefore mean that it is not one of the remaining causes of amenorrhea, all of which show special characteristics in blood tests, other than just low levels of serum FSH. The underlying disturbances of physiology are really anything but simple!

## Hyperprolactinemia

**Prolactin** is a hormone produced by the pituitary gland, especially during pregnancy. It prepares the breast for lactation, so that milk production will start once the high estrogen and progesterone levels of pregnancy disappear on delivery of the baby and the placenta. Unlike the other pituitary hormones, which are driven by "releasing factors" from the hypothalamus, prolactin is controlled by an "inhibiting factor" called dopamine. Dopamine can be depressed by a whole range of conditions, although most dopamine shortages are idiopathic, meaning that no known cause can be invoked to explain them. The net effect of depressing dopamine is that production of prolactin from the pituitary goes up. Prolactin has a reflex action on the hypothalamus, decreasing its drive (via GnRH) to the pituitary cells responsible for FSH and LH. Anovulation and then amenorrhea follow.

## Big and Bigger Prolactin Molecules

Not all apparent hyperprolactinemia spells trouble with ovulation. Remember that our measurements of hormones in the blood do not necessarily measure their capabilities. We use immunity molecules called antibodies to detect hormones; they match the target hormone and bind them in a way that is measurable. The part of the hormone these antibodies react to is not necessarily the part that binds to the receptor in the target tissue and that translates into hormone action. (There are assays that detect bioactivity, called "bioassays" or, in the laboratory, "receptor-based assays," but they are difficult and expensive and are used only in sophisticated medical research.)

For most hormones most of the time, this difference between the part of the hormone that binds the antibody and the part of the hormone that binds the hormone receptor does not matter, but for prolactin it can matter dramatically, if innocently. Some people naturally produce prolactin molecules that link together in pairs ("dimers") or in fours ("tetramers"). The molecules, despite their bigger than normal size, function normally. Only one part of the dimer (in the case of "big prolactin") and only one part of the tetramer ("big, big prolactin") binds to each receptor. Everything functions as it should; there is no abnormal milk production in the breasts (**galactorrhea**) and no problem with ovulation. All is normal, that is, until someone measures prolactin with a conventional antibody assay. Each dimer will be measured as two prolactin molecules, and each tetramer will be measured as four prolactin molecules, apparently revealing hyperprolactinemia of two or four times the normal range for people with ordinary sized prolactin molecules. We can distinguish these states using chromatography, another expensive and difficult test. In practice we do not bother. If ovulation is normal by other criteria then an incidental finding of hyperprolactinemia can be ignored.

There are several causes of hyperprolactinemia, all of which need to looked for. Certain drugs can cause hyperprolactinemia, including the maj tranquilizers used for schizophrenia and other causes of psychosis, such chlorpromazine (Largactil); some older antihypertensives (drugs used to low blood pressure), including methyldopa (Aldomet); antiemetics (drugs used control nausea and vomiting), like metoclopramide (Maxolon); and opium d rivatives, such as heroin. The presence of tumors around or in the pituita gland, which stop normal levels of dopamine from being produced or sto normally produced dopamine from getting to all or part of the pituitary glan can also cause hyperprolactinemia. Pregnancy and normal lactation is anoth cause. Reflexes from suckling travel from the nipple to the hypothalamus, de pressing dopamine. Chronic irritations or inflammations of the wall of th chest that mimic the nervous reflexes otherwise produced by suckling const tute still another cause.

The result of each of these conditions is not just the disappearance of th periods due to the elevation of prolactin. Quite often the high levels of prolacti stimulate the production of milk in the breasts, called **galactorrhea**, which therefore an important symptom to convey to the doctor.

## Polycystic Ovary Syndrome

Polycystic ovary syndrome (PCOS), also called polycystic ovarian diseas (PCOD), is a condition in which ovulation is rare and tiny cysts (actually fiv to ten millimeter follicles) accumulate in the ovaries. These follicles contai eggs, but instead of the follicles growing and going on to ovulate, they stall an secrete male hormone into the blood. Thus, there is an imbalance of pituitar hormones and male hormones in the blood that perpetuates the PCOS prob lem. Incidentally, it is important not to think that this condition means "cysts in the conventional sense of biggish, abnormal structures that may require spe cial treatment.

If you have PCOS it usually will have been obvious for years, because of ir regular periods and, often, a tendency to develop acne and an increase in facia and body hair. Occasionally, PCOS first manifests itself during ovarian stim ulation, either for ovulation induction or as part of a **gamete intrafallopia transfer** (GIFT) or **in vitro fertilization** (IVF) cycle (see Chapter 20), whe many more follicles than usual start to grow. The diagnosis of PCOS is mad by finding either a high ratio of serum LH to serum FSH or a high free andro gen index. The high levels of LH stimulate the cells around the follicles to pro duce too much in the way of **androgens** (the male sex hormones, a little o which comes from all normal ovaries). With PCOS the serum testosterone level can be increased, or at least raised toward the upper part of the normal range, whereas other causes of anovulation cause testosterone levels to be low. A woman can have polycystic ovaries (PCO) without showing untoward symptoms. (We call it PCOS—the PCO syndrome—if there is a clinical disturbance, such as irregular periods or abnormal hair growth.) The most sensitive test for PCO is a **transvaginal ultrasound**. The characteristic appearance of PCO is a ring of small to medium follicles around the circumference of an enlarged ovary.

PCO causes various disturbances to ovulation. At one extreme there is amenorrhea or anovulatory bleeding (estrogen is abundant in PCOS). With mild cases, ovulation may be a bit less frequent than normal, but provided that other aspects of reproductive functioning are normal (explained in Chapter 6), fertility might be all right and the condition itself can go undiagnosed for a lifetime. Indeed, PCO is so common that it may be wrong to call it abnormal (see Chapter 3).

When you are not trying to get pregnant, the oral contraceptive pill is very good treatment for PCOS, because it stops the follicles and the male-hormone-producing tissue from accumulating, thus protecting future fertility. It also stops such complications as abnormal hair growth (**hirsutism**); makes periods regular, preventing overgrowth of the endometrium (risking endometrial hyperplasia), and provides contraception (there is always a risk, with so much luteinizing hormone about, that a follicle will grow to the stage at which it might ovulate). If the pill is personally or culturally distasteful, however, the same ends can be achieved by separately administering an estrogen and a progestogen, such as Provera or, if available, the male-hormone-blocking progestogen **cyproterone acetate**.

# Inducing Ovulation

In conditions of amenorrhea or anovulation, there are two reasons why there is generally no point in undertaking **ovulation induction** unless there is an immediate intention to conceive. First, the complications of amenorrhea, such as low estrogen levels, abnormal hair growth, irregular bleeding or endometrial hyperplasia, are more cheaply and more directly dealt with by appropriate hormone treatment. Second, the ovaries may become resistant to the drugs, especially **clomiphene**.

## PCOS Is Often Gene-Based

At least a few cases of PCOS—some investigators think most cases—have an inherited cause. The condition is more common among women with a family history of the syndrome, and men in affected families have a tendency toward premature male-pattern baldness, with early receding of the hairline. The abnormality is thought to be in cytochrome P450, a metabolic unit inside cells responsible for fine-tuning the production of the sex hormones. There is also a small proportion of women with PCOS (about one in 70) who have a more clear-cut abnormality in the production of steroid hormones from the adrenal gland. As a result, the adrenals leak too much male sex hormone. This condition is called "attenuated" or "adult-onset" congenital adrenal hyperplasia (CAH). Adult-onset CAH is related to more severe forms of CAH that manifest at birth with ambiguous genitals (**intersex**), because of excess male hormone exposure in the female fetus, which causes enlargement of the phallus and a joining of the skin over the vagina. These abnormalities of the genitals do not occur in adult-onset CAH. In CAH, as in other causes of PCOS, there is an increase in serum testosterone and the free androgen index, as well as a diagnostic increase in the intermediate steroid **serum 17-hydroxyprogesterone**.

In both the common (ovarian) variety and the attenuated CAH (adrenal) variety of PCOS, there is therefore a strong genetic component. Why does nature allow PCOS to flourish when it appears to be a disadvantage for fertility? First, there are evolutionary advantages to reduced fertility generally, similar to the situation with **endometriosis** (see Chapter 16) and **oligospermia** (see Chapter 9), both of which partly have an hereditary basis. Second, women with PCO will mostly ovulate normally when they are below otherwise ideal weight (a body mass index of less than 20), giving, at least in prehistoric times, the advantage of being able to reproduce in times of famine.

## Bromocriptine

One exception is the use of the drug **bromocriptine** to treat hyperprolactinemic amenorrhea. This drug is so specific for this condition—it precisely mimics the action of dopamine, the natural inhibiting factor for prolactin in the pituitary—that it should probably be used unless there is some reason not to

By lowering prolactin at its source, bromocriptine not only prevents the complications of this form of amenorrhea due to low estrogen, it also prevents the prolactin-producing cells from growing into a tumor of such cells. The treatment can be safely continued for years. Because ovulation nearly always returns quickly, it is often necessary to use contraception (the birth control pill is satisfactory once treatment with bromocriptine has begun).

If given too suddenly, bromocriptine is likely to cause side effects, including dizziness (from low blood pressure), headaches and nausea. It should be started slowly, beginning with a low dosage. If side effects still occur they can usually be avoided by administering the tablets (not the capsules!) by placement in the vagina. Absorption from the vagina, across its moist, mucous surface, is excellent, and, unlike veins from the stomach and intestines, the veins from the vagina do not go first to the liver (where most side effects originate).

Bromocriptine treatment is very effective in hyperprolactinemic infertility. Unless they have other reasons for infertility, up to 40 percent of women taking it do not get a period, because they are pregnant in the first cycle! Only intravenous GnRH treatment approaches it for effectiveness.

# Clomiphene

In other anovulatory conditions, if you are attempting pregnancy, then the drug clomiphene is the first choice to induce ovulation, because it is inexpensive and simple to use. **Clomiphene** is marketed as **Clomid** by Merrill Dow and (in the United States and Europe) as **Serophene** by Serono. It acts by increasing the natural production of FSH, which is deficient in most of the causes of anovulation we are considering here. Clomiphene acts as an antiestrogen, that is, it blocks the effect of estrogen on various tissues. This effectively tricks the pituitary gland into assuming that there is not enough estrogen about, thereby pushing the pituitary into increasing its output of FSH. The increase in FSH needs to be enough to get a group of follicles to grow, after which they reach maturity and ovulate in the way described in Chapter 3. The needed dose of clomiphene ranges from half a tablet (tablets are 50 milligrams) to five tablets a day, always for five days and generally starting between the second and the fifth day of a period. (When there has been amenorrhea, menstruation should be brought on by a course of progestogen tablets.)

Side effects are common with higher doses of clomiphene but not with the lower ones. Such effects include headache, depression, hot flashes (all symptoms of lack of estrogen) and temporary blurring of vision or an appearance of yellow coloration to things. These symptoms have never been permanent.

Clomiphene is probably not a safe drug to take during pregnancy, especially once the embryo's genital tract begins to develop, around eight to ten weeks from the start of the fertile cycle. Although no direct evidence of harm, or teratogenesis, has been reported on human fetuses, clomiphene as an estrogen-blocking drug is very similar in structure to the estrogenic drug diethylstilbestrol (DES), which was widely prescribed in the 1950s for miscarriages. DES is now notorious for having caused deformities of the upper vagina and uterus in female fetuses and of the epididymis and vas deferens in male fetuses. Experiments show that clomiphene and DES do similar harm in pregnant mice. What the drugs have in common, in disturbing these estrogen-sensitive events in the embryo, is prolonged attachment of the drug to the estrogen receptors, distorting the normal sequence of events in the development of the relevant organs and tissues.

Because it has been seized on by some writers, I should stress that there is no practical possibility of enough clomiphene remaining in the body through the time of ovulation and into pregnancy for there to be a risk of these harmful effects when clomiphene is taken to induce ovulation. Apart from being metabolized and excreted, clomiphene is so bound to existing receptors that even if some were to stick around this way, there would be negligible amounts free to cross into the fetus weeks after the last administration. But these data do serve to warn that it is important not to use clomiphene in amenorrhea without first ruling out pregnancy.

Precautions should be taken to be certain that a woman is not pregnant before clomiphene is prescribed. Because ovulation precedes a period by two weeks, it is possible for pregnancy to complicate a naturally resolving case of amenorrhea without a woman having had a period. This is why, if there is an absence of periods, we bring on a period first, using a one-to-two-week course of a progestogen that is probably innocuous in pregnancy, such as 5 milligrams per day of medroxyprogesterone acetate (**Provera**). If there is a question about pregnancy, a **pregnancy test** can be done, although it is possible for a woman to have a very early pregnancy without showing a positive test result. If, however, her serum progesterone is measured, it can reveal if she has ovulated, so that natural period can then be expected before the clomiphene is started; the serum progesterone and the pregnancy test can then be repeated if the period seems too light or too unusual to rule out pregnancy.

Unwanted antiestrogenic effects, especially with higher doses of clomiphene, can spoil the drug's beneficial effects. Some actions of clomiphene linger well past the useful rise in FSH, interfering with the production of mucus in the cervix, which spoils sperm transport, or jeopardizing the normal growth of the endometrium, made apparent by periods getting lighter (see Table 10.1). Pregnancy will happen in about 50 percent of patients who respond to clomiphene by ovulating over the course of six to nine months; of these pregnancies, about 20 percent end in miscarriage. The reason for the lack of successful outcome despite ovulation is thought to be the unwanted estrogen-blocking effects of the drug, namely an inhibition of the normal estrogen-driven growth of the lining of the uterus, or endometrium, and an inhibition of the development of cervical mucus that can readily be penetrated by sperm.

If clomiphene does not work then we have two further options for stimulating ovulation. We can substitute gonadotropin-releasing hormone (GnRH) in cases where this hormone is lacking (it will work in all cases of anovulation except PCOS and ovarian failure), or we can directly inject follicle stimulating hormone when it is absent. FSH is really the only option for PCOS when clomiphene fails, except in the occasional case of overactivity of the adrenal gland, when we can sometimes suppress the adrenal gland with a synthetic corticosteroid drug such as dexamethasone.

## Pulsatile GnRH

To use the FSH-regulating hormone GnRH clinically, we have to administer it in the way it is produced by the brain, namely, in spurts directly into the blood system. To do this, we load the GnRH into a portable, battery-operated, electronic syringe driver, preset to administer an exact amount of drug intravenously every 60 to 90 minutes for about two weeks (that is, for the normal length of a follicular phase). It is a wonderfully effective, if inconvenient, treatment, with no appreciable risk of ovarian overstimulation (see Chapter 11) and no substantial risk of multiple pregnancy. The rate of ovulation, with properly chosen cases of amenorrhea, is 100 percent (there is not much in medicine you can say that about!) and the chance of pregnancy, if there are no other reasons for infertility, is up to 40 percent per month.

The GnRH stimulus to the pituitary gland to produce FSH has to be in pulses but it need not be cyclical. The monthly pattern of the ovarian cycle (see Figure 3.2 in Chapter 3) is governed solely by the ovary. Thus, the role of GnRH, although indispensable, is just facilitatory. To get this effect clinically we therefore administer GnRH into a vein. Special precautions need to be taken to change the intravenous site every four or five days, or at the first sight of in flammation of the vein. Because of the small risk of infection, some doctors pre fer to administer pulsatile GnRH under the skin (subcutaneously), but it is no well absorbed there and treatment often fails. For the GnRH to work it needs sharp upward then downward profile in the blood. If it is administered unde the skin, this profile is blunted and it may not work. (GnRH should not be use in patients with heart murmurs because of the hazard of bacterial endocarditi a condition in which bacteria grow on heart valves.)

# Gonadotropin Treatment

The other option if clomiphene fails is to stimulate the ovary directly with fol licle stimulating hormone. Like GnRH, FSH also cannot be given by mouth, an it must be injected daily, generally intramuscularly into the arm or buttock o subcutaneously with the newer highly purified FSH preparations, for about th two weeks it takes a follicle to develop.

During the 1960s and 1970s and up to about 1985, human FSH in som countries was removed directly from pituitary glands obtained at autopsie. Some of these glands, tragically, had been infected before death with a "prion (a nonbacterial, nonviral infective agent) that causes Creutzfeldt-Jakob diseas (CJD), an irreversible, deadly brain degeneration (see Chapter 11). Five wome in Australia, out of about 2,000 women treated, contracted CJD, and there ha recently been an extensive, government-sponsored investigation there into th previous use of FSH.

Until very recently the method of preparation of FSH used the urin of women who had been through menopause and is thus called huma menopausal gonadotropin (hMG). It consists of a mixture of FSH and LH and is available as Humegon and Pergonal (FSH plus LH mixtures produced respectively, by Organon and Serono) or as Metrodin (pure FSH after LH ha been removed, a Serono product). These preparations still contain contaminat ing proteins of a nonhormonal nature, proteins that are responsible for the dis comfort the injections can cause and that occasionally elicit allergies. These side effects are not experienced if such proteins are removed, as in Serono's Metrodir HP (HP for "highly purified"). They are also absent from FSH made through gene technology, known as recombinant FSH (rFSH), preparations of which are now being marketed by Organon and by Serono (see the box "A Bureaucratic Brouhaha").

The same FSH preparations are used in GIFT and IVF to increase the pro portion of follicles that grow and ovulate. Using hMG to induce ovulation in

The amount of luteinizing hormone in Humegon and Pergonal varies, although its effect is usually slight; it does not last long in the body, probably less than an hour, and hMG is an injection that is given daily. Because preparations of hMG, to comply with published pharmaceutical standards, have had to contain 75 units of LH activity for every 75 units of FSH activity, both of its manufacturers have apparently added variable, small amounts of hCG to make up for any lack of LH. We really do not need extra LH activity in the body, and we do not want significant amounts of hCG, which, although it acts precisely like LH, has a much longer survival time and could have unwanted luteinizing effects on the follicle before ovulation.

Because Organon admitted to their use of hCG to standardize the LH activity of hMG preparations, Humegon was deemed to be in breach of pharmaceutical standards and was thus off the market in Australia for a year or two while its registered official description was altered. Organon then bought Serono's Pergonal at a number of different places round the world, analyzed it carefully, and discovered that Serono had been doing the same! The irritating aspect of all this is that we do not usually want either the LH or the hCG. (Serono has Metrodin on the market, from which the LH has been removed and has no added hCG;

Organon has marketed Normegon, with an FSH:LH ratio of 3:1.)

Meanwhile, Serono has marketed its highly purified FSH (Metrodin HP, or in the U.S., **Fertinex**), which consists of Metrodin with not just LH removed but also a group of other proteins normally excreted in urine (and for many years an included by-product of the extraction processes used for obtaining hMG). These miscellaneous proteins could be responsible for an allergic reaction in sensitized people and seem to be in large measure responsible for the discomfort produced by these injections. As well as using Metrodin HP in hypersensitivity states, it means that the drug can be administered subcutaneously, that is, under the skin.

Both Organon and Serono have now successfully synthesized FSH from scratch using recombinant gene technology. **Recombinant human FSH** ($r$hFSH) has been shown to induce completely normal follicle growth (pregnancies have resulted). When mass produced, $r$hFSH (or simply $r$FSH) will completely remove the need for a human source for FSH, and it will be highly appropriate to deliver it under or through the skin. Organon and Serono both began to have their $r$FSH available in some countries during 1996, but it is uncertain whether the competition between them will mean a fall in price any time soon.

To induce ovulation, we typically start with 150 to 225 units of FSH each day, increasing the dose if necessary to get a rising level of serum estradiol, which we monitor frequently, getting the result back on the same day the blood test is taken. Once the level reaches a concentration of about 1,000 picomoles per liter, or about 400 picograms per milliliter (a picogram is one-thousandth of a nanogram, which is one-thousandth of a microgram, which is one-thousandth of a milligram, which is one-thousandth of a gram!), we perform a transvaginal ultrasound to see how many follicles have been produced that are contributing to the estrogen being measured. The number of follicles that grow depends more on the number of responsive follicles that are there at the beginning of FSH injections than on how much FSH is given; it is largely an all-or-nothing effect.

If we are inducing the development of follicles for **superovulation** (that is, for **assisted conception**; see Chapter 20), we want a larger number of follicles to get to about 1.8 to 2.0 centimeters in diameter than if we were inducing ovulation in an anovulatory patient destined for natural intercourse. If the number of follicles is too high, we gradually reduce the daily amount of FSH, mimicking the sorting out that occurs in natural cycles as FSH levels fall during the follicular phase (see Chapter 3). If the number of follicles is way too high, we may have to stop altogether and, in consultation with the woman concerned, cancel the cycle; sometimes, by decreasing the FSH, we lose all the follicles, and the cycle is then also canceled.

Ideally, one follicle will reach maturity (1.8 to 2.0 centimeters diameter on ultra-

preparation for getting pregnant naturally is tricky at the best of times, because of the risk of stimulating too many follicles and having a multiple pregnancy, but the accumulation of very many little follicles that occurs in PCOS makes the use of hMG even trickier for this condition—sometimes 20 or more follicles grow in each ovary!

When bromocriptine, clomiphene or GnRH is used to induce ovulation, the normal feedback relationships between the follicles in the ovary and the FSH-producing cells in the pituitary gland are more or less maintained. This means that there is little increased risk of twins or higher-number multiple pregnancies such as triplets or quadruplets. It also means that there is little risk of serious enlargement of the ovaries, known as **ovarian hyperstimulation syndrome** (see Chapter 11). This, however, is not true of treatment with FSH.

## The Nitty Gritty of hMG and hCG (concluded)

sound scanning) in natural intercourse ovulation induction cycles, whereas between five and ten follicles will do so for an assisted conception cycle, such as IVF or GIFT. To achieve these different aims, it is common with ovulation induction to leave several days between the last injection of FSH and the injection of hCG; this is called "coasting," and it causes the less fully mature follicles to fall by the wayside (that is, to become **atretic**). This minimizes the risk of a higher-number multiple pregnancy. With superovulation for assisted conception, such coasting is usually counterproductive, reducing the number of healthy eggs obtained.

Once the follicles are mature, we start the process of ovulation itself by administering hCG in a dose usually of 5,000 to 10,000 units. We know that ovulation will take place from follicles more than 1.5 cen-timeters in diameter 38 hours later. Thus, for natural sexual intercourse we usually give the hCG during the afternoon, in preparation for intercourse the following evening. For assisted conception we first fix the time at which we want to carry out the follicle aspiration procedure (for egg pickup), then count back 36 hours to time the hCG injection, giving an hour or two in reserve in case there are delays.

Smaller doses of hCG (1,500 to 2,000 units) are often given four days and eight days after the initial ovulating dose of hCG, to maintain drive to the corpus luteum, so that it (or they, if there is more than one corpus luteum) will produce adequate progesterone for long enough for pregnancy to become established—at which time hCG from the pregnancy itself will stimulate the corpus luteum and rescue it.

When FSH injections are used, the ovaries are stimulated directly. The only feedback that operates is what we get from monitoring. We check on the appropriateness of the doses by measuring the estrogens the follicles are producing (as **serum estradiol**) and by doing transvaginal ultrasounds to compare how many follicles are producing the amount of estrogen we are measuring. We therefore use these tests to limit the amount and duration of FSH, trying to get just one or two follicles to the point of ovulation. Ovulation itself, including the final 38 hours or so of immediately preovulatory changes in the follicle, is triggered with an injection of **human chorionic gonadotropin** (hCG), which acts like LH and is marketed as **Pregnyl** by Organon and **Profasi** by Serono (see the box "The Nitty Gritty of hMG and hCG" for more details on the treatment).

Even with the best of monitoring, however, too many follicles can reach maturity than is safe, and either the ovulation cycle that has been induced will need to be canceled (a waste) or a last-minute suggestion might be made to carry out an assisted conception procedure such as GIFT or IVF. This is especially likely for ovulation induction for PCOS, in which response to FSH is all too easily excessive.

# Untreatable Anovulation: Primary Ovarian Failure

Anovulation is generally one of the best-treated forms of infertility, but there are exceptions. As described in Chapter 5, it is only when there are no responsive follicles in the ovaries that ovulation cannot be induced with the hormones or drugs described above. This happens in **primary ovarian failure**, meaning that the ovarian failure is not secondary to a problem mediated by the pituitary gland. The diagnosis is pointed to by serum FSH levels that are high, particularly if this has been the case on more than one occasion.

The diagnosis of primary ovarian failure (also called **premature menopause**) will be the case in 5 to 10 percent of patients under the age of 40 investigated for absent periods and absent ovulation. It may have been suspected by the experience of menopause-like symptoms, including hot flashes. The younger a patient with primary ovarian failure is, the more likely it is that there will be an abnormality of the chromosomes to account for it, which is detected by performing a **karyotype** of the white blood cells, ovarian tissue or both. Identifying an abnormal karyotype, however, often has little point, because reproduction is prevented, and it is usually dispensed with (outside research or special family studies) for all but the most inquisitive of patients and doctors. It is enough to cope with knowing that ovulation will never be possible without having to contend with the thought that one's chromosomes are not normal.

A **biopsy** of the ovary can sometimes help, because it can reveal a complete absence of follicles (true premature menopause), the presence of many unstimulated follicles (the "resistant ovary syndrome") or, rarely, an inflammation of the follicles due to antibodies produced by the body against its own tissues ("autoimmune oophoritis"). Although eggs are still present in the last two of these three conditions, there is no treatment available (see the boxes "Special Case #1: The Resistant Ovary Syndrome" and "Special Case #2: Autoimmune

## Special Case #1: The Resistant Ovary Syndrome

**Primordial follicles** in the ovary (discussed in Chapter 3) start to grow for reasons that seem to have nothing to do with FSH; it is not until the **secondary** or **tertiary follicle** is a millimeter or two in diameter that it becomes sensitive to FSH. This means that there is an opportunity for things to go wrong that will frustrate FSH despite the presence of many primordial follicles. We know that a local peptide growth factor called activin is involved in the initial development of primordial follicles, but its production has not yet been studied in patients with resistant ovary syndrome.

The presence of many follicles, all resistant to FSH or, more accurately, follicles that are not developing to the point at which they become sensitive to FSH, can be due to a number of abnormalities, by no means all understood. Treatment, for the moment, involves trying to sensitize the blocked follicles, using estrogen in an attempt to get them to grow to the point where they will respond to FSH. This

means we do not give estrogen and progestogen together (this would be like being on the birth control pill); instead, we give a small dose of estrogen, say ethinyl estradiol (Estigyn), 10 to 20 micrograms, or Premarin, 0.3 milligrams, per day for four to six weeks, interspersed with medroxyprogesterone acetate (Provera, which is the least likely of the easily administered progestogens to put an embryo in inadvertent jeopardy), 5 milligrams per day for two weeks. With such estrogen treatment—but probably also without it—perhaps 10 to 15 percent of women with resistant ovary syndrome sooner or later have a pregnancy.

There is rapid progress being made in understanding what primordial follicles require to grow, as well as in being able to develop eggs from such follicles in vitro. One or another approach means that we might soon be able to expect a reliable treatment for the resistant ovary syndrome for the young women who presently receive this diagnosis.

Oophoritis"). In each case, a shortage of estrogen production from the ovaries means that medical complications are likely to happen eventually, comparable to those that follow menopause (such as a loss of calcium from bones and an increased risk of heart disease), but at a younger age. It is important to prevent these complications by using estrogens, to which a progestogen tablet needs to be added (for 11 days or more per month) to keep the endometrium from overresponding and overgrowing.

There is a class of diseases in the body called autoimmune diseases, in which the body's immune system mounts an attack not on foreign proteins but on the body's own tissues. Examples include attacks on the joints (rheumatoid arthritis), the skin and the muscles (dermatomyositis), the arteries (polyarteritis nodosa), the liver (autoimmune hepatitis) or many tissues at once (a disease called **systemic lupus erythematosus**). The same can be true of the ovary in autoimmune oophoritis.

In its early stages autoimmune oophoritis causes painful enlargement of the ovaries, visible on transvaginal ultrasound. An ovarian biopsy, taken at **laparoscopy**, will reveal inflammatory cells attacking the follicles, many of which may be cystic. There is a chance, still mainly theoretical, that early treatment with drugs that suppress the immune system, such as cortisone and stronger drugs, might reverse the process, but because it is a rare condition there has been too little experience with them to know. The end result is true premature menopause, with loss of all follicles. Sometimes the only relief from the pain it causes is to remove the ovaries at operation.

It is usual to look for various tissue antibodies in primary ovarian failure because autoimmune oophoritis might not manifest itself until it has run its course completely and all the follicles have been burned out by the immune process. In addition, autoimmune oophoritis tends to occur in association with some other specific autoimmune diseases of various glands. Special antibodies can be looked for in the blood to predict the later development of serious disease, which can therefore be anticipated and treated before harm is done.

The other antibodies usually looked for include thyroid antibodies, which produce an underactive thyroid, or hypothyroidism; adrenal antibodies, which cause the adrenal glands to fail, with weakness, low blood pressure and, often, increased skin pigmentation; islet-cell antibodies (the islets of the pancreas produce insulin, so these antibodies anticipate diabetes), and gastric parietal cell antibodies, stomach cells that produce "intrinsic factor," which is needed for the lower intestine to absorb vitamin $B_{12}$ (deficiency of $B_{12}$ causes pernicious anemia and degenerative disease of the spinal cord). Although we do all these tests routinely, they are rarely positive.

# Other Serious Causes of Anovulation

The careful physician will consider whether or not there is a potentially dangerous tumor in every case of amenorrhea, but especially if there is hyperprolactinemia or if there is no obvious reason for the amenorrhea, such as weight loss or PCOS. Tumors affecting ovulation can grow in or above the pituitary gland, best revealed by a **CAT scan** or **MRI scan** of the pituitary gland and hypothalamus, or on the ovaries or adrenal glands, suspected on hormone testing and confirmed by imaging with a transvaginal ultrasound, or a CAT scan or MRI scan of these organs. Occasionally a hormonally active tumor in one or the other ovary will be evident only by localizing the production of a high amount of a hormone, such as estradiol, testosterone or **androstenedione**, to the affected ovary by **selective catheterization**, and sampling the ovarian and adrenal veins to assay these hormones.

If the serum prolactin is more than about twice normal, then it is especially important to look for a tumor in the pituitary gland. If the tumor is small, not distorting the bone that contains the pituitary gland, it is called a microadenoma; if it is bigger than about one centimeter, it is a macroadenoma. In either case, drug treatment with bromocriptine is the treatment of first choice, because it will shrink the tumor. Remember, however, that irrespective of the size of the tumor, bromocriptine will cause fertility to return very quickly. Because prolactin-producing tumors are likely to grow during pregnancy, it is not usually wise to allow pregnancy to occur before a macroadenoma has shrunk to the size of a microadenoma. Even then, complications from sudden growth or hemorrhage into the tumor (with compression of a surrounding structure such as the optic nerve) can occur during pregnancy, which requires urgent bromocriptine or surgery (performed through the back of the nose) to take away the effects of the pressure.

# "Post-Pill" Amenorrhea

It is commonly believed that the birth control pill can stop periods for months after its discontinuation. It is now known that this is not true—the effect of the pill wears off in days. The confusion began in the 1960s and 1970s, when not all the causes of amenorrhea were understood. In particular, the effects of weight loss on the periods was not appreciated until the late 1970s, after Dr. Rose Frisch from the Harvard School of Public Health drew attention to it in a series of careful studies and publications. We know now that virtually every instance of amenorrhea that arises when the pill is stopped comes about because one of the above conditions has developed coincidentally but has been masked because the pill will cause periods in anyone with a sensitive uterus and endometrium. The estrogen and progestogen in the pill drive the uterus directly, irrespective c what the pituitary and ovary might otherwise have been doing.

There is no relation, incidentally, between periods disappearing while o the pill and periods not occurring after the pill is stopped. "Pill amenorrhea," a absence of periods while on the pill, is simply an exaggerated manifestation c what every pill user knows, namely that periods are lighter while on the pil This is because the progestogen in a pill cycle stops the endometrium from get ting thicker much earlier than in the natural cycle; progesterone in the natura cycle does not take effect until after the first two weeks. About 10 percent c women get extremely light or absent periods while taking the pill. Apart fron losing the reassurance that there is no pregnancy, no harm comes from the pe riods being absent in this situation.

This is as good a place as any to dismiss the notion that the pill should b stopped for several months before attempting pregnancy in order to "get it ou of the system" (as if it were a poison). This advice is foolish. The pill, as demon strated by the bleeding that follows when a woman stops taking it, is out of th system within a few days. At least one condition that can jeopardize the chanc of getting pregnant—endometriosis—is usually suppressed on the pill, an stopping the pill for several months in favor of an alternative contraceptive ca be just long enough to allow endometriosis to become active again and spoil th chance of pregnancy.

In the next chapter we will focus on what can go wrong with ovulation in duction, before we move on to some of the other specific causes of and treat ments for infertility.

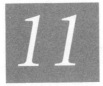

# Complications with Gonadotropin Stimulation

The dangers associated with inducing ovulation with gonadotropin treatment especially multiple ovulation induction (**superovulation**) for **assisted conception** (see Chapters 9 and 20), are dominated by the risk of overenlargement of the ovaries. The condition that can result is **ovarian hyperstimulation syndrome** (OHSS). Other aspects of gonadotropin treatment that cause concern, neither of which have definitely been proved, include the possibilities of cancer and birth defects.

# Ovarian Hyperstimulation Syndrome

It is normal for the ovary to produce fluid in the abdomen (the **peritoneal cavity**) as a follicle grows. It is normal for the ovary to bleed at **ovulation**, and it is normal for a **corpus luteum** to form in the ovary and to become cystic in the second half of the cycle, the **luteal phase**. Pain can accompany ovulation and the formation of a cystic corpus luteum. **Premenstrual tension** can cause bloating, irritability, depression and breast pain. When the ovaries are stimulated to increase the number of follicles, all these events (and often their symptoms) are usually greater in degree than you would expect in a natural cycle.

There is no sharp distinction between the expected and the unexpected when the ovaries are stimulated. It is a matter of degree. The signs and symptoms usually get worse if there is successful conception, because the natural production of **human chorionic gonadotropin** (hCG) will then be added to the injected hCG that has stimulated the ovaries up to that point. In our experience of more than 10,000 stimulations at Sydney IVF and Royal Prince Alfred Hospital, we would estimate that about one in 30 stimulations are accompanied by enough pelvic pain in the luteal phase to cause a woman to want to rest in bed for a day or more (mild OHSS). In about one in 200 stimulations, rest in hospital results, mainly for observation and to enable us to give adequate relief of discomfort or pain (moderate OHSS). In about one in 1,000 stimulations there is enough fluid in either the abdomen or the chest to be of serious medical concern (severe OHSS).

The main symptoms of dangerous degrees of hyperstimulation are difficulty in breathing and vomiting or diarrhea. Breathing difficulties are caused by fluid in the abdomen or the chest and are relieved quickly by aspirating excess fluid surgically (local anesthesia is used). Removing fluid this way, or losing fluid through vomiting, can cause dehydration, which if not recognized and not treated promptly can lead to thickening of the blood and to thrombosis. These

## Twisted Ovaries

Torsion of the ovary causes a sudden onset of severe continuous pain, usually accompanied, equally suddenly, by nausea and vomiting. A very useful study from Dr. Gabriel Oelsner and others at the Chaim Sheba Medical Center in Israel has shown that most cases can be treated by simply untwisting the ovary, even if the torsion is of more than a day's duration. Of 40 patients over a ten-year period, 14 were treated this way at **laparoscopy**, avoiding the need for major surgery as well as saving the ovary. Torsion can happen without a prior major degree of hyperstimulation, and it is more common if pregnancy has occurred.

are serious consequences. Strokes and even deaths have occurred in some centers. The enlarged ovaries can bleed, especially if they are traumatized in any way.

Why do some women get severe OHSS while others, with either larger ovaries or higher hormone levels, do not? It is clear that the fluid that accumulates is not coming directly from the ovaries. It is also clear that it is not a direct effect of high hormone levels on the tissues. A recent study from Monash University in Melbourne may point to an answer. Dr. Neil McClure and others have reported in *The Lancet* that a protein is being produced in the ovary called "vascular endothelial growth factor," which increases the permeability of capillaries to fluid. If the question of why some women produce too much of this factor compared with others is still obscure, we might soon have a more reliable way of predicting the occurrence of this complication.

The ovaries will always recover completely from hyperstimulation, as long as they are not operated on and removed. Operation is rarely necessary for hyperstimulation. One situation in which it *is* necessary is when the enlarged ovary rolls around and twists on its blood supply—a phenomenon known as torsion. Unless torsion is recognized and treated quickly, the ovary may not recover.

# Ovarian Stimulation and Cancer

There is no direct evidence linking cancer to ovarian stimulation with follicle stimulating hormone (FSH), but there are suspicions of an association. There are three particular areas of significant concern.

One reason to suspect that there could be a significant cause-and-effect relationship between excessive ovulation and ovarian cancer is that it is known that pregnancy or prolonged use of the oral contraceptive pill, both of which inhibit ovulation, protect against its later development. In the case of the pill, its use for 10 years or more *reduces* the risk of ovarian cancer after menopause to about one-fifth of the incidence if the pill was not taken. It is therefore plausible that repeated multiple ovulations caused by repeated cycles of FSH treatment increase the risk of ovarian cancer. This is not the same as saying that these hormones are carcinogens or are the *cause* of the cancer (for example, in the way cigarette smoking causes lung cancer). What is likely is that the risk of cancer of the ovary depends in some way on the total number of ovulations a woman has had; ovulating 10 eggs at once would then amount to 10 months' worth of risk from single ovulations.

Some women at particularly high risk of ovarian cancer, because of similar cancers in their family, have chosen to have the two ovaries removed surgically after menopause (the procedure can nowadays be done at laparoscopy). The best protection against ovarian cancer after menopause, short of such a radical step as surgical removal, is to have regular checkups, and presently the best way of examining the ovaries, before or after menopause, is with **transvaginal ultrasound** and to have a special blood test done, a **serum CA125 antigen** level. The cost-effectiveness of screening the general population for ovarian cancer this way has not been demonstrated, but for people with special concerns it is likely that such examinations will accompany Pap smears and breast examinations after menopause as routine screening maneuvers. Meanwhile, research is continuing on other blood tests that might indicate early ovarian cancer.

Breast cancer is the most common cancer of women during the reproductive years, especially if there is a family history of it at a young age. It is also more common among women who have not had children. Therefore, there is a significant risk of it coinciding with infertility treatment, and the high levels of estrogen and progesterone that go with stimulating the ovaries (and which also go with pregnancy) could cause a cancer that is already there to grow more quickly. For these reasons ovulation induction or assisted conception should not be undertaken, particularly by an older woman, if there is an unresolved suspicion of breast cancer, such as a recently discovered breast lump.

Cancer of the cervix is another common malignancy in young women. Although it is not caused or aggravated by ovulation induction or by pregnancy, treatment of it during pregnancy is difficult. Be careful to stay up to date with your cervical smears (Pap smears). Do not assume that because you are having procedures done vaginally that checkups of the cervix are being carried out. A smear for cancer will not usually be taken during ovulation induction or assisted conception treatment unless you specially ask for it to be done.

Ovarian cancer is usually a tumor in older women, but about ten ovarian cancers in women who had or were having ovarian stimulation (ovulation induction) have been reported in the medical literature. In some of these cases the cancer clearly preceded treatment and was therefore a coincidence. The reported frequency is still no higher than might be expected by chance, considering the huge numbers of treatments with gonadotropins that have been conducted around the world since the early 1960s. Nonetheless, the association needs further research and, like breast cancers that are already there before treatment, ovarian cancers can grow much more quickly during ovarian stimulation and during pregnancy.

# Ovarian Stimulation and Birth Defects

In Australia, the National Perinatal Statistics Unit (NPSU), which for many years has collected data on birth defects in the Australian population, cooperates with the Fertility Society of Australia to publish the birth outcomes of all pregnancies that happen as a result of **in vitro fertilization** (IVF) and **gamete intrafallopian transfer** (GIFT). Although providing this information is voluntary for the 26 or so IVF units in Australia, all centers or units take part.

In 1987 Dr. Paul Lancaster, who heads the NPSU, suspected that there could be a slight increase in birth defects after IVF. Given that miscarriages are more common in infertile women in general but are particularly so in those conceiving with clomiphene, which was routinely used with gonadotropins to stimulate the ovaries for IVF in the 1980s, Dr. Lancaster's proposal might not have been very surprising. Of special concern was a possible several-fold increase in major deformities of the nervous system called neural tube defects, which comprise anencephaly, an absence of development of the brain and not compatible with survival, and spina bifida, a serious defect of the spinal cord producing paralysis and a lack of bowel and bladder control.

Curiously, on the other hand, no cases of cleft lip or palate (one of the mo: common birth abnormalities) occurred after IVF for quite a number of years. it is legitimate to suspect, just on the basis of statistics, that IVF caused neur tube defects, then it is equally justified to conclude that IVF protected embryc against cleft lip and palate. I point this out just to show the dangers of jumpin to conclusions from limited data. So many different birth defects are known tha it was inevitable, just by chance, that some of them would be more common an some less common than expected. In both cases, further experience has not sur ported the original conclusions. Cleft lip or palate has since happened. It ha also been established that there is in fact no increased chance of neural tube de fects after ovulation induction or assisted conception.

# Creutzfeldt-Jakob Disease

In the 1960s and 1970s several governments established national programs in which thousands of pituitary glands were removed at all sorts of autopsies. Th primary purpose was to secure growth hormone for the treatment of childre: with growth hormone deficiency. Another purpose was an opportunity to sav on the high cost of human menopausal gonadotropin (hMG) and to extract th gonadotropins, as a mixture of FSH and luteinizing hormone (LH), to yield product called **human pituitary gonadotropin** (hPG). All appeared to go wel until the 1980s, when several patients who had been treated with growth hor mone in different parts of the world, including the United States, developed rare brain disease, known as Creutzfeldt-Jakob disease (CJD), which, onc symptoms of dementia appear, is inexorably and rapidly fatal. In Australia (bu curiously not in other countries so far), five women who received hPG fo amenorrhea related to FSH-deficiency developed CJD and died.

CJD has not been reported to occur from the forms of gonadotropin usec therapeutically today for ovulation induction and assisted conception. There i: also no reason to suppose that women who are being treated this way with hor mones extracted from urine run such a risk. We are all reminded, however, tha much treatment for infertility is new and powerful. As in all areas of medicine we cannot always be sure of the longer term downsides to the treatment we car make available. Physicians need to be aware of the uncertainties that are in volved, and these uncertainties need to be shared with patients before decisions are made on treatment. We will take up communicating properly with your physician in Chapter 26.

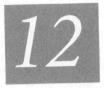

# Blocked
# Fallopian
# Tubes

When the fallopian tubes are blocked, sperm cannot reach the ovulated egg. Complete infertility, or **sterility** (the subject of Chapter 5), is inevitable. But a fallopian tube might be only partially blocked, or one tube can be blocked while the other tube is open. Such partial or mixed blockages reduce the chance of the sperm and egg getting together, bringing about **relative infertility** (the subject of Chapter 6). They can also trap an egg that does get fertilized, sometimes causing an **ectopic pregnancy** (see Chapter 14).

Tubes can be blocked from birth, as in **congenital** tubal obstruction, although this is rare; from inflammation (**salpingitis**); and from intentionally cutting, tying or clipping the tubes for **sterilization**. In this chapter I talk about salpingitis. I also talk about **peritubal adhesions**, which are fine sheets of scar tissue like plastic wrap enveloping the tubes and ovaries that impede the working of the tubes. How to stop them from forming or, if they are being treated, how to stop them from growing back, is discussed in Chapter 13. For really seriously damaged fallopian tubes, those beyond help with microsurgery, in vitro fertilization is needed and is discussed in Chapter 20.

## If You Have Forgotten Chapter 3

Remember that each **fallopian tube** (see Figure 3.5 in Chapter 3) is about 10 to 12 centimeters long and consists of a outer, wide and thin-walled part, the **ampulla**, and an inner, much narrower, more muscular part, the **isthmus**. The isthmus connects to the narrowest part of all, the **interstitial segment**, which passes for one to two centimeters through the wall of the uterus to join the cavity of the uterus. The tube is lined by two kinds of cells: **secretory cells**, which produce mucus, glucose and other substances important for nourishing the egg and embryo; and **ciliated cells**, which bear tiny hairlike structures, the **cilia**, beating in the direction of the uterus and carrying the still-sticky **cumulus mass** (the mucus-like blob inside which the egg is released from the follicle) down the ampulla, toward the junction between the ampulla and the isthmus.

It is at the fallopian tube's **ampullary-isthmic junction** where fertilization takes place. The fertilized egg stays at the junction for two to three days before the tubal isthmus loses its dense secretions and the muscle in its wall relaxes, enabling the early embryo, now rid of its cumulus cells, to reach the uterus. The hormone that causes these changes in the tube is **progesterone**.

A woman should be aware that if she has just one ovary it will normally take over completely from the one that is lost, ovulating every month instead of what on average would have been every second month before. Generally, she will not run out of eggs and go through **menopause** any earlier, as the rate at which eggs are lost by **atresia** (see Chapter 3) is also halved. Thus, the menstrual cycle generally stays the same.

### ... but Two Ovaries and One Tube

If there are two ovaries, whether the tubes are normal or not, they will *tend* to take turns at ovulating from one cycle to the next. Exceptions happen, and one ovary may dominate the other over longer periods of time, especially if part of one ovary has been significantly removed. Obstruct just one tube and pregnancy will take, on average, twice as long to happen. Thus, depending on the strength of a woman's underlying fertility and the amount of time left to get pregnant, one blocked tube may or may not be important.

There is also a risk of ectopic pregnancy in the blocked tube, because sperm can get out of the open tube, swim across to the other side and fertilize an egg headed for the blocked tube. Before IVF made it wise to retain as much ovarian tissue as possible for egg pickups (see Chapter 20), we sometimes intentionally removed an ovary next to a hopelessly blocked tube if the other tube and ovary were normal, paradoxically but effectively doubling **monthly fertility**, the monthly chance of pregnancy. Such a "paradoxical ovariectomy" can still occasionally be useful for improving fertility in special circumstances.

### ... and One Ovary and Opposite Tube Can Spell Trouble

If a woman has just one ovary (one having been removed for, say, a serious ovarian cyst), and the only tube available happens to be on the *other* side, conception is quite unlikely (only a handful have been reported in the medical literature), and quite a number of the pregnancies that do occur turn out to be ectopic ones. **In vitro fertilization** (IVF) or **gamete intrafallopian transfer** (GIFT) is a good option in this instance (see Chapter 20).

The tests use to diagnose and to evaluate the severity of tubal disease, the **hysterosalpingogram** and **laparoscopy**, as well as the new technique of **falloposcopy** (used to assess the lining of the tube), are all described in Chapter 4. The complicated combinations of one or two ovaries with tubes that are not completely blocked are common (see the box "One Ovary Can Be Okay ...").

# Salpingitis and Tubal Adhesions

Salpingitis means inflammation of the fallopian tube (the Latin for which "salpinx"). Inflammation may reach the tube from within, that is, from t uterus, as with sexually transmitted diseases, including **chlamydia** and gono rhea. The **acute salpingitis** that follows can be without symptoms, and clinica silent and unsuspected, as is often the case with chlamydia, or it can be accor panied by peritonitis (inflammation of the **peritoneal cavity**), with pain, te derness, fever and a vaginal discharge. These symptoms should be quick checked by a physician and often require admission to a hospital for treatme with intravenous antibiotics.

Inflammation can also reach the tube from its outside, by the spread, for e ample, of inflammation from a neighboring organ such as the appendix (see t box "Expending the Appendix"). When this happens, most of the damage is c the outside, often sparing the delicate structure of the inside of the tube.

## Expending the Appendix

Appendicitis rarely affects the fallopian tubes unless the inflammation is severe and an abscess has formed in the pelvis and involved the tube and ovary. To stop this from happening is good reason for surgeons erring on the side of caution and removing the appendix early. If the appendicitis does involve the tube and ovary, it is usually just the right side of the abdomen that gets caught up in the inflammation and the adhesions that follow.

More general peritubal adhesions arising from neglected or advanced appendicitis are rare in the United States and most Western countries, where good surgeons and hospitals are easily and quickly available. It is true that many appendixes are removed that turn out to be normal, but for fertility this is better than a general policy of operating only when the diagnosis is absolutely certain.

What can be less fortunate, however, is mistaking a painful (usually right-sided) **ovulation** for appendicitis, operating, finding the appendix to be normal, then removing the appendix as well the "cyst" on the ovary (in reality a normal **corpus luteum**). This will cause peritubal adhesions, not from the appendicitis or the appendectomy, but from the incautious surgical assault on an ovary, one that almost always in these circumstances deserves to be left alone.

If acute salpingitis occurs in the presence of an intrauterine contraceptive device, the IUD should be taken out. IUDs can occasionally introduce an infection into the uterus when they are inserted. This is most uncommon (it occurs in fewer than 2 percent of insertions). More often, the presence of an IUD makes the uterus and tubes less resistant than they normally are to sexually transmitted diseases acquired at a later date. Salpingitis in the presence of an IUD, as without it, can be acute or chronic. Whereas salpingitis usually affects both tubes more or less equally, salpingitis in the presence of an IUD can be asymmetrical, affecting one side disproportionately.

Because of these considerations, IUDs are best used for contraception in women who have had children, who are in stable, single-partner relationships and who do not want the intervention or the permanence of a tubal ligation for sterilization.

The tube and ovary can become separated by new tissue, referred to as peritubal adhesions if they surround the opening of the tube and periovarian adhesions if they enclose the ovary. Think of an **adhesion** as a sheet of scar tissue. If you shaved off the skin over the tips of your two index fingers and held your fingers together long enough, an adhesion would grow between them to join them. When the organs in the abdomen and pelvis lose their single-cell-thick lining and continue to lie close together, they become joined by an adhesion. The same can happen when scarring of the tube follows surgical operations in the pelvis for other conditions, resulting in postsurgical adhesions.

Adhesions can also block the outer end of the tube as a result of **endometriosis** (see Chapter 15), especially when the neighboring ovary is affected. Rather less often, the tube can be blocked by endometriosis of its wall, usually in the middle part of the tube, a location for a blockage that is different from what we see resulting from salpingitis.

In the best of all these cases, the tube itself is spared from harm and the peritubal adhesion is like plastic wrap, enveloping tubes and ovaries and stopping egg pickup by the fimbrial end of the tube. Microsurgery (discussed in Chapter 13) can then be particularly helpful.

**Chronic salpingitis** can result either from repeated episodes of acute (or short-term) salpingitis or from the sort of infective organisms that elicit only a

## Salpinx, Hydrosalpinx and Pyosalpinx ...

The word "salpinx" is Latin for "tube," here specifically the fallopian tube. A hydrosalpinx is a tube blocked from previous inflammation at the outer end and months or years later is filled with watery fluid. A **pyosalpinx**, the worst villain, is an acutely inflamed and blocked tube filled with pus; it sometimes subsides with antibiotics, becoming a hydrosalpinx, and it sometimes ruptures and forms an abscess in the pelvis, much like a burst appendix, and then usually needs an operation to drain it and the abscess. A pyosalpinx can represent a tube infected for the first time, if the infection has gone untreated, or it can represent a hydrosalpinx that has become reinfected.

A hydrosalpinx can have a particularly perverse and harmful effect on getting pregnant, whether the opposite tube is normal and a couple is trying naturally or whether IVF treatment is being performed. How it does this has only been properly appreciated since 1994, when no fewer than three articles were published that showed that women having IVF had a much lower chance of getting pregnant if their **transvaginal ultrasounds**, the technique used for monitoring IVF treatment (see Chapter 20), disclosed a hydrosalpinx (or two hydrosalpinges) forming as the time for egg pickup got closer. What happens is that the high amount of estradiol coming from the ovary at this time both stimulates production of more water in the tube and constricts the isthmus of the tube, trapping the fluid in the now swelling hydrosalpinx. Then, after ovulation and fertilization, while an embryo from either the good tube on the

long-term chronic inflammation. In many parts of the world, tuberculosis is the most common cause of chronic salpingitis and also one of the most common causes of sterility.

A tube acutely infected but treated promptly with antibiotics can recover completely, with no damage done. If the infection is repeated or goes untreated, the inflammation becomes chronic. All of the tube's normal functions are disrupted: the hairlike cilia are lost; the muscle of the tube's wall is disorganized; the secretions needed to nourish the embryo are spoiled; and the tube itself nearly always gets blocked. The blockage can be mostly at the outer, **fimbrial end**, resulting in a **hydrosalpinx**, or mostly at the inner end, close to the uterus, involving the isthmus and/or the interstitial segment of the tube. Depending on how much damage there is and where, the tube might still work once the blockages are removed with microsurgery.

## Salpinx, Hydrosalpinx and Pyosalpinx ... (concluded)

other side or from the IVF transfer is waiting in the uterus to implant (see Chapter 3 for the details), the rising levels of progesterone coming from the ovary relax the isthmus, allowing the watery fluid to pour down through the uterus, often washing out the waiting embryo or embryos. The woman may experience fluid escaping through the vagina at this time.

This perfidious process accounts for not a few cases of persistent failure to conceive with IVF and needs to be overcome, by removing the tube surgically, by opening it with microsurgery (see Chapter 13), or perhaps by placing a clip on the isthmus at laparoscopy. Such a clip will not do anything for the hydrosalpinx except cause it to be swollen all the time, but it effectively prevents the fluid entering the uterus and compromising the implantation process.

### ... and Salpingitis Isthmica Nodosa

**Salpingitis isthmica nodosa** is the fairest character of the group of inflammations, but an enigmatic one. The name means that it is an inflammation of the tube, but there are none of the usual inflammatory white blood cells visible to the pathologist. It affects the isthmus and nearly always does so on both sides. It feels (and later looks) lumpy, or nodular. It is best diagnosed with a hysterosalpingogram, which reveals tiny side channels off the main channel of the isthmus—which itself may be open or, later in the disease process, blocked. The operation to correct it is a tubal anastomosis, after the abnormal part of the isthmus has been cut out.

A properly functioning tube is most likely if the blockage is in the isthmic or interstitial part of the tube. The microsurgery required to correct the blockage is then the same as that carried out for the reversal of most sterilization operations, a **tubal anastomosis**. Pregnancy rates of up to 70 percent can be expected from overcoming these inflammatory blockages. Fimbrial blockages are more damaging; the microsurgery operation to reverse it is a **salpingostomy**. If there is still a small opening in the fimbrial end, the damage to the tube is typically a lot less than if the tube is completely blocked; the microsurgery for this less severe situation is called **fimbriolysis**. When the tube is blocked at both its ends, there is usually disruption along the whole length of the tube and microsurgery rarely helps. Evaluating the tubes for microsurgery is a very specialized field. Before I make a final decision on whether or not to recommend an operation, I often want to know what the tube looks like inside, by a hysterosalpingogram, a falloposcopy and a salpingoscopy, an outside, by a laparoscopy (see Chapter 4).

Depending on the extent and severity of damage to the fallopian tubes, the best remedy may be careful microsurgical repair of the tubes (the subject Chapter 13). Remember, however, that it was because microsurgery of the tube even in the hands of an excellent microsurgeon, has poor results when damage to the tubes has been extensive that IVF came to be invented as an alternative

# Microsurgery of the Fallopian Tubes

In Chapter 12 we looked at how the fallopian tubes can become blocked. Thi chapter describes the details—and the limitations—of the operations that a available for overcoming tubal blockages.

# Salpingolysis and Fimbriolysis

**Salpingolysis** is the microsurgical operation for cutting out adhesions from th tubes, usually with a fine electrocautery needle. Electrocautery uses a high volt age electric current to evaporate tissue at the point of a fine surgical needl **Fimbriolysis** is similar but refers to removal of adhesions from the tube's del cate fimbrial end, near the ovary.

These surgeries can, in principle, be done either at an open operation, a **lap arotomy**, or at **laparoscopy**. Special skills are needed in either case. Laparoscop has the advantage of a short hospital stay, but the operation is technically muc

## What's in the Knife?

Electrocautery has the advantage over the more ordinary cutting of tissue with scissors or scalpel in that bleeding is well controlled by switching the pulsing, high voltage cauterizing current from a cutting frequency to a coagulating frequency and back again. Some surgeons have experimented with laser beams to cut the adhesions, especially during laparoscopy. Laser surgery has not been shown to have advantages over electrocautery, whereas the laser equipment necessary is a lot more expensive and difficult to use.

The way in which the adhesions are cut does not matter in order to prevent adhesions from regrowing, provided they are cut out accurately. The other mainstays of modern microsurgery include careful control of bleeding, avoiding unnecessary trauma to the peritoneal serosa, constantly irrigating the exposed tissues with warm salt solution to stop them from drying out and meticulously sewing back together any gaps in the peritoneal serosa (if this can be done without tension). Unfortunately, care and surgical skill alone are not enough to stop adhesions from returning, whether the operation was laparoscopy or laparotomy.

more difficult and usually takes longer; there is less drying out of tissues than with laparotomy, but unexpected difficulties with the operation are less readily dealt with. Laparotomy is a more difficult procedure in terms of recovery, but it is more accurate and generally quicker. The advantage between the two has not been decided.

In either approach, salpingolysis and fimbriolysis are made more accurate by using the enlargement provided by the laparoscope itself or, during a laparotomy, the operating microscope, which has a magnification of about 6. This allows the surgeon to see exactly where the adhesions are attached, then to cut them free a millimeter or so from the healthy tissue.

Microsurgery for treatment of peritubal or perifimbrial adhesions is a worthwhile operation in most cases in which the tubes are open and there are adhesions on each tube. When there are adhesions on only one tube, conception takes longer because, on average, ovulation will occur into the working tube only half the time, doubling the time it takes to get pregnant, but often within the expected time, so many such women will never be aware of reduced fertility. Whenever adhesions are mild or mainly on one tube, the gynecologist recommending operation will be taking into account many things other than the anatomy of the ovaries and tubes, such as the duration of the infertility, the contribution of other infertility factors, perhaps the result of a falloposcopy (see Chapter 4), the age of the woman and her wishes in relation to **in vitro fertilization** (IVF) or **gamete intrafallopian transfer** (GIFT) and her feelings generally regarding an operation.

# Salpingostomy

The operation in which a new opening is made in a tube completely blocked at its outer, fimbrial end is called a salpingostomy, or sometimes a neosalpingostomy. (If the tube is open but the fimbriae are stuck together with fine adhesions then the operation is a fimbriolysis.) Carrying out a salpingostomy that gives the maximum chance of success, given the damage the tube has suffered, requires a surgeon with a great deal of experience with tubal microsurgery. The most must be made of what fimbrial structures remain. The ultimate result of the operation, however, is out of the surgeon's hands. The scarring and thickening of the tube's wall, the loss of the **cilia** (the fine hairs on the cells that propel the egg) and the coexistence of other places of blockage along the tube will all

## Salpingostomy: The Details

An operating microscope is used once a small opening has been made at what the surgeon senses is the point where the fimbriae have come together. After this the operation involves dissecting between the folds of the tube as seen from the inside. In some cases the result is dramatic—the fimbriae themselves can be freed and the tube soon looks almost normal.

In other cases there are adhesions between folds in the tubal lining, the tube's wall is too thick and there may be several complete blockages in the tube resulting in cystic spaces that cannot be made to communicate with each other and therefore need to be excised. In these cases the tube can usually be made to stay open, but the opening that is constructed is contrived, often limited in mobility and usually lined by very damaged tissue. Once the tube is open, its damaged tissues do tend to recover, but the process takes years rather than weeks or months, and in the meantime there is more frustration and disappointment. Of the pregnancies that do occur when the tubes are so damaged, one-quarter take place in the tube itself because the fertilized egg gets stuck (an ectopic pregnancy, discussed in Chapter 14); another quarter miscarry because of the poor nutrition the tube offered those early embryos that did reach the endometrial cavity.

still be there after salpingitis has been cured and a blockage cleared. This damage continues to reduce the tube's ability to transport eggs, sperm and embryo after a technically successful salpingostomy leaves the tube open and reasonabl close to its ovary.

On average, only 5 to 10 percent per year of the women undergoing salpin gostomies have a pregnancy that leads to a baby. The results are better if the lin ing of the tube has been well preserved (see **falloposcopy** in Chapter 4). The re sults are worse than this for women with badly damaged tubes and for wome who have had a previously unsuccessful attempt at the operation. For mo women, one cycle of IVF provides a better chance of pregnancy than a year waiting after salpingostomies, but because an untreated hydrosalpinx can itse cause treatment with IVF to fail, it is now becoming common again for suc damaged tubes to be submitted to salpingostomy while still intending to hav early treatment with IVF (see the box "Salpinx, Hydrosalpinx and Pyosal pinx ..." in Chapter 12).

When the coating of the peritoneal cavity, the serosa, is injured, as it inevitably is to some extent during any pelvic operation, the blood on its surface soon clots. This superficial clot causes nearby organs to stick together, at least temporarily. Normally the clot dissolves in about six hours. The wandering cells of the peritoneal cavity, the **macrophages**, form a protective coat over the raw and exposed peritoneal tissues. Any blood clot that is still left three days after the operation begins to form scar tissue. If there is no blood clot left three days after operation, there will be no adhesions.

There is still some doubt about where the new peritoneal serosal cells come from, but it does not matter much. The important point is that the new serosa lining the peritoneum is fully formed by eight days after an operation, except for those areas where a blood clot was left undissolved and which by eight days is already well on the way to forming scar tissue between organs, such as the tube, the ovary, the uterus and the intestines. This scar tissue is thus the adhesion. Prevent the scar tissue from forming and you prevent adhesions. The more often the scar tissue (the adhesions) has been operated on, the more likely it will regrow—and they will be tough, thick adhesions rather than delicate, filmy ones.

Surgeons have long contrived to influence the outcome of peritoneal healing in favor of repair instead of scarring. To be sure, if we were to use drugs to completely stop blood from clotting or scar tissue from forming, we could stop adhesions, but for someone who is recovering from an operation neither of these extreme maneuvers is acceptable. Surgeons in the 1940s, for example, showed that anticoagulants were effective in stopping adhesions only if they were kept going for dangerously long times after the operation and in dangerously large amounts. We need something that either sticks around locally for three days, encouraging the clot to dissolve, or keeps all the surfaces apart for the eight days it takes all the serosa to reform. For now, we only have the means for the second option.

### Early Laparoscopy

Eight to ten days after the microsurgery, after the serosa has healed, we can do a laparoscopy. During the laparoscopy we push apart any early points of adherence between the tubes and ovaries or other organs. This separates the very early scar tissue, on its way to forming an adhesion, and allows a few days for islands of new serosal cells to have another chance at linking up and completing the job of healing the peritoneum. Several different groups of infertility surgeons around the world, including some in Sweden, Holland and the United States, as well as myself, have shown that carrying out such an early ("second-look") laparoscopy is effective in diminishing eventual adhesion formation.

Enough "third looks" have been done to know that adhesions are usually much reduced by the maneuvers at the second look and often have been prevented altogether. Professor A. F. Haney of the Duke University Medical Center in North Carolina has begun new, detailed studies of second looks in mice. The aims are to introduce a reevaluation of optimum timing after microsurgery and to prompt proper evaluation of the procedure's efficacy in the difficult financial setting of U.S. managed-care health programs. The reluctance of surgeons (and health maintenance organizations) to accept second-look laparoscopies may be overcome by the recent development of **minilaparoscopes**, instruments just a few millimeters in diameter that can be used in an ambulatory care setting without general anesthesia (see the box "Minilaparoscopy—For a Minilook" in Chapter 4).

### Surgical Adhesion Barriers

There are a number of products on the market that can be used during an operation to form a barrier between organs. Some dissolve and thus can be left inside the body; others do not, so, depending on where among the pelvic organs they are used, they may need to be removed at the second-look laparoscopy. The dissolvable adhesion barrier with which there has been the most experience is **Interceed** (made by Johnson & Johnson), a material woven from fibers of modified cellulose. After being placed over abdominal surfaces where the serosa is likely to have been damaged, it dissolves in about eight days into simple sugar molecules, which are then absorbed by the body and metabolized. In the meantime, the cloth keeps the covered surfaces apart while the serosa reforms. Controlled trials have shown Interceed to be effective in reducing or (sometimes) preventing adhesions, but an adhesion-free result is not guaranteed, and in my opinion a second-look laparoscopy is still advisable.

The nondissolvable product available is **Goretex** (the same stuff that some ski clothing is made from). Goretex has a long history of use in cardiac surgery, where it is used to permanently replace the serosa around the heart when adhesions there are troublesome after inflammation or repeated operations. Its credentials in infertility surgery are not as good. If it is used between the tube and ovary (not clinically tested so far in published controlled trials), it obviously needs to be removed after eight days, when the serosa has healed; removing it during laparoscopy is possible. If it is used on other surfaces, such as the uterus or the side of the pelvic peritoneal cavity, it can in principle be left, but studies on its usefulness are still limited.

# Preventing Adhesions

By reading up to this point, you know that adhesions are a menace to fertility. They can also cause pain from cramping of the intestines and from closely confining the process of ovulation. The hunt for ways of stopping adhesions from forming or reforming after operations has been accompanied by some research, a lot of speculation and a bucketful of snake oil—magic remedies that are all promise and do not deliver the goods. The way adhesions form is interesting (see the box "Adhesions or Healing"). The only way to stop them from growing back after they have been cut out is, first, to operate very carefully with microsurgery; second, to carry out a laparoscopy eight to ten days after the microsurgery, detaching adherences before they become adhesions again; and third, perhaps use one of the new adhesion barriers made from woven, dissolvable material.

Not every infertility surgeon is convinced about the wisdom of the early second-look laparoscopy for stopping adhesions from growing back. There is a good deal of "out of sight, out of mind" thinking about surgery for adhesions. I believe that these few paragraphs here will be the most controversial in the book among some infertility doctors. On the positive side, there is now not much doubt that it is effective in at least reducing adhesions. On the negative side, it is another operation and still no guarantee that adhesions will not return.

One thing I can say for sure is that if adhesions are going to grow back they do so straightaway. A surgeon who tells a patient that she has just six months to get pregnant after being "treated" for adhesions is misleading the patient badly. It is an unfair and self-serving thing to say. Sure, if you do get pregnant quickly the surgeon probably did a good job and gets your thanks, but if you are not pregnant in that time, the surgeon has made it your fault. You had six months and you did not try hard enough! The fact is that adhesions, if they are going to grow back, do so soon after the operation, probably before you have even thought about having sex. By not regularly doing early laparoscopies, most surgeons cannot know how often their operations fail to relieve adhesions.

# Tubal Anastomosis

Removing a blocked part of the fallopian tube and then rejoining the freshly open ends is called **tubal anastomosis**. It can be done for tubes blocked intentionally (for sterilization) or accidentally (from salpingitis).

## Previous Sterilization

Blocking the fallopian tubes intentionally has become a most popular form of permanent contraception. It is not this book's job to discuss the different way this can be done, but it is a fact of life that at least 2 percent of women will, for one good reason or another, change their minds. Study after study has shown that in practice no amount of counseling at the time of sterilization can predict this group. Losing one or more children through accident or disease is not something anyone expects, nor do many people, at the time the tubes are tied, expect to divorce and then remarry.

Thus, it is important that all sterilization operations be done in a way that is both effective and reversible with microsurgery. This means limiting the part of tube that is removed, tied or squashed to a centimeter or two, preferably in the region of the **isthmus**. **Fimbriectomy**, which means removing the **fimbrial end** of each tube, has the highest failure rate, is the most hopeless to reverse with microsurgery and can be followed by complications after menopause. Thus there are many good reasons why fimbriectomy should not be chosen as a sterilization operation.

The word "anastomosis" means "a join." Tubal anastomosis is thus the operation in which a blocked or diseased part of the fallopian tube is cut out and the healthy two ends of the tube on each side of the removed bit are sewn back together. The sutures we use for tubal anastomosis are less than one-fifth of a millimeter in diameter, with a tiny needle to match (see Figure 5.1a & b in Chapter 5). The tube is brought back together with sutures in two layers, the muscle layer just outside the tube's inner lining, and then the **serosa**, the outer lining of the tube. The details of the operation depend on just where and how much tube has been lost. With accurate surgery, done at high magnification (typically 10x to 16x), the risk of a later pregnancy being an ectopic tubal one should be less than 2 percent and the risk of miscarriage no higher than for women of the same age with normal tubes.

The success rates for microsurgical sterilization reversal can be the highest of any form of infertility surgery. Pregnancy rates among the best surgeons are between 80 and 90 percent. For women who are still under about age 38 and have fertile husbands, it is rare not to get pregnant. Therefore, IVF is rarely needed. The time between the sterilization operation and its reversal is not important, apart from the effects of increasing age. One patient I operated on had her tubal ligation at the time of her (second) cesarean section at the age of 19; she was 42 when the tubes were rejoined and 43 when the baby was delivered. (This differs from the situation of **vasectomy reversals**, in which there is

The most common and simple form of anastomosis is from isthmus to isthmus on each side of the blockage (see Figure 5.1a & b in Chapter 5). Typically, five or six sutures will be used in the muscle layer. The chance of the tube remaining open and functional should be almost invariable.

If the junction between isthmus and ampulla is missing after the sterilization operation, the joining will inevitably be between two parts of the tube with different diameters, the narrow isthmus and the wider ampulla. The opening in the ampulla is then made as small as practical, but this form of join still works provided that the sutures (typically from six to eight in the muscle layer) are accurately located around corresponding parts of each freshened tube's circumference.

The trickiest anastomoses are between ampulla and ampulla. Many sutures (often 10 to 15) are needed. Because the wide ampulla has a very thin muscle wall it tends to collapse in on itself. Too few stitches means narrowing at the site of the anastomosis and a risk of a later ectopic pregnancy. Because the ampulla operated on has more chance of sticking to the ovary, which lies alongside it, than anastomosis operations closer to the uterus, we often carry out an early second-look laparoscopy to check for adherences after this kind of anastomosis, whereas it is not usually necessary after the others.

What kind of sterilization operation would the infertility microsurgeon choose for the very best chance of reversing it successfully? My choice would be a single Filshie clip on each tube, placed about two or three centimeters from the uterus, where the isthmus is getting a little bit wider, but before it becomes ampulla.

strong negative correlation between the time elapsed and the chance of successfully fathering a pregnancy. The reason for the difference is men's development of **sperm antibodies** after vasectomy.)

# Isthmic Salpingitis

The same operation of tubal anastomosis can be used if the tube is blocked in the region of the isthmus not because of a sterilization operation but because of previous salpingitis. In some cases, the condition that causes this kind of blockage is the condition known as "salpingitis isthmica nodosa" (see the be "Salpinx, Hydrosalpinx and Pyosalpinx ..." in Chapter 12). In this conditio there is thickening of the wall of the tube due to tiny outgrowths from the in side of the tube; it feels lumpy when touched with the fingers during an oper tion, as if it has little nodules in it. These nodules connect with the tube itse and can cause an ectopic pregnancy before the disease process completely bloc the tube.

In other cases of salpingitis the tube is blocked at the isthmus or in its in terstitial segment, where the tube passes through the wall of the uterus, simp by scar tissue. Traditionally, the same microsurgery operation, tubal anastomo sis, is used to overcome it, although if the blockage is deep in the wall of th uterus, it can be particularly tricky for surgeons not especially experienced wit this operation at this difficult site.

Overall, up to 70 percent of women with these forms of salpingitis-relate tubal blockage can expect to conceive in the 12 months following the operatio if the tubes remain open and if there are no other infertility factors. This is no quite as good as the chance of pregnancy after sterilization reversal, because th tube has been damaged more generally than it would have been just from ster ilization, but is still good enough to be a very real alternative to IVF.

# Tubal Canalization

If the damage from salpingitis of the isthmus is particularly limited, a nev method of treatment has recently become available, with quite some publicit in the media. This is the procedure of **tubal canalization**. Dr. Amy Thurmond a radiologist from Portland, Oregon, has become famous by advocating the use of a catheter or a probe made of wire to push through and thus open a block age in the isthmus or the interstitial segment of the tube, close to the uterus.

The procedure is done vaginally, through the cervix and the cavity of the uterus. In practice a variety of tubal catheters and probes can be made use of fo this procedure (and it is sometimes automatically done if you have a fallo poscopy). The catheter or wire first needs to brought to the point at which the tube enters the cavity of the uterus. This can be done either during hysteroscopy (so that the opening of the tube is actually seen while the catheter is passed into it) or at X-ray, while a hysterosalpingogram is attempted. The procedure is mod erately painful, more so than with the usual hysterosalpingogram, although the pain should be brief.

Dr. Thurmond has not always been able to reproduce the good results she has had at home with this technique in other countries. This discrepancy means that all the patients with tubes apparently blocked this way are not equally suitable for the procedure. There seems little doubt that her approach works well for cases of "tubal spasm" or with blockages from "plugs of secretion." But there is doubt that these apparent blockages are, in fact, real or permanent blockages. I have found the technique especially useful when a tubal anastomosis has for some reason become blocked.

Being a new form of treatment there is still debate among infertility specialists about the proper place of tubal canalization procedures. Undoubtedly part of the problem in evaluating it is that many of the cases treated this way by some radiologists have not been properly investigated first. I personally doubt that true tubal blockages, especially if they extend over a centimeter or more, are best treated this way instead of with microsurgery.

# 14

# Ectopic
# Pregnancy

A pregnancy is **ectopic** (out of its usual place) when an embryo implants in location that is not the optimal one—the cavity of the uterus, well away from the fallopian tubes and well away from the cervix. Ectopic pregnancies are found in the fallopian tubes, the ovaries, the cervix and even in the abdomen Pregnancies in strange corners of the uterus also can misbehave.

# Tubal Ectopic Pregnancies

Most ectopic pregnancies are found in the fallopian tubes and are called "tuba pregnancies." Most of these, in turn, are located in the outer part of the tube (the **ampulla**; see Chapter 3). Less often they occur in the narrow, inner part of the tube (the **isthmus**) or even in the **interstitial segment** of the tube that passes through the wall of the uterus (an interstitial or "intramural" pregnancy).

## Symptoms

The classic tubal pregnancy first makes its presence felt by causing discomfort, then pain, low in the abdomen or pelvis, often (but not always) localized to one or the other side. There can be symptoms of early pregnancy, such as nausea and tenderness of the nipples. A period might or might not have been missed; there can be some irregular, dark bleeding, or a period might simply seem to be lingering on. If the ectopic pregnancy has been bleeding internally, there can be a general feeling of faintness, perhaps with spells of dizziness. There can be a local feeling of discomfort in one or the other shoulder. The pain is felt in the shoulder because the internal bleeding irritates the undersurface of the diaphragm, nerves from which enter the spinal cord with those that come from the shoulder, and the brain mixes up the messages.

## Signs and Tests

When the doctor carries out an examination, the abdomen can be sore to the touch low down. Nearly always there is tenderness on one or the other side on vaginal examination; pain on one side when the cervix is gently pushed each way is typical. If the tubal pregnancy has burst through the tube's wall and there is bleeding, the pulse can be either fast (from blood loss) or slow (a reflex from

A blood pregnancy test gives a simple yes or no, an answer the lab can provide very quickly. It does not measure the actual level of the pregnancy hormone human chorionic gonadotropin (hCG) but signals whether it is present in serum at a level greater or less than 50 units per liter (u/l). There is a tiny amount of hCG present in everyone's blood. It is such a basic hormone for human tissue to produce that our body's cells, many years after being derived from those present when we were early embryos, never completely forget how to make a bit of the hormone, and they do, in a tiny amount), but the concentration in serum is much less than 10 u/l.

In the early stages of a pregnancy, before the missed period, hCG will be detectable in blood at a concentration greater than 10 u/l, but perhaps not high enough to show up in a simple pregnancy test. To detect it, a **serum quantitative hCG** needs to be ordered from the pathologist. Likewise, if serial measurements are to be done, the same test should be ordered twice, at least two or three days apart (when with a normal pregnancy hCG should double). It is best for serial measurements to be done in the same lab, for strict consistency of method.

bleeding into the abdomen), but in either case there will be low blood pressure (that is, "shock").

A blood **pregnancy test** will almost always be positive. Characteristically, measuring **serum hCG** sequentially fails to show doubling of **human chorionic gonadotropin** (hCG) levels every two to three days, which is the way hCG goes up in a normal pregnancy. The **serum progesterone** level will be lower than for a normal pregnancy. (These last two tests, although they distinguish an abnormal pregnancy from a normal one, do not themselves discriminate between an ectopic pregnancy and an **inevitable miscarriage**.)

The other test the doctor will arrange is a **transvaginal ultrasound**. This is sensitive enough to show what ultrasonologists call "free fluid" (in this case, blood) in the abdominal or pelvic cavity or, sometimes, among the echoes to one or other side of the uterus, to reveal the pregnancy itself (occasionally with a detectable fetal heart beat).

If left to nature, some tubal pregnancies will abort themselves out the end of the tube and everything settles down (a **tubal abortion**), in which case no further treatment is usually needed. Some ectopics stop growing and gradually

fade away as the tissue dies and gets absorbed. Others, however, keep growing
and if not treated rupture the tube, usually with considerable internal bleeding—a surgical emergency.

The most dangerous place to have an ectopic pregnancy is in that part of the
tube that passes through the wall of the uterus (an interstitial or intramural ectopic). Considerable growth is supported by the surrounding tissue of the
uterus until—ultimately and dramatically—rupture occurs, usually involving
main branch of the artery to the uterus. Fortunately, interstitial pregnancies are
among the least common of ectopic pregnancies and are plainly visible on
transvaginal ultrasound.

## Options for Treatment

The first thought that comes to mind if you have had trouble getting pregnant
and an ultrasound shows the distressing picture of an apparently healthy pregnancy in the tube is why the pregnancy cannot be shifted from the tube to
the uterus. In the August 1994 issue of the *British Journal of Obstetrics and
Gynaecology* there was a report of just such a case and apparently a successful
one. The gynecologist at St. George's Hospital, London, responsible for the report was, upon investigation, unable to support his claim; the article has been
retracted by the journal, and the disgraced gynecologist has been barred from
further medical practice in Great Britain.

If the pregnancy cannot be saved, usually the tube can be. Drug treatment
with methotrexate nowadays ensures this (see the box "Active Treatment of
Ectopics Without Operation"). A **laparoscopy** should otherwise be the first line
of treatment if pain persists. If the tube has not ruptured, it is usually possible
to remove the pregnancy sac from the tube without requiring **laparotomy**. The
procedure in which the tube is slit open to reveal the pregnancy is called a **salpingotomy**; the tube is then left open after the pregnancy has been pulled or
washed out to heal naturally. Such laparoscopic surgery is still not available
everywhere but expertise with it is spreading fast. Sometimes during laparoscopy the pregnancy will be seen to have ended already, with a tubal abortion. In either event the patient can generally leave the hospital that evening or
the next day. Whether with methotrexate or with laparoscopy, it is essential to
keep the patient under observation with serial measurements of serum hCG levels, making sure that they fall promptly and consistently (if they do not, the ectopic may persist and in time bleed again).

If the clinical situation with a tubal pregnancy deteriorates, perhaps with
collapse from internal bleeding, an operation becomes urgent. Depending on

the circumstances, a laparotomy is then carried out as soon as possible. If clinical conditions are less urgent, a laparoscopy may be performed first to confirm the diagnosis and perhaps to enable laparoscopic treatment. During the laparoscopy or laparotomy a decision will need to be made on whether to conserve the fallopian tube by performing a salpingotomy and just removing the pregnancy sac or to remove the tube itself (a **salpingectomy**). This decision is rarely easy to make unless there is obviously too much bleeding for conserving the tube to be safe or if the patient has had enough ectopic pregnancies to want no further risk of it. Factors that bear on the decision include the previous condition of the tube, the chance of later repairing it microsurgically, the hope for future natural pregnancy, the apparent condition of the other tube and whether the tube has contained an ectopic pregnancy before. It should rarely be necessary—and it is certainly very undesirable—to remove the ovary along with the tube, even though it may be bleeding from a **corpus luteum** that has been disturbed.

Not all ectopic pregnancies need surgery of any kind. When symptoms are few, the same kind of close watch that is used after salpingotomy can be kept to see if a small tubal pregnancy will resolve itself without treatment.

## Active Treatment of Ectopics Without Operation

Cells in the tissues of an embryo and the **trophoblast** that surrounds the embryo grow quickly. This means that, like cancer cells, they can be rather selectively stopped in their tracks by drugs that focus on preventing fast-dividing cells from multiplying. These drugs are called "cytotoxic" drugs. One such drug is methotrexate, which can be given to kill an ectopic pregnancy, leaving the embryo and the trophoblast to be absorbed by the body. The methotrexate is either given alone at a moderate dosage or in a very high dose that is reversed some hours later with the administration of folinic acid, which specifically antagonizes methotrexate's lethal effect ("folinic acid rescue"). Although various authors have reported injecting methotrexate or other drugs directly into the ectopic pregnancy by ultrasound-guided needle, this seems to be less reliable. It is important to follow the progress of the ectopic pregnancy with ultrasound and with serial measurements of serum hCG to make sure the drug treatment has been effective.

# Ectopics in Exotic Places

Aside from the unwelcome excitement of experiencing an ectopic pregnancy when you are on vacation or business a long way from home, risking lack of proper medical care, there are locations for ectopic pregnancies within the body that cause them to behave differently from those in the fallopian tube.

## Ovarian Ectopic Pregnancy

An ovulating egg may be fertilized while still in its **follicle** and then get stuck there. Such an **ovarian pregnancy** accounts for about one in 200 ectopic pregnancies. It can be hard to distinguish during laparoscopy from a bleeding corpus luteum (the structure that forms after a follicle has ovulated). The treatment has usually involved surgery to remove the ovary, but in early cases that are not bleeding, drug treatment with methotrexate is probably the best first choice.

### Pregnancy in the Abdomen

In parts of the world where surgical treatment is not available, the clinical situation when a tube ruptures from an ectopic pregnancy can deteriorate to the point of serious collapse and death. Sometimes it nevertheless settles, and, rarely, the pregnancy may keep growing—now in the **peritoneal cavity**.

I managed such a case in New Guinea. The woman believed she was normally pregnant, experiencing movements of the fetus as it grew. It was not until the fetus stopped kicking (and died) at 36 weeks that she sought medical help. A laparotomy revealed the truth, after an X-ray showed where and how the baby was lying, and I delivered a 2.8 kilogram baby from the cavity of the abdomen, saw that I would experience a lot of difficulty detaching placenta from the loops of intestine and decided to leave the placenta to be absorbed, which it did without further complications.

## Cervical Ectopic Pregnancy

Pregnancies that develop in the wall of the cervix, or **cervical pregnancies**, can also be a diagnostic puzzle. They are rare and, to confuse matters, typically have the appearance of a cancer of the cervix. The correct diagnosis may not be made until a biopsy is taken in the operating room. The blood supply to such a pregnancy is greater than to a malignant tumor. Characteristically, bleeding begins during the surgical excision process and will not stop easily. Tying off the major arteries to the uterus, or even a hysterectomy, may be necessary to stop the bleeding. If bleeding does stop quickly after taking the biopsy, the diagnosis may not be made until the biopsy is examined by the pathologist; a further operation or drug treatment with methotrexate should then be undertaken.

# "Slightly Ectopic" Pregnancies

Within the cavity of the uterus there are locations for an embryo to implant that will cause problems for the embryo and the mother-to-be. These are not truly ectopic pregnancies, even though they are in the uterus, but because of their position in the uterus complications are more likely.

## Placenta Previa

If the embryo attaches to the lining of the uterus, the **endometrium**, in the lower part of the uterus, the placenta will get in the way of the fetus during labor, a condition called "placenta previa." Cesarean section may be needed for the baby to be delivered safely.

## Angular Pregnancy

On the other hand, the embryo may implant just on the side of the uterus where the tube joins it, in a narrow, constricted part of the uterus called the "angle" of the uterus. A pregnancy here is called an **angular pregnancy**. It is more likely to miscarry, as I explain in Chapter 7, often after the woman has experienced cramping pain on the side the pregnancy is located. Occasionally the wall of the

Strictly speaking, a cornual pregnancy is one located in one horn of a **bicornuate** ("two-horned") **uterus** or in a **unicornuate uterus** (see Chapter 18). If the horn is of good size a relatively normal pregnancy and delivery may follow, perhaps prematurely, and will more likely than on average be a breech birth. If the horn is small, and particularly if it does not communicate with the main part of the uterus, then sooner or later it will rupture, like an interstitial pregnancy; surgery is needed as soon as the condition is diagnosed.

The term "cornual pregnancy" is also loosely used to include angular pregnancies and interstitial tubal pregnancies. The distinction is more than academic, because an angular pregnancy may go to full term, whereas an interstitial pregnancy will rup-

ture if not treated promptly. The two conditions can be distinguished during laparoscopy by observing to which side a structure called the "round ligament" is pushed. (The round ligament is a cord of tissue that in the embryo runs from the ovary down to the groin, pulling it down from the abdomen into the pelvis, and is an easily recognizable structure in the adult pelvis.) If the round ligament is pushed outward, it means the pregnancy is in the uterus; if pushed inward, the pregnancy is in the tube. Both may need surgery if the wall of the uterus looks set to tear, but an angular pregnancy—as is also true of a true cornual pregnancy—can often then be treated by **vacuum curettage** through the cervix rather than operating on it through a formal, open laparotomy.

uterus is so stretched by the growing pregnancy that it ruptures, the way an interstitial pregnancy does. Early angular pregnancies and interstitial pregnancies can look the same on transvaginal ultrasound, lying in a space apparently separate from the cavity of the uterus. Usually, however, with further growth the angular pregnancy settles into the cavity properly and will go to term. The placenta, imbedded in the angle of the cavity, can get stuck, or be "retained," and might have to be removed manually.

# What Causes Ectopic Pregnancies?

When it comes to explaining them, ectopic pregnancies are like miscarriages in the frustration they cause the patient and the gynecologist. We know what tends to cause them, but, with the exception of fallopian tubes that have obviously been damaged (see Chapter 12) and perhaps those that occur while taking a **progestogen**-based contraceptive, we often cannot pin down the cause in a particular instance.

To be sure, the **relative incidence** of ectopic pregnancies (compared with the number of normal pregnancies) has increased in many Western societies over the past 30 years or so because of the wider occurrence of chronic salpingitis caused by **chlamydia** and gonorrhea acquired venereally, by sexual intercourse (see Chapter 12). In addition, those rare pregnancies that do occur despite normally effective contraception (intrauterine devices and progestogen-based contraceptives, such as the minipill and implants under the skin such as Norplant), are more likely to be ectopic, because they are less effective at preventing tubal pregnancies than they are at stopping pregnancies in the uterus.

## Damaged Tubes

Chronic salpingitis or a previous surgical repair of the tube increases the risk of an ectopic pregnancy from less than 1 percent of pregnancies to 10 or 20 times that frequency. After **tubal anastomosis** (to reverse a **sterilization** procedure) the risk is about 2 percent of pregnancies, a rather low figure, because the health of the tube on each side of the place at which it has been joined is usually normal. With operations for more serious disruption of the tube, such as **salpingolysis** and, especially, **salpingostomy** (see Chapters 12 and 13), the risk is much higher, up to 25 percent or more of pregnancies.

## Hormone Disturbances

The human fallopian tube is very sensitive to hormones, as described in Chapter 3. **Estrogen**, produced by the maturing follicle, causes the tube to secrete mucus, which would normally be protective against an implanting embryo. After ovulation, under the influence of **progesterone** from the developing corpus luteum, this mucus quickly disappears. This is the probable reason why progestogen-based contraceptives, should a breakthrough conception occur, are associated with an increased chance of ectopic pregnancy.

On the one hand, human embryos are especially invasive compared with those of other animals. On the other, the human fallopian tube has much less protective mucus than the tubes of other animals. These two facts both contribute to the high frequency of ectopic pregnancies in humans as compared

## Wrong-Side Ectopic and Heterotopic Pregnancies

Gynecologists have long observed that during an operation for an ectopic pregnancy there is a corpus luteum on the opposite side of the location of the tubal pregnancy. This does not necessarily mean that the egg traveled across the pelvis to get into the tube. Rather, the signals a tubal pregnancy sends that it is there (its production of hCG) can be marginal, perhaps not enough to stop menstruation and a further ovulation—perhaps more often than not from the opposite ovary. (This, incidentally, is one reason why the woman with an ectopic pregnancy may not seem to have missed a period.)

Sometimes there can be one or more pregnancies in the uterus and one or more pregnancies in the tube, a condition called **heterotopic pregnancy**. In this case it is possible that there was a second ovulation, perhaps a day or two after the main ovulation, with sperm still around to fertilize the egg, but with a tube that has lost its will to resist the intrepid, if straggling, embryo. In cases of tubes damaged by salpingitis, one embryo can make it safely to the uterus while another gets caught somewhere in the tube. When this picture is revealed on transvaginal ultrasound, early operation to remove the pregnancy in the tube can mean that the one in the uterus is saved.

with other species. Monkeys are in between; they occasionally get ectopic pregnancies. Rabbits and mice, with not-so-invasive embryos and with heaps of mucus on the surface of the tube's cells throughout their ovarian cycles, never do, even when pre-embryos that have been stripped of their **zona pellucida** (which adds to the fertilized egg's side of the lubrication needed for transport) are intentionally placed in the tube during experiments.

If, while progesterone is going up after ovulation, the pre-embryo's transport down the tube is interrupted, the tube will have lost much of its lubricating mucus and its resistance to implantation. This can happen in three ways: an adhesion in the tube from previous salpingitis; a delay in the release of an egg from the ovary, or the egg being lost by the tube on the side of its ovulated ovary, to be picked up later, by chance, by the tube on the other side.

With the morning-after pill (**postcoital contraception**, for example using two birth control pills in the morning and night after unanticipated sex), there is a small but increased chance of ectopic pregnancy. Although this has been attributed to high estrogen levels keeping the tube blocked with secretions, it seems to me at least equally plausible that it is a late ovulation that has released the egg, which is then fertilized by remaining sperm. By this time the tube is well and truly under the influence of progesterone or progestogens (which are present in the pill).

Similarly, the increased risk of tubal pregnancy with ovulation induction, particularly with **follicle stimulating hormone** (see Chapter 12) and with **in vitro fertilization** (IVF) or **gamete intrafallopian transfer** (GIFT), which also has been attributed to high levels of estrogen, also can be explained by a later ovulation under progestogenized conditions. If there are lingering sperm about (which, given the usually excellent mucus in the cervix, there often are), an egg ovulated by a small follicle a day or two after the GIFT procedure could be a perfect candidate to be fertilized late and to cause trouble.

## Assisted Conception

The risk of an ectopic pregnancy in the tube is higher after either GIFT or IVF, on top of the effects of the hormone disturbances we have just been talking about. With GIFT, the risk is about 6 percent of pregnancies. The reason may be unsuspected disease of the fallopian tube, which is discussed further on). IVF, even with transfer of fertilized eggs to the uterus rather than to the tube, or **zygote intrafallopian transfer** (ZIFT), can also result in an ectopic pregnancy, even if there is only a stump of tube left after, say, salpingectomy. If the tube itself is still present but is blocked only at its outer, **fimbrial end**, the risk is significant. The reason for these ectopics may be that IVF embryos are always transferred with a few small bubbles of air (necessary to stop them drifting up or down the transfer catheter and getting lost). The embryos probably stick to these air bubbles, which in general may be a good thing, because they keep them up in the uterus rather than following the catheter back into the mucus of the cervix (and into oblivion). But the same air bubbles can float up into what is left of one or the other tube, carrying the hapless embryo with it. If the tube is normal this probably happens quite often, and can advantage the embryo, which then reenters the uterus perhaps when it is better prepared for the embryo. If the tube is not normal, however, it has little driving power to return it to the uterus.

## Fertility After Ectopic Pregnancies

The question of fertility after an ectopic pregnancy is a difficult one. Few modern clinical series have been published, and the medical literature on the subject

## The Perils of Selective Reporting

When it comes to doctors or scientists reporting medical or scientific outcomes in the journals that comprise the medical literature, it is part of human nature to spend more effort reporting good results than bad ones. True, a note of optimism lubricates the human spirit, of both patients and physicians, but I can think of no clearer area than ectopic pregnancy where this tendency to report often small series of good results and to postpone reporting bad or even average results has so distorted the medical literature. If there were some way of making sure that all results were reported, as is now the case, for example, with IVF and GIFT outcomes in Australia and the United States, this bias would disappear. For the time being, however, it persists and it is only with time (and with particularly large, contradictory series described in the medical literature) that we will get the true picture. That picture is that successful pregnancy after one ectopic pregnancy is not rare, but after two, whether in the same tube or in opposite ones, a normal pregnancy in the uterus is decidedly uncommon, whatever method (short of removing both tubes) has been used for treating the tubal pregnancy.

suffers from enthusiastic reports at the expense of more average results (see the box "The Perils of Selective Reporting"). Keeping options—and damaged tubes—open always runs the risk of a further ectopic pregnancy. Ironically, as ectopic pregnancies have come to be diagnosed earlier and as surgical methods have improved, more women get pregnant again, but the proportion of those pregnancies that are ectopic again is also higher. The probable reason for this paradox is that, in the past, results of surgery were mostly poor (no pregnancy) and only occasionally very good (normal pregnancy).

What tests should be done after a tubal pregnancy? If the patient is planning to try and get pregnant again naturally, then a full investigation of both fallopian tubes is wise. At minimum, I would suggest a **hysterosalpingogram**. Nowadays we are performing **falloposcopies** to also look down inside the tubes. These tests are described in Chapter 4.

# 15

# Endometriosis– Symptoms and Causes

Endometriosis is the name given to the condition in which tissue resemblin the lining of the uterus (the **endometrium**) grows where it should not, in loca tions other than in the uterus itself. It affects the lining of the pelvis and ab domen (the **peritoneal cavity**), including the surfaces of the pelvic and abdom inal organs.

# What Does It Look Like?

To the gynecologist or surgeon looking inside the abdomen (at a **laparotomy** o a **laparoscopy** carried out for one reason or another), endometriosis typically has a dark brown appearance, in the form of spots or cysts. This color come about because it bleeds each month at about the same time that the lining of the uterus menstruates. Because the blood has nowhere to go, it gets stuck in the tis- sues, dries out and goes dark. If the endometriosis forms a cyst in an ovary (it happens to about one in eight women with endometriosis), the semifluid mate- rial in the cyst is rather like chocolate in its color and texture, which gives rise to its usual description as a "chocolate cyst."

The tissue most affected by endometriosis is the **serosa** of the **peritoneum,** which is the one-cell-thick, smooth membrane that lines all of the pelvic and abdominal cavity and its organs (see Chapter 12), together with the soft sup- porting tissue just under the serosa. The peritoneum can be affected anywhere, even under the diaphragm, but in general the closer the peritoneum is to the ovaries the more likely it is to be affected by endometriosis. Behind the uterus, the surface of the bladder and the ovaries themselves are all areas commonly affected.

In 1986 my friend and colleague Professor Peter Russell, a pathologist in Sydney, helped me to study a range of abnormal appearances in the peritoneal cavity to work out what they were. We took biopsies of more than 160 such le- sions. The great majority turned out to be endometriosis. We published our re- sults in the *American Journal of Obstetrics and Gynecology,* and from this time on gynecologists have recognized what we called "nonpigmented endometriosis." This is early endometriosis that has not developed yet to the point of bleeding and thus does not have a brown color. Researchers at the Gasthuisberg University Hospital in Leuven, Belgium, are now showing that these nonpig- mented lesions can be just as chemically active as, or more active than, more typical pigmented endometriosis, secreting substances capable of disturbing re- productive function.

# How Common Is It ?

In the past about one in 100 women had very troubling symptoms of endometriosis, including severe pain and abnormal bleeding bad enough to lead to an operation, but endometriosis is a lot more common than this. Often it causes minimal or no symptoms; many women have it without ever knowing about it. If it is not causing symptoms there is no need to worry (unless it is discovered by accident, perhaps in someone very young, who might be likely to develop symptoms as she gets older). Among women in their thirties whom I have operated on to rejoin tubes to reverse a sterilization operation, about 20 percent have had some endometriosis, whether they have symptoms or not. In women I investigate with a laparoscopy because they are having trouble getting pregnant, the incidence is about 40 percent. This makes endometriosis very common—too common, strictly speaking, for us to be justified in calling endometriosis "abnormal." Nonetheless, it is undoubtedly a major cause of symptoms and suffering in women—women who want treatment to relieve them.

# What Symptoms Does It Cause?

The symptoms that suggest endometriosis include pain, in the form of painful periods (**dysmenorrhea**) and painful sexual intercourse (**dyspareunia**), and abnormal bleeding, particularly **premenstrual spotting** and, later, heavy periods (**menorrhagia**).

## Pain

Dysmenorrhea should be suspected as being caused by endometriosis if it gets worse instead of better as a woman grows out of her teens, if it starts to last longer than the first day of menstruation, or if it is increasingly felt in her back. The pain of dysmenorrhea can be caused by endometriosis bleeding as the endometrium does at menstruation, but with congestion and trapping of blood in the endometriosis tissue. More often, the same hormones, the endometrial **prostaglandins**, that cause normal, first-day menstrual cramps are released by the endometriosis at menstruation time, making the cramps coming from the uterus worse and more persistent. Note, however, that menstrual cramps,

## Is the Pain Really Endometriosis ?

Not all pelvic pain or back pain in women is due to endometriosis. Pain that is felt during a period or soon afterward is the most typical of endometriosis pain. The pain can be spasmodic, but really only at period time. It can be accompanied by diarrhea and pain evacuating the **bowel**, but again really only around period time, except perhaps in particularly severe cases of endometriosis affecting the tissue that lies between the vagina and the **rectum**, in which case the endometriosis can be easily felt by the doctor on vaginal examination. More than a few hours of pain at **ovulation** can come from endometriosis affecting the ovary.

Spasms of pain—rising knife-like then abating—*must* come from a muscular tissue that is contracting in an involuntary way inside the abdomen. The organs a woman has that have such involuntary muscle tissue in them are the uterus, the fallopian tubes and the intestines. Spasms at times other than around period time and ovulation are almost always coming from the intestines, that is, the bowel. Because endometriosis is so common, very many women whose

pain is actually caused by abnormal contractions of the bowel and/or heightened sensations of pain from the bowel (together known generally as **irritable bowel syndrome**), have their conditions labeled endometriosis and go through an extraordinarily frustrating time with their doctors trying to get relief from their symptoms through treatments that will work only for endometriosis.

**Premenstrual tension** (PMT) is another condition whose symptoms are commonly confused with those of endometriosis. PMT symptoms usually precede the period (although some women feel emotionally at their worst toward the end of menstruation). Many women with endometriosis have both PMT and the symptoms of endometriosis. Unless the patient and her doctor distinguish them carefully, treatment of one condition without the other will inevitably result in much dissatisfaction. (To be sure, this is one major reason hysterectomy has a bad name, because despite what hysterectomy does for symptoms of endometriosis, it does nothing for the cyclical symptoms of PMT.)

especially in teenagers, can be severe without endometriosis being present nonendometriosis dysmenorrhea, even though distressing, usually becomes less severe once a woman is in her late teens or early twenties, especially after a pregnancy and childbirth.

A common site for endometriosis is on or below the ligaments that support the uterus from behind, at the level of the cervix, and which lie just below the ovaries. These ligaments are the uterosacral ligaments, running from the sacrum (the lowest part of the backbone) to the uterus, and endometriosis affecting them is one reason why dysmenorrhea is often felt in the back. Because these ligaments are located behind and to the sides of the uppermost part of the vagina, pain with sex (dyspareunia) is another symptom of endometriosis; it is characteristically felt deep inside the vagina, sometimes particularly after a period, when the endometriosis will have become congested. The dyspareunia can be felt from the time of first intercourse or it can develop in sexually active women who previously had no symptoms during sex. If scarring occurs in the uterosacral ligaments from the repeated irritation and bleeding each month, the uterus can be pulled backward, producing a retroverted uterus that can make dyspareunia worse.

Nevertheless, many women with endometriosis will have no significant pain. Need they worry? In general, no. Having endometriosis is not like, say, having a positive PAP smear. Rarely does it lead to complications if it is not causing pain.

## Abnormal Bleeding

Premenstrual spotting or premenstrual staining is the most characteristic symptom of endometriosis. (I will not abbreviate this to PMS, because it has nothing to do with premenstrual tension syndrome; let us call it PMSP.) Periods start in a quite definite manner for most women. It is usually abnormal to have spotting or staining—whether fresh or dark in character—that lasts more than about 12 to 24 hours before menstruation begins properly. The association between PMSP and endometriosis was discovered in 1980 by Dr. Anne Wentz and her colleagues in Memphis, Tennessee. We have since found that even a small amount of spotting or staining, sometimes separated from the actual period by several days, correlates with the presence of endometriosis in more than 80 percent of patients, a surer correlation than for either dysmenorrhea or dyspareunia, both of which can have other causes. This strong association was true both for infertile women and for women who had been referred for reversal of a previous sterilization operation. PMSP is therefore an important clinical symptom, but PMSP is especially interesting scientifically because it may be a clue to explaining the fourth symptom of endometriosis, **infertility**, which we will get to shortly. In the absence of a desire for fertility,

PMSP is rarely a troublesome enough symptom to require investigation and treatment.

Bleeding between periods, however, can be substantial enough to be troublesome. It is not always clear, however, whether such bleeding is due to endometriosis or to a hormone imbalance associated with abnormal ovulation particularly in the case of teenagers and older women.

## How Do I Know If I Have Endometriosis ?

There are three common ways endometriosis prompts you to see your doctor. Teenagers usually go because they have very painful periods, sometimes with bleeding between them or with spotting before the periods. After visits to several doctors, each of whom might be reluctant to take the symptoms seriously, laparoscopy will be decided on, and the endometriosis will be revealed.

The most common way that endometriosis is discovered in women in their twenties or thirties is during tests when they are having trouble getting pregnant. Just how important the endometriosis actually is in causing the infertility varies a lot. In general, the more substantial the endometriosis, and the more other symptoms that exist, such as increasing pain or premenstrual spotting, the more likely it is to be an important factor behind not conceiving.

Endometriosis will most likely be discovered in women in their thirties or forties if they are developing heavy and painful periods, troublesome enough for them to see their doctor. Among the tests that will usually be done is a **trans vaginal ultrasound**, which might show some other causes for the symptoms (such as **fibroids**, an **endometrial polyp** and, sometimes, **adenomyosis**), but which will *not* reveal endometriosis unless there is a cyst visible in the ovary. A woman having an ultrasound for these symptoms should make sure that it is done during or just after a period, so that the ultrasound appearance of a normal **corpus luteum** is not mistaken for an endometrioma (or vice versa); just at the end of a period is the best time to have this test.

Thus, the diagnosis of endometriosis can sometimes be suspected if there is an abnormal cyst seen on transvaginal ultrasound, but it can also be strongly suspected if a careful vaginal examination reveals nodules, often tender, below or to the side of the cervix. (I should say, however, that detecting the signs of endometriosis in young girls is more difficult, because vaginal examination, except gently, under anesthesia, is usually not an option.) Confirmation comes by looking for it and seeing it during laparoscopy. That same laparoscopy can often be used to treat it (see Chapter 16).

# What Causes Endometriosis ?

Many diseases and disabilities are the result of both hereditary and environmental causes acting together. Endometriosis is no exception.

## Inheriting Endometriosis

Professor Joe Leigh Simpson, now of the Baylor College of Medicine in Houston, Texas, but in 1980 at Northwestern University in Chicago, studied the families of 123 women with proven endometriosis. Nine of their 153 sisters (over age 18) and 10 of 123 of their mothers also had diagnoses of endometriosis. This means that of the first-degree relations there was particularly substantial endometriosis in 19 of 276 women—a prevalence of 17 percent. Furthermore, only one of 104 sisters of the patients' husbands (sisters-in-law) and only one of 107 husbands' mothers (mothers-in-law)—nongenetic relations used as a **control group**—had endometriosis of the same severity. Therefore, a patient with a **positive history** of endometriosis among her closest relations is about seven times more likely to have endometriosis. This substantial increase in **relative risk** of endometriosis if there is a mother or sister with endometriosis is consistent with it being inherited by the interplay of several genes.

## Environmental Influences: Ovulations and Menstruations

We know that different women are at different inherited risk of developing endometriosis, but there is also a special risk factor for endometriosis apart from this **congenital** tendency present from birth. This is a woman's total number of ovulations and menstruations.

Two things happen in these cycles that may be very important in the development of endometriosis. First, with each ovulation, the ovaries pour huge amounts of hormones, especially **estrogens**, into the abdomen. If there is tissue there that is potentially even a little bit sensitive to estrogens, it will respond and grow. With each ovulation there is another chance of this happening.

Second, all women who menstruate and who have fallopian tubes that are not blocked will bleed backward during their menstrual period, out through the fallopian tubes and into the abdomen. Menstrual blood, coming as it does from an endometrium that has come apart and is all set to regrow over the next few

## Endometriosis and the Modern Woman

From a functioning reproductive point of view, modern women are special not just because they tend to have children later than their predecessors but also because it is only in rather recent times in our history and prehistory that women have spent more than a few months of their reproductive life ovulating and menstruating. Over the past 100,000 years or so, women typically spent their reproductive years either pregnant or breast-feeding their infants. The nine months of each pregnancy and the two or more years of (unsupplemented) breast-feeding that followed each pregnancy stopped the ovaries from ovulating. If each weaning was soon followed by another pregnancy, then the normal human female condition, biologically, was, and arguably still is, to ovulate and to menstruate not more than 10 or 20 times in a lifetime. (There is more on this in Chapter 2.)

days, is presumably stacked full of growth factors and other things that the endometrium uses to rebuild itself. It could even contain some viable endometrial gland cells. With each menstruation another opportunity is available for abnormal growth. Modern women, who have many more ovarian and menstrual cycles than their ancestors, even those in prehistory (see the box "Endometriosis and the Modern Woman"), are now sharing the effects in the form of endometriosis.

Thus, we have two variables so far as to why some women get endometriosis early, some get it late and some never get it at all. We have the likelihood that women can have a varying genetic susceptibility to endometriosis, and we have this "environmental" variable, the number of a woman's ovulatory menstrual cycles.

Thus, it is the accumulating effects of ovulatory menstrual cycles that explains how the prevalence of endometriosis increases with age and increases in women who delay having children. It is also clear from the genetic influences why some women develop endometriosis at a young age, whereas other women never develop it at all. It can cluster among close relatives for genetic reasons, but many affected people have no affected relatives (sisters or daughters are still more likely not to develop it). Once it is present, continuing ovulation and/or menstruation usually makes it develop further.

## Environmental Pollution Too ?

There are indications that endometriosis is becoming more and more common for reasons beyond the social circumstances that have increased the experience of ovulation and menstruation. Part of the increase, for sure, is that many women are postponing having children. Doubtless, too, we are more likely to diagnose it than in the past; far more laparoscopies are done to investigate pain and infertility than before. We are also now aware of nonpigmented endometriosis, which a decade ago was often missed.

But the possibility remains that there might be other environmental factors that have changed over the last generation or two, just as there seem to be more environmental contributions to **oligospermia** in men (see Chapter 9). Recent discoveries in monkeys have pointed the finger at an industrial pollutant, the

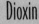

### Dioxin

In Chapter 2 we discussed the occurrence of endometriosis in monkeys and apes, but it is rarely severe. Researchers at the Harlow Primate Laboratory in Madison, Wisconsin, have been studying dioxin's long-term effect on reproduction in female rhesus monkeys. In a systematic study that started 15 years ago, the Harlow researchers began feeding 16 monkeys small amounts of dioxin in their diet. This addition to their diet was continued for 4 years. Unexpectedly, 6 to 10 years later three monkeys died of debilitation—apparently from endometriosis. Tennessee gynecologist Dan Martin operated on the surviving monkeys and was staggered to find that there was severe endometriosis in most of the monkeys given the highest dose of dioxin (25 parts per trillion). A smaller group of monkeys was given 5 parts per trillion and some had moderate to severe disease. The monkeys given no dioxin had no endometriosis or only the mild form normally found in monkeys anywhere.

Several studies are now under way to correlate levels of dioxin and related chemicals in women with the presence of endometriosis. If the association is confirmed, the search for other environmental toxins, and how they operate on an internal tissue, will be on. Its importance for women of the future, as well as for our understanding of endometriosis today and what causes it, would be immense. (See Chapter 9 for dioxin's possible role in oligospermia.)

poison dioxin, but we will need more definite information to be sure (see th
box "Dioxin"for details of the studies so far).

## How Does Endometriosis Develop ? Does It Spread ?

One theory on the way endometriosis gets going, the so-called implantatio
theory, first developed by gynecologist John A. Sampson of Albany, New Yor
in the 1920s, has it that live cells from the endometrium in the uterus are she
into the menstrual flow. With passage of menstrual flow back out through th
tubes, surviving cells are said to attach themselves to the serosa near the ends c
the tubes to produce endometriosis. Further shedding from these "implants
then results in further implants, and so the endometriosis gets more extensive
Just how often this might happen is causing a lot of debate.

### Implantation or Metaplasia ?

Peritoneal tissues close to the ovaries in the developing female embryo give rise to specialized hollow structures, the **Müllerian ducts** (discussed further in Chapter 18). These hollow pipes grow as the **fallopian tubes** from the peritoneal cavity immediately next to the ovaries; they meet in the middle to form the uterus and below it the cervix, and then connect with the lower vagina.

We know that in adult life tumors of the surface of the ovaries and the peritoneum close to the ovaries can mimic development of the lining tissues of these Müllerian-derived organs. Often these cancers differentiate in the same way and at about the same time in many locations in the pelvis. Endometriosis has nothing at all to do with cancer, but perhaps the peritoneum in some women retains the memory and capacity to develop into these Müllerian tissues. The result would consist of a series of conditions—all of which we do in fact find—ranging from "endosalpingiosis" (growth of tissue like that of the fallopian tube, or salpinx) to "endocervicosis" (growth of tissue like the lining of the cervix), as well as endometriosis, which is the most common and most important of the three possibilities. These observations underlie the metaplasia theory for endometriosis. Controversy between proponents of the implantation theory and the metaplasia theory continues.

Endometriosis is sometimes found in women who were born without a uterus or vagina (a condition discussed in Chapter 18), and thus have never menstruated.

The other main theory on how endometriosis gets started and develops is the **metaplasia** theory, by which the body for some reason determines that there are patches of sensitive tissue in the abdomen, or peritoneal cavity. These patches, it is thought, then respond either to the repeated huge amounts of estrogen with every ovulation, or they respond to repeated exposure to menstrual blood with every menstruation and the growth factors it presumably contains. Metaplasia then involves the peritoneal tissues undergoing a metamorphosis from simple serosa to having the structure of endometrium. Any apparent spread of endometriosis, according to this theory, is just the slower development of some patches in comparison with others.

Traditionally, it is the implantation theory that has captured the imagination, especially in North America—to the point that each lesion of endometriosis has come to be called an "implant." Since we have recognized the early, nonpigmented lesions of endometriosis, many gynecologists are becoming

## Implantation or Metaplasia ? (concluded)

This means that implantation of menstrual cells is not *necessary* in the causation of endometriosis. In addition, probably every woman with open fallopian tubes who menstruates will shed endometrial cells out through the tubes into the abdomen each month, but not every woman gets endometriosis. This means that implantation of endometrial cells is not *sufficient* to cause endometriosis.

In science, a theory that is neither necessary nor sufficient is not usually a particularly strong theory. This was the belief of Emil Novak, probably America's greatest gynecological pathologist. Novak died in 1957 convinced that endometriosis was a metaplasia much more often than his contemporaries were prepared to concede, despite earlier attempts by two of Sampson's implantation-theory disciples, Roger Scott and Richard TeLinde, to get him to change his mind.

Still, there are cases of endometriosis that are more difficult to explain by metaplasia than implantation. The most striking is the occurrence of endometriosis in scars in the abdomen after operations done during pregnancy to open the uterus and remove the fetus (an operation rarely done nowadays). For some peculiar reason, such scar endometriosis complicates about one in 50 such operations in the middle three months of pregnancy, but it happens much more rarely after cesarean section, a comparable operation, in the last three months.

convinced that endometriosis only very uncommonly spreads from one locatio to another, previously normal, location.

Unlike cancer, which spreads and spreads, most cases of endometrios once the lesions have matured, remain reasonably restricted to the same loc tions throughout a woman's menstrual years. This is not to say that cysts of e dometriosis in the ovary do not often grow back after being removed, but, f example, if a woman has had 20 years without endometriosis cysts in the ovar it is rather unlikely that the cysts will suddenly start developing.

## Mild or Moderate Endometriosis and Infertility

Severe endometriosis distorts the tubes and ovaries so much that it is not hard to imagine why fertility fails. With more moderate endometriosis, however, the tubes and ovaries are usually completely normal. What is going wrong?

Recent speculations center on two things. First, there are cells wandering about the body called **macrophages**, which surround and ingest all sorts of debris that one way or another gets into the body. There are many macrophages in the peritoneal cavity (probably because in women the peritoneal cavity, via the tubes, uterus and vagina, is open to the outside environment). Macrophages, for example, ultimately dispose of sperm cells that get into a woman's body. In endometriosis, these macrophages are known to be particularly aggressive and are called activated macrophages. Activated macrophages may get into the fallopian tubes and dispose of sperm before they have had a chance of getting to the egg. This is one way endometriosis probably works in decreasing fertility, especially in a woman whose partner has a low sperm count or low sperm motility (see Chapter 9). Activated macrophages also produce a variety of chemicals called "cytokines" that have been shown, in the laboratory, to interfere with sperm motility and with the survival of embryos. Cytokines are also capable of causing normal tissues to bleed, perhaps explaining the premenstrual spotting that endometriosis often causes.

Second—and this is still speculative—we know that the endometriosis that is associated with infertility is located very superficially in the peritoneal cavity, just on the peritoneal surface, the serosa. This is different from endometriosis that is causing pain, which is more likely to be several millimeters deep, growing into the underlying tissues. (These conclusions

# Endometriosis and Infertility: Chicken or Egg ?

How ironic! A woman is more likely to have endometriosis if she delays having her first baby (because of all those ovulatory menstrual cycles over the years), but once endometriosis is there it contributes further to not getting pregnant.

## Mild or Moderate Endometriosis and Infertility (concluded)

have been reached recently by Dr. I. A. Brosens and his colleagues at the Gasthuisberg University Hospital in Leuven, Belgium.)

We also know that superficial endometriosis has glands that secrete mucus, just as the endometrium in the uterus secretes mucus in the second half of the menstrual cycle. This mucus, if it were to specially adhere to the **fimbrial ends** of the tubes (responsible for attracting the mucus-surrounded egg, called the **cumulus mass**), could stop the egg from entering the tube, with the egg more likely either to remain within the follicle or to float into oblivion in the abdomen. What is the evidence that this might be taking place?

Researchers have been working on endometriosis in hamsters. Hamsters, like mice and rats, do not develop endometriosis naturally, but they can be made to develop it by grafting endometrial tis-

sue into their peritoneal cavity. The hamsters with endometriosis induced this way (but not normal hamsters) have shown a coating over the surface of the fimbrial ends of their fallopian tubes when looked at with great magnification using scanning electron microscopy. This is just what one might expect if secretion of mucus from the endometriosis was getting in the way of ovulating eggs at the ends of the tubes.

We also know from extensive experience among women with endometriosis that when we put lots of sperm directly into the fallopian tube (getting around a low sperm count), and we also put three or so eggs directly into the tube (getting around any possible problem with egg pickup by the tube's fimbrial end), we have a very high chance of the woman getting pregnant. This is the procedure known as **gamete intrafallopian transfer (GIFT)**, discussed in Chapter 20.

There are also special puzzles. Every experienced gynecologist knows of som paradoxes that just do not appear to make easy sense. On the one hand, treati the mildest forms of endometriosis rarely seems to be followed quickly by pre nancy. On the other hand, there have been examples of substantial endomet osis in which pregnancy has happened quite quickly. It is like saying that curi a mild form of a disease is more difficult than curing a severe case. How do v explain these paradoxes?

The key to understanding endometriosis and infertility is to realize that it not like having blocked tubes, not ovulating or having no sperm. Unless t scarring that sometimes goes with it blocks the tubes (accounting for no mo than 5 percent of women with endometriosis), there is always a chance of ge ting pregnant; it is a cause of **relative infertility**, not **sterility** (see Chapter 1)

Instead, experience (and theory) is consistent with endometriosis gradual decreasing fertility as it becomes more extensive, or as it becomes more acti in whatever the way is that it gets in the way of conception (see the box "Mi or Moderate Endometriosis and Infertility"). In practice, however, the futu chance of getting pregnant naturally, as with most of the reasons for decrease fertility, depends more on the length of time a couple has been trying and th woman's age than it does on the "dose" of the particular infertility factor that h been discovered.

Paradoxically, the more severe endometriosis is, the more likely it is that er dometriosis is the chief explanation of a couple's infertility and that successf treatment will be followed by pregnancy. The arithmetic of this paradox is e plained in Appendix A. Briefly, because we do not understand or cannot poir the finger at all the reasons why normal fertility varies between different cor ples, the more dramatic the cause for infertility that is found, the more likely is that it will be the only cause, and that treating that particular recognized cau will lead to conception.

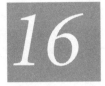

# 16

# Endometriosis–Treatment

In this chapter I describe the various ways endometriosis can be treated—sup pressing it, destroying it or ignoring it—and concentrate on relief of symptom The symptoms of endometriosis and how endometriosis comes about are di cussed in Chapter 15.

# Treatment—If or When?

If endometriosis is not causing symptoms, especially if it is not causing significan pain or infertility, it might not need treatment at all. It will probably disappea after menopause, when it stops being stimulated by ovulation or menstruation There are two main exceptions to this noninterventionist medical policy: whe endometriosis is discovered in a teenager and gentle suppression of it is pruden to be sure of conserving fertility in the future; and if there is a chocolate cyst o the ovary (see Chapter 15) and suppression is important to prevent the cyst from getting bigger and risk bursting. Remember that not everyone with endome triosis will have impaired fertility; until fertility has been put to the test, no on can know for sure whether the endometriosis will be important in this regard.

There are three main strategies for treating endometriosis that is causing, o likely to cause, symptoms: withdrawing the hormone support endometrios

**Table 16.1**  **Treatment Options for Endometriosis[1]**

| Hormonal | Destructive | Symptomatic Only |
|---|---|---|
| Progestogens[2] | Laparoscopy diathermy | NSAIDs[3] |
| Danazol | Laparoscopy laser | Oral contraceptives |
| GnRH-agonists[4] | | Assisted conception |
| | | Presacral neurectom |
| Ovariectomy | Laparotomy excision | Hysterectomy |

[1]The further down the table, the more substantial the intervention.
[2]The progestogens used most often are medroxyprogesterone acetate (Provera, made by Upjohn) and norethynodrel (Primolut N, made by Schering).
[3]Abbreviation for "nonsteroidal antiinflammatory drugs," which include aspirin, mefenamate (Ponstel, made by Parke Davis–Wellcome), naproxen sodium (Naprosyn, Naprogesic, both made by Syntex) and ibuprofen.
[4]The GnRH-agonists available include goserelin (Zoladex, made by ICI), leuprolide (Lupron, made by Abbott) and nafarelin (Synarel, made by Syntex).

depends on from the ovaries; removing or destroying the abnormal endo-metriosis tissue, and/or ignoring the endometriosis itself while concentrating on alleviating the symptoms it is causing.

# Strategy #1: Stopping Ovulation

The drugs used to suppress ovulation and cause endometriosis to regress have the advantage of neither requiring anesthesia nor involving the ordinary haz-ards and discomfort of an operation. The drugs are taken usually for a mini-mum of six months, during which time there is no possibility of pregnancy hap-pening (because ovulation intentionally does not take place). After the drugs are stopped it takes four to six weeks for normal cycles to return. With time, if preg-nancy does not happen, the endometriosis will become active again. For their infertility, or for long-term control until fertility is to be put to the test, women in their teens or twenties usually choose drug treatment, because for them time is not as critical a factor for getting pregnant as it is, say, for women with infer-tility in their late thirties.

## Progestogens

Drug treatment of endometriosis originated from the observation that en-dometriosis often regresses in those women who get pregnant despite it, an ef-fect attributed to the main pregnancy hormone **progesterone**. There are several synthetic progesterone-like drugs (**progestogens**) available to mimic progesterone's effect. Dr. Robert Kistner of Boston began treating endo-metriosis with **medroxyprogesterone acetate** (MPA; trade name Provera) in the late 1950s. **Norethynodrel** (NET; trade name Primolut N) is also well tolerated and effective. MPA or NET are the hormone drugs I would choose for a woman if she has endometriosis diagnosed years before pregnancy is wanted; the maintenance dose can be very small, with no side effects. The hor-mone drugs we usually prescribe for shorter (less than six months) courses of treatment, however, are a little more powerful. They include the male hor-mone derivative **danazol** (Danocrine) and a new class of substances called **GnRH-agonists**.

# Danazol

Danazol works in several ways at once. It stops the production of estrogen a*
progesterone in the ovaries, decreasing the amounts of these hormones in t'
blood, and, more importantly, in the peritoneal fluid. Second, it blocks the r
ceptors to those hormones in responsive tissues, which means that the end
metrium, as well as endometriosis tissue, cannot respond to whatever sm;
amount of estrogen is still circulating. Menstruation therefore gives way
**amenorrhea** (absent periods) during treatment, although some breakthrou;
bleeding is not rare. Third—and probably because of danazol's resemblance
male sex hormones—danazol stops the **pituitary gland** from trying to cor
pensate for the inactivity of the ovaries by increasing its production of **follic
stimulating hormone** (FSH).

## Danazol Mischief

Thin women generally tolerate danazol better than fatter women, because danazol often stimulates the appetite. Danazol can also increase weight through fluid retention. It is an anabolic steroid and develops the muscles. Muscle cramps can occur during the first few weeks of treatment. About 5 percent of patients on the drug soon develop a rash, usually on the face and upper body; although the rash resembles an allergic reaction, allergy is probably not its cause because it subsides with continued treatment.

Because of danazol's relationship with male sex hormones, it is common for women to experience an increase in facial hair during treatment, and acne can be troublesome. Although these reactions subside after treatment is finished, other rarer reactions may not. Enlargement of the clitoris occurs in about 1 percent of women taking the drug; a noticeable change should mean stopping the danazol because an increase in size can be permanent.

Do not take danazol if you sing. Women who sing as a career or for their own pleasure should never take danazol because sensitive testing shows that *most* women who take danazol will have some measurable change in the voice. A semitone loss in vocal range would not be noticed by or be particularly important to many women, but the loss may be critical for a singer, who needs not just the best vocal range but also needs to have confidence in the full power of her voice over her range.

Because of its three-pronged action, danazol has been a little more effective at suppressing endometriosis than the progestogens, but the main advantage of danazol is its comparative lack of breakthrough bleeding. I often use a short course (two to three months) of danazol to stop the periods effectively before switching to a progestogen.

Danazol must not be taken during pregnancy, because it causes abnormalities of the genital organs in female fetuses (of a kind described in Chapter 18 as **intersex**). To prevent the possibility of such deformities, a course of danazol should start only at the time of a normal menstrual period, following a pregnancy test if there are doubtful circumstances. If there is the slightest doubt that ovulation is suppressed in a sexually active woman, for example, with low doses of danazol, a barrier method of contraception or an IUD should be used. Danazol's side effects are generally slight, especially with short courses of treatment, but they sometimes can be serious (see the box "Danazol Mischief").

# GnRH-Agonists

The **GnRH-analogs** are drugs that are similar to the body's natural **gonadotropin-releasing hormone** (GnRH; see Chapter 3), which the **hypothalamus** produces to stimulate the pituitary gland. **GnRH-agonists** mimic the action of GnRH and **GnRH-antagonists** block its action (see the box "The Long, Short and Ultrashort of GnRH-Agonists" in Chapter 20). GnRH-agonists first stimulate the pituitary but then soon exhaust the pituitary of its follicle stimulating hormone (FSH) and luteinizing hormone (LH). This means that the ovaries are also stimulated briefly, but as FSH and LH levels fall they shrink from lack of support, and withering with the ovaries are the tissues that depend on the ovaries' hormones, including those affected by endometriosis. This class of drugs, recently introduced to gynecology, has found an important place in reversibly removing the influence of the ovaries. In addition to being useful for endometriosis, we use GnRH-agonists for **fibroids** and **adenomyosis** (see Chapter 17) and for controlling the pituitary during ovarian stimulation with injected FSH for **assisted conception** (see Chapter 20).

GnRH-agonists can be administered in several very different ways, probably equally effectively: first, by daily injection under the skin using a very fine needle (such as **leuprolide**, trade name Lupron); second, by the several-times-a-day inhalation of a nasal spray (such as **nafarelin**, trade name Synarel), the drug being absorbed by the nasal mucosa to reach the pituitary gland through vascular channels in the intervening brain tissue; or third, by monthly depot injection (of, for example, **goserelin**, trade name Zoladex).

Removing estrogen, specifically **estradiol**, is our intention when we use GnRH-agonists, and a lack of estrogen is precisely the basis of their common side effects, just as if it were menopause. In the short term, within a month or two of starting, hot flashes are common, and there can be night sweats. Headaches and loss of libido are much more common with GnRH-agonists than with danazol, but weight gain and increased body hair are rare.

Over a six-month course, the estrogen deprivation produced by the GnRH-agonists causes calcium to be lost from the bones—similar to the situation after menopause. The bone loss is mostly temporary, recovering over six to twelve months after the treatment ends. The loss of bone can be prevented by giving a small dose of estrogen and progestogen at the same time—a maneuver called "add-back." Because ovulation and the levels of estradiol in the abdomen are still so dramatically lowered, the small amount of estrogen given with add-back does not stimulate the endometriosis. In addition, all the GnRH-agonists release a small amount of histamine, which can cause an annoying rash; an antihistamine can be tried to alleviate the rash.

Over a term longer than six months (the information comes mainly from men who have undergone years of treatment with GnRH-antagonists for cancer of the prostate gland), more bizarre side effects might come to light. The fact is that the natural hormone GnRH is found not just in the hypothalamus, from which it drives the pituitary gland, but all over the brain and the spinal cord, in places where we have no idea of its role and no idea of what the effects of GnRH-agonists might be (except, so far, that they are not obvious). Some men on very long-term treatment, however, have developed nervous-system side effects, including dementia and paralysis. Whether these developments are truly complications of treatment or whether, in these usually old people, they are a coincidence is not certain, but when things go wrong and a patient is on a drug, the drug is always the first suspect. No harmful effects have been obvious in several newborn babies delivered after GnRH-agonists were inadvertently used during early pregnancy, but it is the agonist's possible interference with the functioning of normal GnRH in the developing brain that means that GnRH-agonists should be avoided during pregnancy.

The effectiveness of the GnRH-agonists is such that the main side effect of treatment is from the inevitable lack of estrogen (see the box "GnRH-Agonist Mischief"). Like danazol, GnRH-agonists should only be started when we can be sure there is no pregnancy.

So far, the strategy of "quieting down the ovaries" for endometriosis has been what we call "medical," meaning that it uses drugs; this is in contrast to a "surgical" strategy, which implies an operation.

## Surgical Removal of the Ovaries

**Ovariectomy**, the surgical removal of the ovaries, has an important place in the overall scheme of endometriosis treatment, and for the same reason as drug treatments. The endometriosis that is left behind after the operation is deprived of its support. Both ovaries need to be removed to get the effect, and the operation is rare without an accompanying **hysterectomy** (see below). Removing both ovaries is important not just for treating left-behind endometriosis but also for removing the source of symptoms of premenstrual tension (PMT), when PMT is part of the problem and when surgery is being undertaken for endometriosis.

# Strategy #2: Removing Abnormal Tissue

The best time to destroy small areas of endometriosis is when it is diagnosed during laparoscopy. The effectiveness of treatment with **electrocautery**, or vaporization using a laser, is restricted by the closeness of other organs and the risk of damage to them, particularly the ureters, which carry urine from the kidneys down to the bladder, and the intestines. Special experience is needed in performing this treatment. At the least, the gynecologist diagnosing endometriosis during laparoscopy usually needs to remove the fluid normally present in the peritoneal cavity to be able to see all the candidate tissues deep in the pelvis, and a second or third instrument may be inserted to lift loops of bowel away from the affected peritoneum to allow safe destruction of endometriosis tissue. If the endometriosis is either widespread or deep, then laparoscopic treatment becomes a very specialized, time-consuming treatment, for which great experience is required.

Operations for endometriosis must enhance fertility if they are to serve their purpose. This seems an obvious statement, but remember that **adhesions** (see Chapter 13) are a considerable hazard after any operation in the pelvis. The last thing we want is for adhesions to replace the endometriosis as the cause of not getting pregnant.

Laparotomy for endometriosis, the formal opening of the abdomen, usually with a horizontal scar just above the pubic bone, is followed by cutting out the endometriosis lesions, and then closing with sutures the resulting gap in the peritoneal serosa. Because endometriosis often affects the ovaries or the peritoneal tissues close to the ovaries, adherence of the ovaries to underlying, operated-on peritoneum is almost inevitable, after even the most careful operations to excise the lesions. If adhesions can be avoided, especially by early postoperative laparoscopy to treat adherences as they form (see Chapter 13), pregnancy rates after surgery are generally better than after drug treatment. Furthermore there is, practically speaking, little delay before the effects of treatment are experienced. "Conservative surgery" (meaning not involving hysterectomy or ovariectomy), with excision of endometriosis tissue either during laparotomy or, depending on the gynecologist's experience, during laparoscopy, is therefore the ultimate option for women with symptoms in whom drug treatment has not worked, and it is often the main option for older women.

A short, preliminary course of danazol or progestogen for two or three months before the operation is regarded by many endometriosis surgeons to be useful for consolidating endometriosis lesions and improving the chance of removing *all* the abnormal tissue successfully. In general, the use of ovary-suppressing drugs is avoided just after the operation, because they will give a contraceptive effect just when everyone's feeling most optimistic about achieving pregnancy. But if aggressive-looking endometriosis has not been completely removed, there may be no alternative to using danazol, a GnRH-agonist or a progestogen for several months after the operation.

The more substantial the endometriosis, the more successful an operation will be in improving fertility, provided all the endometriosis can be excised and an adhesion-free result is gained. The nature of each operation is as varied as the distribution of the endometriosis, and more than the usual amount of surgical and gynecological experience is needed to obtain good results consistently. The expectation of pregnancy after technically successful treatment varies according to age and according to the couple's length of prior infertility. As a rough approximation, about 40 to 60 percent of couples conceive within 18 months after the operation and about 30 to 50 percent do so within 18 months of finishing a course of danazol.

Gynecologists should be aware of the results of their own operations and not rely on the published results of others in advising operation for treatment. Insist on finding out what these results are for your gynecologist before you choose an operation over medical treatment.

# Strategy #3: Suppressing Symptoms

Endometriosis is not ordinarily a dangerous condition in the sense that it might lead to cancer. It usually leaves its mark through one or several symptoms, such as pain, abnormal bleeding or infertility. In young people it is important to bring endometriosis under control to stop it from causing more symptoms later. For older women, however, in whom the endometriosis has taken many years to develop, a treatment approach directed purely at the symptoms may be best. In this regard, the oral contraceptive pill is safe and diminishes both bleeding and period pain (dysmenorrhea); it may also control painful intercourse (dyspareunia). **Nonsteroidal antiinflammatory drugs** (NSAIDs) may be all that is needed to control dysmenorrhea (see Table 16.1). When there is severe and intractable pelvic pain, some gynecologists favor the operation called presacral neurectomy, a dissection and division of the nerves coming from the pelvis where they join together, just in front of the sacrum.

**Gamete intrafallopian transfer** (GIFT) and **in vitro fertilization** (IVF) (see Chapter 20 on assisted conception) work at least as well with endometriosis as they do with any other cause of infertility, provided endometriosis is not causing cysts of the ovaries. Going straight to this approach is popular among women in their thirties and forties. Remember, however, that the ovarian stimulation that is usually part of assisted conception will stimulate the endometriosis more than natural ovulations, even though it would be suppressed by a successful pregnancy.

Hysterectomy, without removal of the ovaries, is no more likely to diminish endometriosis than tying off the fallopian tubes (which, as it turns out, is of no help at all), but hysterectomy reliably stops abnormal bleeding and dysmenorrhea. If a woman is past wanting to have children and has endometriosis or premenstrual tension that is driving her to distraction, hysterectomy and ovariectomies, followed by **estrogen replacement therapy** (ERT), can be a good strategy. Special information and precautions are needed before choosing a hysterectomy for relief of symptoms (see the box "Hysterectomy: Between a Rock and a Hard Place"), but I hope that by my providing the medical facts you can understand the ambiguous experience of others and can make a decision on a firm medical basis.

## Hysterectomy: Between a Rock and a Hard Place

Entire books for laypersons have recently been written about hysterectomies—especially how to avoid them. Why do some women intensely regret having an operation that to other women has meant peace and relief from symptoms? Obviously, a hysterectomy is not an option for someone intent on retaining the potential for having children. Equally obvious is that there is no question about the place of hysterectomy for serious disease of the uterus when there is no alternative satisfactory treatment available. Where is the balance?

There are two reasons why removing the uterus has a place in the treatment of endometriosis. First, the uterus is the source of bleeding and period pain, both of which are symptoms that inevitably respond to hysterectomy. Second, the presence of the uterus complicates estrogen replacement therapy (ERT) after the ovaries have been removed, because a progestogen must be taken in addition to the estrogen to prevent **endometrial hyperplasia**. And progestogens, in turn, have uncomfortable side effects that can mimic the very symptoms that led to the hysterectomy. Thus, when a radical operation is planned for either endometriosis or premenstrual tension (or both), it is the removal of the ovaries that is actually therapeutic; the uterus is removed so that ERT can be used without needing progestogens.

Still, you might ask, won't ERT cause the endometriosis to flare up, especially in the absence of progestogens? The reason why 95 percent or more of the time it does not is that endometriosis depends so much on especially high levels of estrogen that come directly from the ovary during ovulation. Take the ovaries out and this cannot happen. The amount of estrogen that gets to any remaining endometriosis through the bloodstream during ERT is very, very small in comparison.

# Fibroids and Other Uterine Problems

For all its central importance for pregnancy, the **uterus**, or womb, is the least likely place to cause trouble with getting pregnant. The uterus ordinarily ages well. Experience with the donation of embryos from younger to older women has shown that the decline of fertility that takes place as a woman gets older owes much more to what happens in the ovaries than to what happens in the uterus. The uterus can keep responding to **estrogen** and **progesterone** long after these hormones have stopped coming from the ovaries.

When things go wrong in the uterus, however, they are often serious for fertility. Overcoming pathology here can be a special challenge, and the possible problems are quite a few. The glandular lining of the uterus, the **endometrium**, can be disturbed by inflammation (**endometritis**), distorted by scar tissue (**intrauterine adhesions**), displaced by small tumors (such as **endometrial polyps**) or depreciated by losing its function (**endometrial atrophy**). Disarray of the muscular wall of the uterus, the **myometrium**, can come from benign tumors (**myomas**, or **fibroids**) and from disruptions in which the glands of the endometrium grow in among the muscle fibers (**adenomyosis**).

Abnormalities of the uterus that are present at birth are discussed in Chapter 18. For the information contained in this chapter, remember that **acute** means short-term and **chronic** means long-term.

# Disruption of the Endometrium

In terms of regenerative powers and acceptance of implanting embryos, the endometrium is rather forgiving. Nonetheless, infertility can result: if there is a general disturbance that seriously inhibits its response to normal circulating levels of estrogen and progesterone; if there is a space-occupying lump that stops the front and the back of the endometrium from effectively trapping the implanting embryo; or if there is a substantial constraint on an implanted embryo and its placenta from expanding its contact with the mother's blood stream.

## Endometritis

Not to be confused with **endometriosis** (see Chapters 15 and 16), endometritis means inflammation of the endometrium, usually from an infection. To a pathologist, acute endometritis means a rapidly developing, usually short-term inflammation and is generally part of an overwhelming infection caused by

In parts of the world where tuberculosis is still common, tuberculous endometritis is one of the most frequent causes of absent periods, or **amenorrhea**. Western special- ists, however, come across it rarely. The infertility tuberculosis causes also comes from damage to and blockages of the fallopian tubes—tuberculous salpingitis.

**chlamydia**, gonorrhea or a pus-forming organism such as Streptococcus. The fallopian tubes commonly carry the brunt of the sepsis, as **acute salpingitis**. There is pain, fever and a purulent discharge through the cervix. The treatment of such an acute infection is usually given in a hospital, with antibiotics administered intravenously.

Chronic endometritis, on the other hand, is long term and more insidious. There are often no symptoms. So little is known about it and its persistence from one cycle to the next that medical opinion is not unanimous on when or how it should be treated. The diagnosis is usually an incidental one, made during a **hysteroscopy** or a **biopsy** of the endometrium, such as during **curettage**. Some cases, at least, are due to Mycoplasma, an organism common in the vagina, which gains access to the uterus through the cervix; it is sensitive to the antibiotics tetracycline and erythromycin, both of which are used to treat it, with a course of treatment for both male and female partners in order to stop reinfection.

## Intrauterine Adhesions

Partial or complete obliteration of the cavity of the uterus with scar tissue is a serious consequence of carrying out a curettage in circumstances in which it is difficult for the endometrium to regrow. In most clinical conditions that require curettage (a "curette"), the endometrium is in no danger. Only the surface layers are removed and normal endometrium grows back in one cycle. It might even be beneficial for fertility. The two situations when it is dangerous to curette the uterus are also, unfortunately, the times when there is little other option, usually after a recent pregnancy: when retained bits of placenta cause bleeding a few weeks after the birth of a baby (called a "secondary postpartum hemorrhage"); and when a **missed abortion** occurs and an unexpelled fetus and trophoblast lie fixed in the uterus, more and more compact and harder and harder to budge. In these two circumstances there is both a shortage of estrogen (the production of it by the ovaries still being suppressed by the recent pregnancy) and a likelihood of infection by bacteria, conditions that jeopardize the endometrium's ability to regrow after the curettage. In some instances, the raw and damaged endometrium does what two opposite and damaged surfaces anywhere else in the body would do—they grow into each other with scar tissue.

If the periods do not return (amenorrhea) after the pregnancy tissue has been removed but the woman is ovulating, the condition is known as **Asherman's syndrome**. The syndrome is caused by blockages in the cavity of the uterus by scar tissue or adhesions, leading to destruction of the endometrium. Treatment for this consists of painstaking separation of the adhesions and often needs to be repeated several times. For the treatment to work, the adhesions need to be separated while the endometrium (or what is left of it) is under the influence of estrogen; an **intrauterine device** (IUD) or something similar, such as a small balloon catheter, can be left in the uterus to keep surfaces apart, and probably separate new adhesions when it is pulled out.

The outcome of treating intrauterine adhesions depends on how badly the endometrium has been damaged and on how well it recovers. Endometrium that has been badly damaged can be beyond recovery and result in permanent endometrial atrophy. If treatment is successful to the point of a return of menstruation (especially if periods are as heavy as before) and if the fallopian tubes are open, another pregnancy is usually possible. Such a pregnancy, however, has a greater chance of ending early as a **miscarriage** or as **premature labor**. More seriously, the placenta of the new pregnancy can grow deeply into the wall of the uterus (called "placenta accreta"), and might not come loose after the fetus or baby has been delivered. The result can be bleeding that is sometimes unstoppable short of an urgent hysterectomy.

# Endometrial Polyps

Polyps, as the name suggests, are benign tongues of tissue that seem to grow in the endometrium (as in other parts of the body) for no good reason. Symptoms include heavy periods and bleeding between periods (including **premenstrual spotting**) as well as infertility. The infertility probably comes about because fluid in the endometrial cavity pools around it or to one side as the front and back surface of the endometrium press together (see the box "Thirst for the Embryo" in Chapter 4). The still free-floating embryo, ready to implant, can find itself in this pool of fluid, with none of the intimate contact with the endo-metrium that is the first step in its implantation.

The diagnosis is suspected at **transvaginal ultrasound** (polyps cause irreg-ular thickening and heightened echoes in the endometrium) and is confirmed during hysteroscopy. Thorough curettage has been used for treatment in the past, but it often misses the polyp; resection of it through the hysteroscope is re-liable. After treatment, polyps quite often grow back within a year or so.

# Disruption of the Myometrium

The muscular wall of the uterus, or myometrium, plays its greatest role at the end of pregnancy, when it is time for its coordinated contractions to expel the baby. It is usually quiet when it is under the influence of progesterone, which it should be soon after ovulation, during implantation and during pregnancy. The two main abnormal conditions we encounter in the myometrium, fibroids and adenomyosis, often have little or no effect on fertility, but they can lead to dis-turbance of an embryo or fetus once pregnancy is under way.

## Fibroids

Fibroids, known technically as "myomas," are benign lumps of muscle tissue growing in or from the myometrium. The closer they are to the endometrium, the more likely they are to cause symptoms, such as heavy bleeding, dysmenor-rhea and infertility (see the box "Mapping Myomas" and Figure 17.1). Fibroids are best diagnosed before operation with transvaginal ultrasound.

The surgical operation for a fibroid that leaves the surrounding uterus in-tact is called a **myomectomy** and conserves fertility. For submucous fibroids, protruding into or lying in the endometrial cavity, the operation can often be done during hysteroscopy, using a special instrument that shaves the fibroid away, strip by strip; this operation is a day-stay hospital procedure, and there are no stitches. For intramural fibroids, lying within the wall of the uterus, an open operation, or **laparotomy**, is usually necessary; the uterus is incised, the fibroid or fibroids are shelled out (they usually grow with a compressed capsule around them and come out like peas from a pod), and the uterus is repaired in layers. If a myomectomy involves dissection of the wall of the uterus, perhaps weakening

Fibroids on the outside of the uterus are called **subserous fibroids**. They can be "pedunculated," on a long pedicle that occasionally can undergo torsion, causing pain and eventual degeneration of the fibroid, or they can be broad-based, a situation that is usually trouble-free unless the fibroid grows to a large size, when it can cause symptoms from pressure.

Fibroids within the wall of the uterus are called **intramural fibroids**. They need to be bigger than a few centimeters or be multiple before they cause symptoms, such as dysmenorrhea and heavy periods and possibly an increased chance of a pregnancy miscarrying and even the prevention of successful implantation of the embryo (infertility).

The fibroid most likely to cause symptoms is one that projects from the myometrium into the endometrial cavity, a **submucous fibroid**. Even a small submucous fibroid can project into the endometrial cavity enough to stop the endometrial surfaces from coming together over the implanting embryo (see the section on endometrial polyps earlier in this chapter), causing infertility, as well as often resulting in pronounced bleeding and cramping pain.

The presence of fibroids and their location is best determined, before operation, with transvaginal ultrasound.

### Malignant Myomas, or Myosarcomas

Cancer is rare in a fibroid. Textbooks say that one in 200 of removed fibroids are malignant, but, with more and more fibroids being diagnosed by transvaginal ultrasound, it is more likely to be about one in 200 *women* who turn out to have a malignant fibroid. The main sign of malignancy before operation, although it cannot be completely counted on, is a fibroid's particularly rapid growth.

it, most obstetricians will recommend that a later pregnancy be delivered by cesarean section. Subserous fibroids, lying outside the uterus, may need no treatment; small ones can sometimes be removed during **laparoscopy**, but large ones require laparotomy.

Sometimes a course of **GnRH-agonists** (see Chapter 16) is used to shrink fibroids, especially large submucous ones, so that they can be more easily treated surgically. Occasionally, instigating GnRH-agonist treatment actually

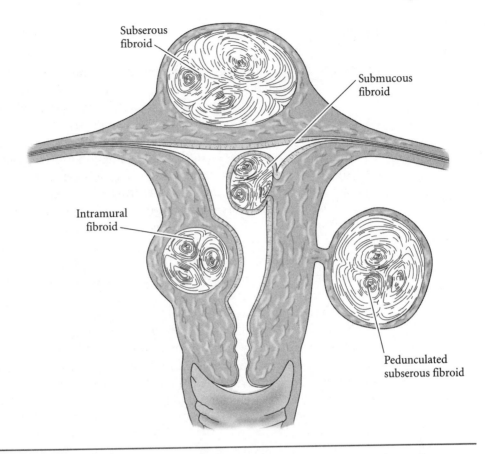

**Figure 17.1**   Fibroids in the uterus. A subserous fibroid can twist and cause pain if it is pedunculated but it does not interfere with fertility. An intramural fibroid can disturb the supply of blood to a developing pregnancy and thus may cause miscarriage. A submucous fibroid affects the lining of the uterus directly and can cause infertility.

precipitates severe uterine bleeding from the fibroid. There is no lasting beneficial effect from these drugs, and the fibroid, after treatment is stopped, quickly grows back to its previous size. GnRH-agonists are not suitable for long-term use, partly because of cost but mostly because of side effects. Although many of the side effects are preventable by "adding back" some estrogen replacement therapy, in the case of fibroids (and unlike when it is used for endometriosis) such an add-back stops the treatment from working.

# Adenomyosis

As the translation from Latin might suggest, adenomyosis is the growth of glands from the endometrium growing in among the muscle of the myometrium. It can be diffuse, generalized or focal, in the form of one or more "adenomyomas." On transvaginal ultrasound, adenomyosis is not always seen; it can cause a generally uneven ultrasound echo from the myometrium. If it is visible discretely, it can sometimes be difficult to distinguish it from a fibroid. Support for a diagnosis of adenomyosis can come from finding an elevation of **serum CA125 antigen** levels (although endometriosis, not uncommonly found in association with adenomyosis, can also cause this test to be abnormal). There are some reports of adenomyosis benefiting from treatment with GnRH-agonist, at least in the short term.

The distinction between a myoma and an adenomyoma is important, because conservative surgery is much trickier for adenomyomas than for myomas. There is no clear separation between the area of muscle containing the endometrial glands—the adenomyoma—and the surrounding normal muscle. Such surgery is usually unrewarding in all but the most limited and focal adenomyomas.

Adenomyosis usually causes pain with periods (**dysmenorrhea**) and heavy periods (**ovulatory dysfunctional uterine bleeding**), as can fibroids. Its contribution to infertility is uncertain. Often the diagnosis is not made until recalcitrant symptoms lead to a hysterectomy and the uterus is examined by a pathologist.

# Abnormalities Present from Birth

A woman can expect to have two **ovaries**, two **fallopian tubes**, one **uterus** (and therefore one **cervix**), and one vagina. The reality, however, can be more complex. To understand what can go wrong—or at least differently—we need to explore how these structures are formed in the female embryo.

# The Müllerian Inheritance

At about eight weeks of pregnancy (eight weeks from the **last menstrual period**, or LMP) the kidneys begin to develop in the fetus. For females, the ovaries then take shape just below them; for males, the testes form there. At this early time the embryo's head has taken shape, and the heart is prominently responsible for the growing circulation. The tail end of the embryo, however, is still rudimentary and rather plastic—able to end up in all sorts of directions.

In females, an open duct—the **Müllerian duct**—begins to form near each ovary, as the tail end of the embryo takes more shape passing over toward the middle (see Figure 18.1). Here it will meet its companion duct from the other side, join, and then grow farther downward, opening into a space formed as a pocket from the skin between the embryo's leg buds; this will later be distinguishable, from front to back, as the urethra, vagina and anus. Where these two Müllerian ducts join, they thicken considerably to form the uterus; the parts of

**Figure 18.1** (right) Development of the Müllerian ducts. These ducts develop in the fetus during the ninth and tenth weeks of pregnancy and form the fallopian tubes, the uterus and the upper two-thirds or so of the vagina. When the tail end of the embryo first forms (side view a), a "cloaca" receives (as it does, for example, in an adult frog) the urinary ducts, the bowel (or "hindgut") and the earliest sex ducts. The "mesonephros" is the embryo's temporary kidney, and its mesonephric duct on each side normally persists only in male fetuses, to form the male sex ducts. The "metanephros" is the permanent kidney. As the tail end of the fetus grows (side view b), the cloaca divides into the rectum in back and the "urogenital sinus" in front; the "metanephric duct" becomes the ureter, connecting the kidney to the bladder; and a new duct grows alongside the mesonephric duct on each side, the "paramesonephric" or Müllerian duct. With further development (front view c), the Müllerian ducts meet and join in the middle before growing down to meet the urogenital sinus, which will soon separate into the urethra in front and the lower part of the vagina behind. In this way the Müllerian ducts form the fallopian tubes, the uterus and the upper part of the vagina. The vulva and lowermost part of the vagina come from the urogenital sinus.

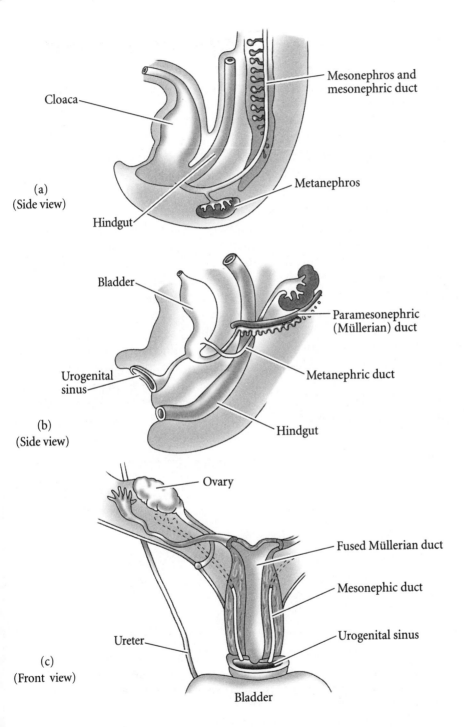

Cloaca

Mesonephros and
mesonephric duct

Metanephros

(a)
(Side view)

Hindgut

Bladder

Paramesonephric
(Müllerian) duct

Metanephric duct

Urogenital
sinus

(b)
(Side view)

Hindgut

Ovary

Fused Müllerian duct

Mesonephic duct

Urogenital sinus

Ureter

(c)
(Front view)

Bladder

Here is how the vagina meets the skin and why you need to have PAP smears to check for early cancer of the cervix. The tissue lining any surface or duct comes in sheets, called "epithelium." Inside the body, epithelium is usually just one-cell thick; on the outside, where there is more wear and tear, epithelium is many-cells thick and said to be "stratified" (the skin is a tough example; see Figure 18.2). The epithelium of the Müllerian ducts, according to this rule, is "simple," or one-celled; the cells are vertical in orientation, like columns, and so the epithelium is referred to as being "columnar." The urogenital sinus, the pouch of skin between the emerging leg buds (see Figure 18.1) and into which passes the bladder, the vagina and the intestine, has epithelium like that of skin elsewhere—stratified squamous epithelium.

Somewhere there must be a meeting of the two, the "squamo-columnar junction." To begin with, this is at the lower end of the vagina, near the vestibule of the vulva (see Figure 18.3a). A woman born with a hymen that has no opening in it (an "imperforate hymen") will have columnar epithelium above and squamous epithelium below the hymen (as shown in Figures 18.2 and 18.3a). Normally, however, the connection between vagina and vulva is complete. Further growth of this region of the fetus proceeds in a curious way—there is slippage of neighboring tissues. The result is that squamous epithelium, rather similar to (but more moist than) skin, slips up to line the whole of the vagina and a variable part of the vaginal side of the cervix (see Figure 18.3b); if it did not, sexual inter-

**Figure 18.2** (right) Collision! The Müllerian ducts are lined by a single layer of surface cells (epithelium), which are column-like or columnar in shape. The urogenital sinus, like the skin generally, is lined by epithelium that has many layers; it is stratified and flat in shape (or "squamous"). Between the two there is connective tissue, which gets thinner and thinner before it disappears, opening the vagina to the outside.

## PAP Smears: You Thought They Were Simple ? (concluded)

course would abrade the vaginal epithelium every time, causing bleeding and damage.

Ideally, the squamo-columnar junction comes to be situated precisely at the opening of the cervix, with the columnar (or glandular) epithelium above it responsible for secreting the mucus of the canal (see Figure 18.3b), but this is rarely the case. Usually it stops short, somewhere between the margin of the cervix and the opening of the canal (see Figure 18.3c). This friable rim of columnar tissue is called, disrespectfully, an "erosion"; it can bleed after intercourse, and as a teenager matures, mildly acid fluid in the vagina causes it to slowly transform into stratified squamous epithelium, like the rest of the vagina. This zone is thus called the "transformation zone," and the normal

metamorphosis of its epithelium from glandular to skin-like is called **metaplasia**. It provides an opportunity for things to go wrong—referred to as "dysplasia," or more modernly "cervical intraepithelial neoplasia" (CIN). Dysplasia (or CIN) can lead to overt "neoplasia," or cancer of the cervix, which almost always arises on the outer surface of the cervix.

The good news is that the transformation zone is easily observed. Wiping the cells off it for examination under the microscope is what a PAP (Papanicolaou) smear is. A positive smear means the presence of dysplastic or early cancerous cells (CIN). Looking at the transformation zone with a microscope is called "colposcopy," which is used to confirm abnormal PAP smears and to judge the effects of treatment of CIN.

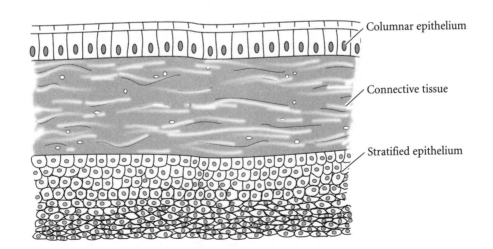

Columnar epithelium

Connective tissue

Stratified epithelium

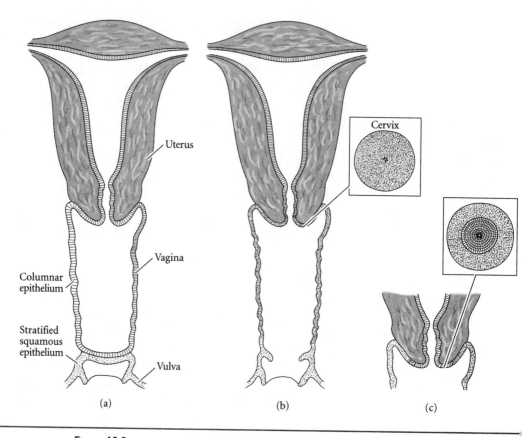

**Figure 18.3** How the Müllerian junction migrates. Before the membrane between the vagina and the outside disappears (a), the upper part of the vagina, like the rest of the Müllerian ducts, is lined by columnar epithelium (see also Figure 18.2). After the vagina has opened (b), the junction between the stratified squamous epithelium of the skin and the columnar epithelium of the Müllerian ducts migrates up the vagina—ideally to the point of opening of the cervix (the "external os"). When this happens, the cervix is completely smooth to look at, with a small opening, or canal, leading up to the uterus (inset). More often than not, the migration is not complete, and the "squamo-columnar junction" ends up on the cervix somewhere (c), leaving a rather fragile, red-colored area around the canal (inset). Because, with time, the exposed columnar epithelium transforms to squamous epithelium, this zone is called the "transformation zone"—the site of interest when a PAP smear is done.

the ducts on each side of the joining become the fallopian tubes. The joined part of the Müllerian duct forms, from top to bottom, the body of the uterus (the uterine fundus), the neck of the uterus (the cervix) and the upper two-thirds of the vagina (see Figure 18.1c, and Figure 3.5 in Chapter 3). The lowermost part of the vagina comes from the skin.

# Congenital Anomalies

Congenital means something you are born with. If something can go wrong in the way the body is put together, sooner or later it will, and a baby will be born with an **anomaly**, or a variation from what is normal. The kidney system is close enough to the developing genital system that anomalies of the two systems often go together. For the Müllerian ducts and the internal sex organs, things may go wrong symmetrically, in which case the kidneys are usually normal; or things may be lopsided, or asymmetrical, in which case commonly there will be a malformation of the kidney system on the abnormal side.

The following accounts are not complete—there is no end to the possibilities and the variations—but I will describe the more common and important conditions a family physician or a gynecologist is likely to come across.

# Symmetrical Malformations

In considering the congenital anomalies, let us start with the symmetrical ones and those that cause obstructions.

## Imperforate Hymen

A transverse barrier across the lower-most part of the vagina can come about as an abnormality at birth or, rarely, after an inflammation in early childhood, causing the bits of a normal hymen to get stuck together. Either way, no one usually knows about the problem until periods are due to start at puberty. As the uterus bleeds, blood accumulates above the blockage and the vagina distends (see Figure 18.4a), causing cyclical episodes of pain that typically get worse each month.

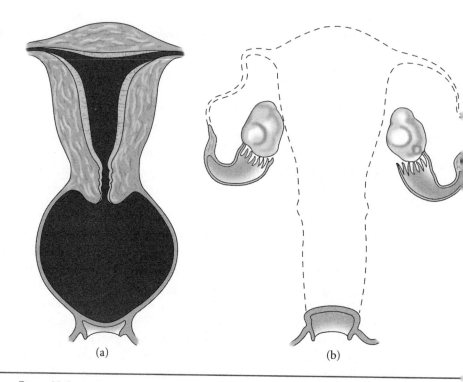

(a)          (b)

**Figure 18.4**  Müllerian atresia: failure of the Müllerian ducts to form properly. Blockage of the lower part of the vagina occurs (a), when the membrane between the Müllerian duct and the outside persists. At puberty, menstrual blood accumulates above the blockage, considerably distending the vagina. (The fallopian tubes and ovaries have not been drawn, but they are normal.) In virtually total failure of Müllerian duct development (b), there is congenital absence of the uterus and vagina. In this case, only the outermost part of the fallopian tubes has formed. Any degree of abnormality between these two extremes is possible.

The diagnosis can be made clinically by seeing a distended, dark membrane where the vagina should be. Carefully feeling the abdomen may reveal a tender lump coming up behind the pubic bone. If an **ultrasound** examination or pelvic **CAT scan** or **MRI scan** has been done, it will point to the distended vagina above the blockage, filled with blood and pushing the uterus upward. Treatment takes place in a hospital, under anesthesia. The offending tissue is cut and the thick, trapped, chocolate-like blood escapes. To stop the hymen from blocking up again, the surgeon makes a cross-shaped incision, cutting off four triangles of tissue between the arms of the cross. Recovery is usually immediate, complete and uneventful.

# Absent Uterus and Vagina

When the uterus and vagina are absent, two ovaries are present and are normal. They start producing hormones and ovulating eggs, and puberty takes place apparently normally. But the Müllerian ducts have failed to form, have failed to join or have failed to meet the lower vagina (see Figure 18.4b). There is no menstruation because there is no uterus to bleed. There may be other reasons, however, why puberty can be interrupted with an absence of menstruation—**primary amenorrhea**—despite apparently normal development of the breasts and pubic hair; these other conditions are associated with failure to ovulate and are described in Chapter 10.

The diagnosis of congenital absence of the uterus and vagina is made clinically by revealing just a dimple, or just firm tissue, where the opening of the vagina should be. An ultrasound or a CAT or MRI scan confirms that there is no uterus, but the ovaries are usually visible, located at the brim of the pelvis. If a **laparoscopy** were to be done (it is not really necessary), the ovaries would be seen to be making **follicles** and ovulating normally, but next to them would be just the beginnings of the fallopian tubes—they peter out toward the middle and there is no swelling where the uterus should be.

A girl with congenital absence of the uterus and vagina will need a lot of understanding and help. She cannot, of course, receive a new uterus, and a vagina will need to be fashioned from the soft and accommodating tissue that is there in its place. She will not be able to have a baby. On the positive side, she has normal ovaries and normal hormones, and there is no physical reason she should not feel every bit a healthy woman. The first priority is to enable sexual intercourse to take place.

There are three ways in which a vagina can be made. The simplest is usually the best. It helps if there is already a dimple in the vulva, but it is not essential. A set of strong, glass dilators is used progressively to push and stretch the skin into the soft space between where the bladder is in front and where the rectum is behind. It is perfectly safe, no damage can be done and no detailed knowledge of anatomy is needed. The dilators will follow the path of least resistance, the right path. Over weeks to months, every time she showers, the woman pushes the dilator upward for a few minutes, gradually stretching the skin to form a vagina.

## An Expensive IVF Baby

I first got to know a particular patient in her teen years, when she had been referred with primary amenorrhea—absent periods despite normal puberty. I confirmed the diagnosis of congenital absence of the uterus and vagina. Satisfactory sexual function followed treatment with dilators. It was after her marriage that I met her again as a patient. She and her husband now wanted their own child.

The surrogacy arrangement (see Chapter 21) she chose was both international and commercial; she rented someone who had a uterus, and she ended up with a baby that was genetically hers and her husband's. Once she had made the decision to go ahead, Sydney IVF and I helped. We stimulated the ovaries (see Chapter 20), the fluid and egg in the follicle were removed by aspiration during a laparoscopy ("egg pickup") and her husband's sperm was used to fertilize her eggs, which were then frozen. She took the fertilized eggs to the United States, where a commercial surrogacy agency had previously introduced the couple to a host mother. After several embryo transfers the host conceived, the baby was born with everyone present and the family of three returned to Australia. With the IVF procedures, the travel and compensation of the surrogate, the bill in 1990 came to about $80,000. The surrogate mother stays in touch. For their second baby, the couple chose to adopt.

Eventually the process will be completed by having sex regularly. For a woman confidence, however, it is best to start treatment well before sex is expected.

The second method is a simple surgical operation called "Williams's operation," after the British gynecologist Arthur Williams who devised it. A short pouch of skin is created surgically in the vulva, pointing backward and open forward. As soon as surgical healing occurs, in about three or four weeks, sex can start. With repeated sexual intercourse, the pouch steadily gets bigger; instead of pointing backward it becomes directed upward—the path of least resistance again—the skin stretching into the proper place for the new vagina. What was ordinary, dry skin becomes moist and very like the normal lining of the vagina.

The third way of producing a vagina is to purposefully dissect the tissue where the vagina should be and then create one artificially, with a skin graft placed over a mold, a procedure called the "McIndoe operation." The effect is immediate, but of all the methods this is the most hazardous. The danger comes from scar tissue forming in what should remain a soft and compliant part of the body. There also is a way of performing this operation with laparoscopy.

## From a Bicornuate Uterus to a Double Vagina

Imperfect joining between the Müllerian ducts from the two sides can produce any degree of doubling. The possibilities range from a short wall dividing the body of the uterus into right and left to complete duplication of the uterus, cervix and vagina all the way down to the vulva, which is always single (see Figure 18.5).

A wall between the right and left sides of the cavity of the uterus is called a **uterine septum**, and such a uterus is a "septate" uterus (see Figure 18.5a). If the septum does not go all the way down to the cervix, it is a "subseptate" uterus (see Figure 18.5b). In either case, there may be no symptoms at all, except for a strong tendency for pregnancies to miscarry, usually in the first three months (see Chapter 8). The most minimal anomaly, really a variation of normal, consists just of a slight downward indentation from the top, or fundus, of the uterus, called an "arcuate" uterus. In each case, the outer surface of the uterus shows little sign of the doubling. The diagnosis is made with an X-ray (a **hysterosalpingogram**) or **hysteroscopy** (see Chapter 4), but needs a laparoscopy to confirm that the outside of the uterus looks single, not double. A septum or subseptum is treated during hysteroscopy by cutting its muscle in the same (flat) plane as the cavity of the uterus (see Figure 18.6); the cut muscle fibers fall away, front and back, and the septum is gone with no scar in the uterus and no deficit of muscle tissue.

A **bicornuate uterus** has the same division of the uterine cavity into right and left, but the outside of the uterus, the fundus itself, is divided into two (see Figure 18.5c). Again there may be no symptoms—until pregnancy. Even then, pregnancies can grow normally, but the abnormal shape inside the uterus means that a breech birth is more common. Pregnancies are less likely to miscarry early than they are with a septate uterus, but miscarriages in the second three months can be common; typically, successive pregnancies reach a more and more mature stage. Because there is no simple operation to correct a bicornuate uterus, one approach, depending on the circumstances, is to anticipate an immature but viable pregnancy with no special intervention. The operation to correct the abnormality—a **metroplasty**—is an open operation done during **laparotomy**, after which it takes a few months for the uterus to heal and before pregnancy should be attempted again.

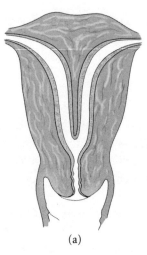

(a)

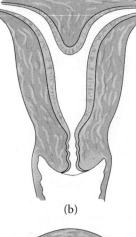

(b)

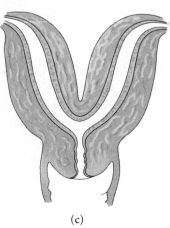

(c)

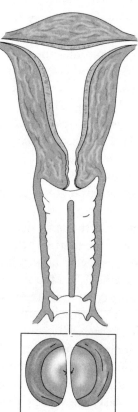

(d)

(e)

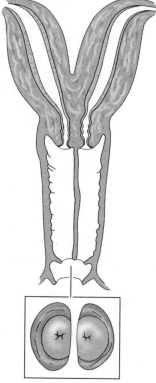

(f)

English gives way to Latin as the more profound duplications of the Müllerian system are described in gynecological textbooks. A "double uterus and cervix," each served by its own normal fallopian tube and ovary, is called a "uterus bicornis bicollis" (see Figure 18.5d). Many women with such a uterus—or with two such uteruses—go through life unaware of a problem. There is a greater chance of prematurity among pregnancies. Occasionally the nonpregnant uterus gets in the way of the pregnant uterus during childbirth. Breech births are more common, again because the effective space available for the baby to move about in has an odd shape. The division of the two uteruses is too great for repair to be feasible, but there is usually no need for it anyhow.

A "double vagina" is not particularly rare (see Figure 18.5e). Sometimes it goes with a double uterus and cervix. The way it declares itself can be startling, though characteristic. Often this is during the teenage years, when a girl begins to use a tampon for menstruation; instead of stopping it, the tampon lets menstrual blood go straight past, down the other vagina. Two tampons fix the problem, but not before some puzzling experiences. Commonly one vagina comes to be preferred over the other, especially with sex. Sex is then sometimes comfortable; sometimes inexplicably it is not. With knowledge, this symptom is straightforward to overcome.

If there is a single cervix and uterus, the septum dividing the vagina into two will stop short of the top of the vagina (see Figure 18.5e). During intercourse sperm will get to the cervix no matter which side of the septum is used for sex. If the preferred side does not communicate with the only functioning cervix, there will be infertility. More complicated is the double vagina that accompanies a double cervix and double uterus (see Figure 18.5f). Conception will only be possible when ovulation takes place on the same side that sex does; most women will not be aware that this will take them twice as long, on average, to get pregnant. If it is troublesome, the wall between such right and left vaginas can be removed by a straightforward operation.

**Figure 18.5**  (left) Müllerian duplications. The Müllerian ducts in these cases have reached the outside, but they have not joined properly (tubes and ovaries are normal and have not been drawn): (a) septate uterus; (b) subseptate uterus; (c) bicornuate uterus; (d) double uterus, single vagina; (e) single uterus, double vagina, also called a "longitudinal" vaginal septum; (f) double uterus, double vagina. In a, b and c the cervix looks normal at vaginal examination and is not shown. In d, e and f the cervix has the appearances shown (insets); note that the cervix is double when the uterus is double.

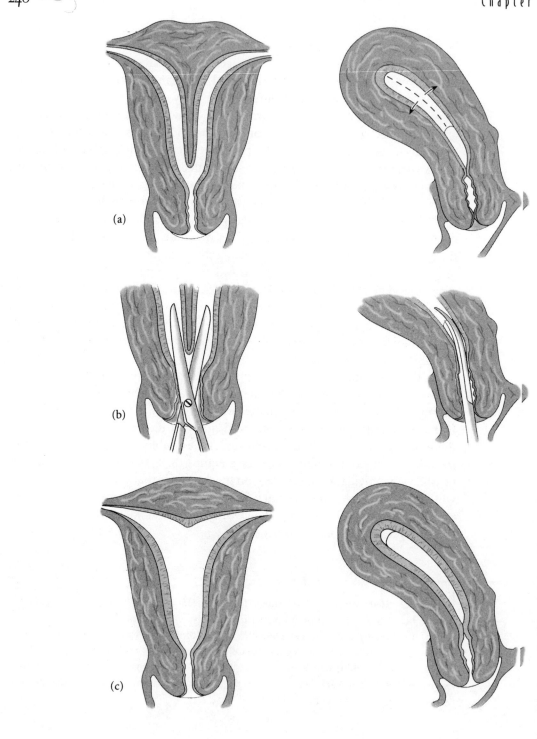

(a)

(b)

(c)

# Nonsymmetrical Abnormalities

With nonsymmetrical anomalies, the two Müllerian ducts not only do not join properly, but one or other side fails to develop as well as the other side. Coexisting abnormalities of the kidney system are common, such as a congenital blockage from kidney to bladder, doubling of the urine collecting system or perhaps a single or a horseshoe-shaped kidney, located lower in the abdomen than usual, perhaps within the pelvis.

## Unicornuate Uterus

With a **unicornuate uterus** there is one uterus and cervix and usually one vagina (all normal-looking so far). On investigation, however, with a hysterosalpingogram or laparoscopy (usually done for other reasons), only one fallopian tube is found to be open (see Figure 18.7a). Development of the fallopian tube on the other side can be variable; the outer, open part is usually there, lying next to the ovary, but toward the middle it either dwindles into nothing (Figure 18.7a), or it expands to a more or less distinct uterus, partly joined onto the main uterus (Figure 18.7b).

Usually there are no symptoms, but, if the rudimentary uterus (or "horn") is unrudimentary enough to have a cavity, pain can be felt on that side during periods; sometimes this is bad enough to warrant an operation for its removal. On average, a woman will take twice as long as otherwise to get pregnant, because conception is very unlikely when ovulation takes place on the closed side. Premature births and breech births are more common, as they are with the bicornuate uterus discussed earlier.

Occasionally a pregnancy will start in the closed side. When this happens it will be because sperm have passed up the open uterus, out along its tube and across the abdomen to the opposite, ovulating ovary, fertilizing an egg just as it

**Figure 18.6**   (left) Treatment for a uterine septum: transvaginal metroplasty: (a) front and side views of a uterus with a septum. The septum is wide-based in the front view, but thin in the side view; (b) special scissors are passed through the canal of the cervix to cut the septum in the plane shown. The same can be achieved with very small scissors at hysteroscopy; (c) the cut muscle fibers pull back into the body of the uterus and the septum disappears.

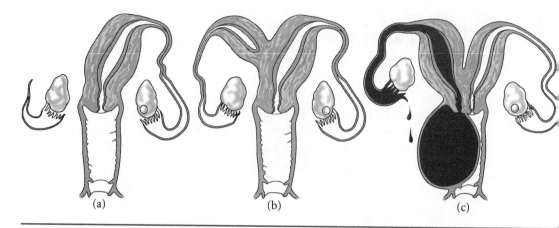

(a)                                              (b)                                              (c)

**Figure 18.7** Asymmetrical Müllerian abnormalities. The Müllerian ducts have not joined properly, and, moreover, the duct on one side has not formed or properly opened to the outside. In a unicornuate uterus (a) the uterus is "one-horned," the Müllerian duct on the opposite side has formed only the very first part of the fallopian tube; in a unicornuate uterus with a rudimentary horn on the opposite side (b), there may or may not be bleeding each month in the rudimentary uterus; in a double uterus and vagina, with one vagina not in communication with the outside (c), blood accumulates in the closed vagina, distending it greatly (unlike the situation in Figure 18.4a, periods occur, so the diagnosis can be missed for some time).

is being picked up by a fallopian tube that leads nowhere. The result is a pregnancy in the tube or in the rudimentary uterus, in effect an **ectopic pregnanc** (see Chapter 14), and sooner or later a surgical emergency.

## Double Uterus and Vagina with One Vagina Blocked

I have seen four teenagers with this distressing abnormality (see Figure 18.7c) There are two tubes and ovaries (as is normally the case), and two uteruses and cervixes (as with a double uterus and cervix). There are two vaginas as well, but not only do they not join, one or the other vagina does not open to the vulva In each case the diagnosis had been missed before the girl had already been op erated on by an uncritical general surgeon and before she had been referred to a gynecologist. But the clinical symptoms and signs were the same with each o the girls and were unmistakable.

At puberty, both uteruses begin to menstruate. As with an imperforate hymen, menstrual blood accumulates in the blocked but distensible vagina, causing increasing pain with each period. As the vagina fills and swells, it pushes the uterus up into the abdomen, producing a bigger and bigger lump, which is eventually noticed clinically, on ultrasound or with a CAT or MRI scan. These features are the same as for an imperforate hymen, except that menstrual periods are taking place, apparently normally and on time; this is the puzzle and a source of confusion. The girls and their parents regard it as a case of bad period pain, **dysmenorrhea**; the examining doctor suspects a tumor in the pelvis, and, all too typically, the general surgeon called in has not seen the condition before, operates, spots a mess and takes something out that would have been best left alone. The correct treatment, under anesthesia, is to make a large opening between the two vaginas for the accumulated blood to discharge. Later, the wall between the two vaginas can be removed completely.

# The DES Anomalies

In the 1950s many pregnant women were given a new synthetic estrogen to try to lessen the chance of miscarriages. This estrogen, diethylstilbestrol, or DES, has left a legacy of uterine and vaginal anomalies that a generation of women now in their forties have had to cope with. These legacies include cancer of the cervix and, ironically, miscarriages. (Read the box "PAP Smears: You Thought They Were Simple?" at the beginning of this chapter, on why PAP smears are necessary, before reading the following box, "DES Disruption.")

Although most women with DES abnormalities are now passing the age of childbearing, the story of DES is notorious; it should not be forgotten by anyone who uses unproven drugs for unproven reasons.

# Girl or Boy ?

There is almost no end to what can go wrong, twixt chromosomes and puberty. This takes us into the highly specialized field of **intersex**, or, as it is known in the United States, **pseudohermaphrodism**.

Diethylstilbestrol binds to estrogen-sensitive tissues for an abnormally long time. It does this in the embryo or fetus after the drug has been swallowed by the mother. This means it disrupts the relationship of ordered growth among the estrogen-sensitive Müllerian ducts. These growth relationships become permanently distorted, showing up years later. In mild cases all that may be anomalous is an unusually large transformation zone on the cervix, from disruption of migration of the squamo-columnar junction. Often, however, this junction between glandular tissue and skin-like tissue will be out on the vagina itself, which is called "vaginal adenosis." Transformation zones (cervical erosions) are much bigger than they otherwise would be, occupying the whole cervix and more. Such out-of-place glandular tissue is more susceptible to cancerous change. The most typical cancer, "clear-cell carcinoma," is not the most common, but it was particularly rare before DES. Numerically, the lead is held by the same cancer of the cervix other people get ("squamous cell carcinoma") and which is screened for with PAP smears and colposcopy (direct microscopic examination of the cervix).

DES anomalies of the uterus and tubes can be subtle. Typically, the cavity of the uterus on a hysterosalpingogram shows a T-shape; the normally seen triangle is pinched in at the sides, and the outer arms of the uterus can also be pinched, making it hard to see where the tube stops and the uterus starts. The outcome of a pregnancy will depend on where in the uterus, or sometimes the tube, the embryo implants. The chance of **miscarriage** (see Chapter 7) and ectopic pregnancy (see Chapter 14) is therefore greater than with a normal uterus, but most affected women sooner or later have a baby. The abnormally shaped uterus does not lend itself to surgical reconstruction.

A hermaphrodite, like Hermaphroditus after his fusion with the nymph Salmacis, has attributes that are both female and male. We speak of a **true hermaphrodite** as one with both ovary and testis—sometimes on opposite sides, sometimes included in the one gland. The end result lies between almost normal male development (perhaps an abnormal testis in a hernia) and almost normal female development (with testicular tissue seen in part of a removed ovary after an otherwise uneventful social history of sex, marriage and children). Anything is possible in between, usually showing up at birth with genitals that are a puzzle.

## Chromosomal Intersex

The chromosome pattern, or **karyotype,** of females is 46,XX and those of males is 46,XY (see Chapter 3). An extra chromosome disturbs the relationship. Nonetheless, the rule is that one or more Y chromosomes determines maleness. The karyotype 47,XYY (a gratuitous Y chromosome) may do little or no harm, but the jury is still out; some say there is a higher chance of antisocial, criminal behavior. The karyotype 47,XXY results in an infertile male with **Klinefelter's syndrome;** tallness is usual, and since no sperm cells are formed, there is infertility.

Karyotypes 47,XXX and 48,XXXX are women who may be normal but might have fewer oocytes and hence may undergo menopause prematurely. The pattern 45,X (a missing sex chromosome) gives a female, but she will be both infertile, from a lack of oocytes and hence **primary ovarian failure** (see Chapter 10), and short (that is, **Turner's syndrome**).

So far, perhaps, this is simple, but it is only a small bit of the Y chromosome that causes the maleness. Suppose just a tiny bit of the Y chromosome gets mislaid? The possibility is that despite a 46,XY karyotype we can have a normal-looking girl and despite a 46,XX karyotype we can have a normal-looking boy. In both these cases the ovaries and testes—the **gonads**—do not form properly and puberty fails, and as adolescents and adults they will be infertile.

## Male Intersex

Suppose now that the testis in an embryo is correctly determined, as planned, by a 46,XY chromosome count. For things to go right, the internal ducts must be sensitive to the male hormone **testosterone;** sometimes they are not, so they disappear. Add to this the fact that the external genitalia—the scrotum and penis—must be sensitive to testosterone's metabolic derivative, **dihydrotestosterone;** if there is complete insensitivity to it, a vagina and vulva form instead, with testes left high in the abdomen. Because the breasts are not sensitive to testosterone, they flourish on the smallish amount of estrogen made by the testes. At birth the girl looks normal. At puberty the breasts develop well. Pubic hair is sparse. Of course, there is no menstruation because there is no uterus (the testes have inhibited the development of the Müllerian ducts normally). The condition is called **testicular feminization,** the children are (and should be) raised as girls, and, because the condition is genetic, sisters can also be affected.

Incomplete degrees of insensitivity to male hormones take all manner of forms. In addition, there is a group of conditions in which tissue sensitivity to hormones is normal but testosterone production is too low. The result can range from the presence of a rudimentary vagina that also receives the bladder to an absent or small penis ("microphallus"), perhaps with the urethra not quite getting to the tip of the penis (**hypospadias**). Assigning boy or girl at birth depends on a judgment as to whether the phallus can be made competent with high doses of hormone cream applied during childhood. Fertility fails in the more severe forms.

### Female Intersex

Almost the same range of appearances can result from problems in the other direction. Suppose, instead, that the ovary does its job (more accurately, there is no testis to impose maleness). The Müllerian ducts form and the external genitalia take the shape of a vagina and vulva. Now, either through nature, in **congenital adrenal hyperplasia** (CAH), or through accidental administration (for example, inadvertently taking **danazol** during pregnancy), there is exposure of the fetus to male hormones. Instead of the internal male ducts being suppressed by absent male sex hormones, they persist. Moreover, instead of an open vulva and vagina, the labia fuse in the middle, attempting to produce a scrotum. We now have ambiguous genitals with a 46,XX karyotype. Surgery helps restore female anatomy, and the result is usually at least workable. Pregnancy is often possible, but may need **ovulation induction** (see Chapter 10).

True hermaphrodism is rare. Much more common is pseudohermaphrodism—patients with either testes *or* ovaries but still ambiguous-looking genitals or with other confusion somewhere between maleness and femaleness. These are the intersex states, which commonly are discovered at birth; occasionally they show up at puberty, when expected maleness or femaleness goes awry. There is no more complicated area in reproductive medicine, and the box "Intersex" discusses the subject at length.

In general, if there is substantial doubt about ascribing gender at birth, "girl" is the safer choice, whatever the chromosomes and whatever the internal glands and organs might suggest, because when it comes to having sex, an absent vagina can be overcome with surgery; the absence of a functioning penis usually cannot be corrected.

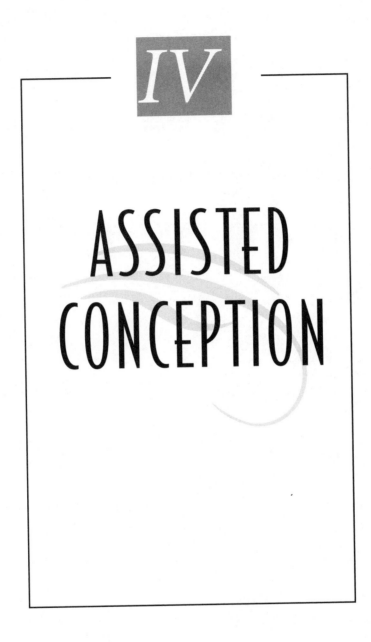

# IV

# ASSISTED CONCEPTION

# Helping Nature a Bit

Sex is important for getting pregnant, so it helps to talk about it. Not everyon
including your partner, however, will want to talk about it to the same extent 
in the same way. But what none of us can get away from is that at some stag
physicians, perhaps nurses and sometimes laboratory technicians, will be shar
ing your knowledge of when and how often you have sex—sometimes even *ho*
you have sex. What has generally been a private matter between the two of yo
can seem to become excruciatingly public.

It would be good if all the professional people you need to talk to about hel
with getting pregnant were always sensitive, neither prudish nor flippant, re
spectful of your personal situation and showed a capacity for empathy. Th
medical care involved with treating infertility, however, is no different tha
other areas of medicine. You will probably encounter a person or several person
relating to you on a very personal matter who will differ in living up to that re
sponsibility. Some will be good at it, some will not. Put simply, you will fin
some people more helpful than others; some will be tactless, crass or rude or ac
in other ways so that you know he or she is not the person for you. Depending
on your personality, you will face these difficulties in one of several ways: with
sad acceptance; with detached understanding and humor; with nonacceptanc
and rudeness or carefully constructed criticism in return; or with nonaccep
tance and a change of physician, pathology laboratory or infertility program
You might even make a phone call to your lawyer or send a note to someone
writing a book on infertility horror stories. Perhaps you might keep open the
option of any one of them at different times and in different circumstances. For
now, let me dispel some myths about sex.

# How to Have Sex

Who am I to tell you how to have sex? Essentially, it really does not matter how
you do it. Use whatever position you both feel comfortable with. Germaine
Greer has written that the most appealing position for many women is with the
man beneath and the woman on top—the opposite of the so-called missionary
position, which has traditionally been prescribed for getting pregnant. Either
of these positions and others can be perfectly satisfactory from the point of
view of reproductive biology. The only requirement is that it is comfortable
and that the ejaculate ends up in the vagina, next to the cervix. The ejaculate
coagulates next to the cervical mucus quite quickly; even if some of the semen

seems to leak out, be reassured that this is not necessarily abnormal and does not always matter.

A woman need not have an orgasm to conceive. Although it is fair to say that nature invented orgasm for a reason, its evolutionary purpose was probably to make sex attractive at times other than ovulation, encouraging bonding between partners. Pleasure with sex has been around at least as long as the monkeys and apes. (There is an intelligent and entertaining book by Meredith Small on the subject.) Even among the apes there are extraordinary differences, for example, between the bonono chimpanzees, who delight in it as often and in as varied ways as possible, and gorillas, among whom it is an uncommon event and takes all of eight seconds. Both species are fertile. If there is one hint I can give, it is that you can best avoid your partner seeing it as a chore by concentrating on enjoying it yourself and your partner's pleasure will look after itself. Recent research, however, shows that an orgasm that follows ejaculation decreases the escape, or flow back, of semen out of the vagina. So, a rather late orgasm might well be a good thing for retaining semen and for getting pregnant—at least when you are having sex around the time of ovulation (see the box "Orgasm and Retaining Sperm").

## How Often to Have Sex

Another question I am asked a lot is how frequently intercourse should take place to optimize the chance of conceiving. In particular, I am asked if it is possible for fertility to suffer from having sex too often. To deal with the second question first, the answer is no. Although we can show that the density of sperm in the ejaculate diminishes with frequent ejaculation, remember that the mucus of the cervix at the time of ovulation is so receptive to sperm that it is the best place for sperm to be—better than in the male ducts awaiting ejaculation.

This is not to say that you should have or need to have sex every day or even twice a day when attempting pregnancy. Every second day during the middle of the cycle is ordinarily enough. With care in timing, it is possible to have sex less frequently and probably have more pleasurable and satisfying sex. Timing sex becomes more important if there is a decrease in the sperm count. When you have sex outside the time of ovulation, of course, it has nothing to do with getting pregnant and everything to do with keeping your relationship pleasant and mutually supportive.

Researchers Dr. Robin Baker and Dr. Mark Bellis of the Department of Environmental Biology at the University of Manchester, England, are quite categorical about it. Female orgasm before ejaculation decreases sperm retention, whereas orgasm after ejaculation can reduce the flowing back of sperm and increase sperm retention. Drs. Baker and Bellis arrived at this conclusion with the help of 35 very cooperative couples—couples who timed and measured their flowback in relation to the woman's orgasm and to the man's ejaculation in 323 copulations. (They also got very similar information from 3,679 women who responded to a nationwide survey.) Specifically, they claim that:

• It makes no difference whether the orgasm happens during intercourse itself or is initiated (by either partner) afterward.

• It should *not* occur more than a minute before ejaculation.

• Extra sperm will be retained if orgasm

happens at any time up to the time that flowback starts.

• Up to a few days, the longer it has been since a previous orgasm, the more semen is retained (I presume this is because the orgasm might be better).

• Orgasm more than a minute before ejaculation reduces sperm retention and increases later flowback.

Whether or not you have a cigarette after sex is up to you, although right now is a good time to say that smoking does decrease fertility, especially in women. How often smoking is the only reason for infertility is not certain, but I do know a couple who conceived within two months of stopping smoking, after about ten years of tests and unsuccessful attempts at treatment. The harmful effect of cigarette smoking is "dose-related"—the more you smoke, the more it decreases fertility.

How important it is to be free of stress is a question I am asked almost every day. Stress can be enough to interfere with

# Sex or Insemination ?

In some circumstances sex consistently fails to deliver the goods. **Impotence** anatomical problems such as **hypospadias**, and physiological malfunctio such as **retrograde ejaculation** are examples of problems with sexual inter proper ovulation (see Chapter 1), but this can be tested for in the usual way (see Chapter 4). If these tests are normal then there is no evidence that the constant worry about not getting pregnant itself interferes with getting pregnant, unless you stop having sex (again, see Chapter 1).

Alcohol has no harmful effects on getting pregnant, at least up to sensible, moderate levels. It will do you and your partner no harm, for example, to have a glass of wine before sex (unless, I suppose, it is in the morning of a working day). I know that I might be putting myself out on a limb with this statement, so I should clarify it. Here are the facts about alcohol. First, no one has shown that small to moderate amounts of alcohol are harmful to any aspect of health. In fact, the reverse is true, for example, in relation to heart disease, in which alcohol has an important protective effect. Second, men on average metabolize alcohol more efficiently than women, so they can generally tolerate somewhat more alcohol than women. Third, overtly intoxi-cating levels of alcohol, especially those that result in a hangover, are harmful to health and to pregnancy (certainly once someone is already pregnant), and nothing I say here should be construed as a license to get thoroughly drunk. Fourth, whether you drink alcohol or not you will not be protected completely from the risk of having a baby with a birth defect, because defects come about from many other causes. Fifth, many people take vitamins A, C and E because they are antioxidants, whereas one of the richest dietary sources of antioxidants is red wine. Last, a lot of quarreling between partners can be avoided by not taking a too restrictive view of alcohol consumption in relation to getting pregnant. Alcohol is not like cigarette smoking, where any exposure is harmful. The medical evidence, as it is available in 1996, is that moderate amounts of alcohol, such as a glass or two of wine, have not been associated with any special hazards—if drinking is followed by going to bed with your usual partner.

course that can be overcome with masturbation, semen preparation in the laboratory and then assisted insemination, usually with "washed" semen placed into the uterus (**intrauterine insemination**, or IUI; see Chapter 9). But is it of any use, given careful timing of either assisted insemination or sexual intercourse, to carry out AIH (assisted insemination, husband) for oligospermia or unexplained infertility?

Apart from these three well-defined disturbances, the usefulness of IU compared with having sex to get pregnant is controversial, despite IUI havin, become a medical industry. With proper timing in regard to ovulation, D Gordon Baker in Melbourne, Australia, and Dr. Michael Hull in Bristo England, among others, have shown in careful and purposeful studies (involv ing **control groups** of couples who had sex normally for comparison) that se: is better than insemination. The Amsterdam study described in Chapter showed that IUI may have the edge if there are more than two million washe sperm available for the insemination procedure. Refer also to Chapter 9 for a account of the limited place there is for IUI in association with injections of **fol licle stimulating hormone** for multiple ovulation induction (**superovulation**)

# When to Have Sex

Humans are not unique among species in pursuing sex for its own sake—w share it as a pastime with monkeys, chimps and dolphins. Evolution has mad it particularly pleasurable, although regimenting it when trying against the odd to get pregnant does lessen its appeal. In women, sex drive or sexual willingnes is not a reliable indicator of fertility, unlike most of the earth's other species. Pleasurable sex is an evolutionary advance. The functional price paid for it i that the female mating instinct (estrus, or "heat," among animals) is no longer synchronous with ovulation or with the chance of pregnancy. A woman's own symptoms of ovulation—and fertility—may be subtle, but they often can be recognized.

For fertility, it is better for sperm to be in the fallopian tube when ovula- tion takes place. The normally ovulated egg is poised to be fertilized as soon as it gets there. Its fertile life is then no more than about 10 to 12 hours, per- haps less. On the other hand, sperm will take just two or three hours to reach the tube and be **capacitated** (see Chapter 3), that is, in a condition able to fer- tilize the egg.

The symptoms that precede ovulation include an increase in secretions in the vagina, when some women will detect particularly stretchable mucus. Once these symptoms disappear, the mucus will have tightened up to keep further sperm out of the uterus. So-called "ovulation pain," or *Mittelschmerz*, in fact precedes ovulation by up to 24 hours; it is therefore a good indication of when to time intercourse (provided it is not so bad that it causes intercourse itself to be painful—a rather cruel situation when it happens).

## Temperature Charting

The **basal body temperature chart** (see Chapter 4) is not a very efficient way to *predict* ovulation. Its main benefit is looking back on ovulation after the event. First, once the temperature goes up, it is too late to conceive, so it is useful in putting an end to an exhausting regimen of sex to get pregnant. Second, a dip in temperature can occur with ovulation, and this can be used as a signal. Third, and most useful, over several months temperature charting will give a woman and her gynecologist an idea of the time in the cycle during which ovulation may occur, providing a general guide to when having sex will provide the best chance of getting pregnant. A temperature chart is not a hormone assay, however, and even the clearest chart can be 24 hours or more off in estimating the day of ovulation. To do better than this means stepping up the technology a notch.

## LH Testing

When a follicle in the ovary is ready, the pituitary gland's signal to ovulate consists of a surge of **luteinizing hormone** or LH (see Chapter 3). The surge usually starts during sleep, about three or four in the morning, and will result in ovulation 36 to 40 hours later. LH enters the urine within a few hours of the start of the surge, where it can be measured using a variety of testing kits bought over the counter in drugstores. The measuring techniques vary a little, but the package insert will explain how the kit is to be used.

The urine sample to test is not the first one when you wake up; that sample will contain the night's accumulated urine. The urine to test is later that morning. If the test is doubtful, test again the same day. A positive result means that ovulation will take place in the next day and a half. Sex that night, and/or the following morning, will be well timed. With this scheme, however, it is best to test the next day as well; if it is still positive, test again that evening. The kits for testing urinary LH are not cheap. To reduce costs by purchasing fewer kits, keep a basal body temperature chart as well, first to show when testing should start (about day 11 for a 28-day cycle; earlier for shorter cycles) and to show when to stop testing, should the LH surge signal have been missed and the temperature be up.

Timing sex this way might not seem to be fun, but it is worth trying to accept the discipline and the challenge with a sense of humor. A seductive dinner once a month, even if timed with a clinical test, can be enticing. Read the box

"Champagne and Candles" in Chapter 25 on how an LH test can help you pla your evening. Should this straightforward approach to timing when to have se not produce a pregnancy (after, say, six months), further help with a more fo mal program of assisted conception becomes the next option and is the subje of the next chapter.

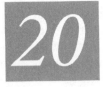

20

# Helping Nature
# a Lot–Assisted
# Conception

$W$hat, exactly, is **assisted conception**? Assisted conception procedures invol
directly manipulating sperm, eggs or embryos, any of which thereby spend
least a short time outside the body before being returned with the aim
increasing the chance of pregnancy during the month or cycle the assisted co
ception procedure is being done. The procedures comprise **assisted insemin
tion** (AI) and **intrauterine insemination** (IUI), as well as **gamete intrafall
pian transfer** (GIFT), **in vitro fertilization** (IVF) and other, newer variatio
involving IVF. In general, these procedures increase the chance of pregnancy b
cause, first, they increase the number of sperm that get to the egg and/or, se
ond, they increase the number of eggs available for fertilization.

Unlike other treatments for infertility that are not likely to be repeated, suc
as surgery for blocked fallopian tubes or prescribing a course of treatment wit
drugs, assisted conception procedures are not intended (at least without furth
intervention) to be effective past the particular cycle or month in which they a
used. Assisted conception procedures can be an alternative or an additional ap
proach to the more traditional, nonrepetitive (and meant to be lasting) ap
proaches to treatment. The correct place of assisted conception and its usefu
ness, compared with the conventional methods of treatment, depends on th
cause of the infertility and also on the patient's own special circumstance
Assisted conception procedures are sometimes the only way infertility can b
overcome. Here, however, at the beginning of the chapter, is a good place t
point out that not everyone will want to go to these lengths to get pregnant.

# The Choice

Assisted insemination (AI) is the procedure in which sperm are delivered int
the **cervix** or into the **uterus** (or into the **fallopian tube** by ultrasound-guide
catheter). AI is useful in only a few circumstances—when there is physical diffi
culty with ordinary sexual intercourse or when there is a specific and localize
problem in the cervix of the uterus that we have to get past. As mentioned i
Chapter 19, experience has unfortunately shown that intrauterine inseminatio
(IUI) using the husband's semen (AIH) is seldom effective for **oligospermi
(decreased sperm counts)** or when there is **endometriosis** or **unexplained in
fertility**, even when accompanied by **superovulation** (multiple ovulation in
duction). Donor insemination (DI), assisted insemination using donor sperm
(previously called "AID"), is described in Chapter 22.

Gamete intrafallopian transfer (GIFT) involves transferring unfertilized eggs and sperm into one or both fallopian tubes. It is probably the best procedure when the fallopian tubes are normal and when there is no reason to doubt that the sperm can, if given the opportunity, fertilize the eggs. GIFT can work even when endometriosis is present (see Chapter 16).

In vitro fertilization (IVF) means fertilization of eggs in the laboratory, literally "in glass" (although nowadays in plastic). The fertilized eggs are then transferred either to the fallopian tubes or, particularly if the fallopian tubes have been damaged, to the uterus. It is the only option for getting pregnant if the tubes are irrevocably damaged or if they have been removed. This is the cause of infertility for which IVF was invented in the 1970s. The second main reason for using IVF is when there is doubt about sperm being able to fertilize the egg. This is the case, for example, with oligospermia, or low sperm counts (especially with decreased sperm motility), when there are **sperm antibodies** present and when two or more GIFT cycles have not led to a pregnancy. When sperm counts are especially low, fertilization will not take place with ordinary in vitro methods. **Sperm microinjection** (SMI) is then appropriate.

# Ovarian Stimulation

Assisted conception based partly on increased egg numbers will generally involve stimulating the ovaries with injections of **follicle stimulating hormone**. Depending on a woman's age, anywhere up to 30 or more **follicles** (each follicle containing one egg) start to develop in each menstrual cycle (see Chapters 3 and 10). Normally, all but one of these follicles are lost on the way. This remaining follicle goes on to ovulate. What the stimulation process does is increase the fraction of eggs that are ready to ovulate, from about one in 30 to about 10 in 30 or more.

## Follicle Stimulating Hormone (FSH)

FSH has to be given by injection, because it is a complicated protein hormone that would be digested and inactivated if given by mouth. The dosage is rather standard: it is not necessarily a case of the more you use the greater the response. The dose needs to be enough to stop the usual competition between

## Clomiphene and Assisted Conception

For many years, **clomiphene** (trade names Clomid, from Merrell Dow, and Serophene, from Serono) was a mainstay addition to FSH regimens for inducing superovulation for assisted conception. First, clomiphene can substitute for FSH for several days at the beginning of the cycle, decreasing the overall cost of stimulation. Second, clomiphene slows down the development of the **endometrium**, which can sometimes be useful in IVF, where embryo development is sometimes slower than it would be naturally. (The retarding of the endometrium is not a normal process in pregnancy, however, and this is one reason why more miscarriages happen when clomiphene is used.) Third, clomiphene also seems to block, to some extent, the pituitary's sensitivity to rising levels of estradiol that signal the LH surge, which in turn causes ovulation to take place. But this effect is incomplete; certainly it is not to be relied on and is one strong reason clomiphene has lost its popularity in assisted conception programs, in favor of the GnRH-agonists. (See Chapter 10 for more information on clomiphene.)

follicles; once we reach this threshold there is not a lot of control possible over the number of follicles that will grow. Remember that using FSH injections does not use up your follicles any faster than they are already being used for development in the ovaries (see Chapter 3). It is possible, however, for the ovaries to become seriously enlarged, to the point of risking complications.

The **ovarian hyperstimulation syndrome**, or OHSS (see Chapter 11), is more common in younger women, who have more follicles ready to respond to FSH, and in women with **polycystic ovary syndrome** (see Chapter 10). Side effects, apart from discomfort from the injections and the sheer inconvenience of having an injection every day, come from the higher estrogen levels than during normal cycles. Some women feel worse, some feel better, all feel different.

## GnRH-Agonists

The **GnRH-agonists** are a group of drugs all closely related to the natural hormone **gonadotropin-releasing hormone** (GnRH), a small amount of which is used by the hypothalamus of the brain to keep the pituitary gland active. Exposure of the pituitary to a GnRH-agonist first stimulates it and then, paradoxically but usefully, inhibits the pituitary. We can make use of both these actions for ovarian stimulation, but the important one is the second; agonists effectively and reliably suppress the LH surge that can (prematurely) start the ovulation process in the stimulated ovaries.

The different GnRH-agonists all work the same way. Those that are available in the United States, Australia and Europe include **leuprolide** (Lupron, made by Abbott), given by daily injection using a fine needle just under the skin; **nafarelin** (Synarel, made by Syntex), given by nasal spray twice a day; **buserilin** (Suprefact, made by Hoechst), given by nasal spray four times a day, and **goserelin** (Zoladex, made by ICI) and **triptorelin** (Decapeptyl, made by Ipsen Biotech), both given as a monthly depot injection and less satisfactory for assisted conception.

When the GnRH-agonist stimulates the pituitary gland, it stimulates the ovaries as well. After a few days it inhibits the pituitary. This is beneficial, because it stops the pituitary from competing with the FSH injections once these are started, typically on about day three of the cycle (sometimes day two; see the box "The Long, Short and Ultrashort of GnRH-Agonists"). The GnRH-agonist effectively prevents the LH surge, so we can continue the stimulation, without the risk of premature or unexpected ovulation, until the follicles are fully developed.

The main side effect of the GnRH-agonists comes from their ability to release histamine in the body, causing an irritating skin rash in susceptible people soon after injection. The GnRH-antagonists (see the box "The Long, Short and Ultrashort of GnRH-Agonists") tend even more to have this side effect. If such a rash is troublesome, it is worth trying antihistamines.

It is probably important that GnRH-agonists not be taken during pregnancy, although women who have been kept on them for the first few weeks of pregnancy have not had babies with obvious abnormalities. GnRH is normally found all over the baby's developing nervous system, so we have to assume that interfering with levels can still turn out to be harmful. For this reason we usually do not start GnRH-agonists until a menstrual period has started. We stop it when ovulation of the stimulated follicles is induced with **human chorionic gonadotropin** (hCG).

# Human Chorionic Gonadotropin

Human chorionic gonadotropin (hCG) is the hormone of pregnancy. We get it by purifying it from the urine of pregnant women. No infectious disease has ever been attributed to the use of hCG. It acts like LH in stimulating the corpus

## The Long, Short and Ultrashort of GnRH-Agonists

GnRH-agonists can be used in assisted conception programs in several different ways. Starting the GnRH-agonist on day two or three of the menstrual period (thus coinciding with and building on the natural start of the ovarian cycle) is called the **short protocol**, and makes use of a flare of FSH activity that follows the first dose or two of GnRH-agonist to get the stimulation of the ovaries under way. Alternatively, we can start the GnRH-agonist many days, even weeks, before FSH injections are started, allowing the pituitary to wind right down and, incidentally, giving great flexibility to timing the expected day of egg pickup, which will be about two weeks after the FSH injections are started. This is the **long protocol**.

One problem with the long protocol is the generation of ovarian cysts along with the developing follicles. These cysts are quite benign. They are either large old follicles without eggs (a "follicular cyst," producing estrogen, or a big **atretic folli-cle**, which produces no hormones) or a cystic and functionless **corpus luteum**. To say the least, they are a nuisance, confusing the picture as to whether they are producing hormones or not. In practice they often lead to cancellation of the cycle of treatment. Researchers in Bristol, England, have shown that such cysts can be prevented from forming by starting a week's treatment with a **progestogen** (such as 10 milligrams per day of Provera) a few days before the start of the GnRH-agonist (for example, on about day 19 of the cycle before the one in which FSH will be given and eggs recovered). Thus, the Provera treatment overlaps the start of the GnRH-agonist administration and thereby possibly avoids the flare of FSH production. Note that the Provera *must* be stopped before injections of FSH start,

luteum to make **progesterone** in early pregnancy (see Chapters 3 and 10), which means we can replace the natural LH surge with an injection of hCG to set into motion the events that will cause ovulation.

The preparations of hCG available include **Pregnyl** (made by Organon in ampules of 500, 1,500 and 5,000 units) and **Profasi** (made by Serono in ampule of 2,000 and 5,000 units). In Australia the usual dose to induce ovulation is 5,000 units, with further doses of 1,500 to 2,000 units on one or two further occasions during the **luteal phase** of the stimulated cycle (see Chapter 10) Because hCG is active in the body much longer than LH would be, it is possible

## The Long, Short and Ultrashort of GnRH-Agonists (concluded)

otherwise there will be two serious problems: the follicles will not respond properly to the FSH, and the endometrium will not develop properly.

It is also possible, in a variation of the short protocol, to stop the GnRH-agonist after just four or five days—the **ultrashort protocol**—without losing control over the pituitary gland. The LH surge will be prevented for at least a week after the GnRH-agonist is stopped. In fact, the pituitary during this time will be even further suppressed than it would have been had the GnRH-agonist been continued up to the induction of ovulation. This ultrashort protocol usually works fine, but there are two possible problems. First, unless the follicles are already well under way by the time the GnRH-agonist is stopped, it may be necessary to increase the dose of FSH at a time when this is rarely necessary with other protocols. The reason for this is

that a woman's own FSH and LH levels become extremely low for a week or more after GnRH-agonists are stopped. Second, should a further dose of GnRH-agonist be given after two days or more without it, the GnRH-agonist will actually induce a second flare of pituitary activity, perhaps including the very LH surge we are trying to stop!

### Antagonizing GnRH Instead

On the horizon is a different type of GnRH-like drug, one that promises to be much simpler to use in preventing the midcycle LH surge. These are the inhibitors of GnRH, the **GnRH-antagonists**. They do not start by stimulating the pituitary, so they can be started later in the cycle, closer to the time ovulation is expected. Only a few doses are needed, over a few days.

to use 10,000 units and then not give further doses, a popular way of administering hCG in the United States.

We know from experience that it takes about 38 hours for ovulation to occur after an injection of hCG. If no GnRH agonist has been used there is a chance that the natural LH surge will have started before the hCG was given, spoiling the cycle if it has not been recognized or if a mistake is made in timing the **egg pickup**. With GnRH-agonist, the LH surge is reliably prevented, so we can first work out the best time for the egg pickup (even, to some extent, the most convenient day), then subtract 36 hours to work out the time to give the hCG injection. We then still have about two hours leeway in either direction, in case the is a problem in performing the egg pickup at exactly the scheduled time.

Injection of hCG can be a more painful injection than follicle stimulati hormone (FSH), because the purer the gonadotropin preparation, the less pa it seems to cause. The time the hCG is given is necessarily at night for an e pickup during the day, and this can be a nuisance. Otherwise, its side effect hyperstimulation, which will not happen with FSH alone, because when hype stimulation is encountered either hCG has been given or an LH surge has tak place. Minimizing the chance of ovarian hyperstimulation syndrome (OHS during assisted conception treatment cycles involving superovulation mea close monitoring of ovarian response.

## Ovarian Monitoring

There is normally an interactive, or feedback, relationship between the pituita gland and the ovary. The pituitary's production of FSH is governed by t ovary's response. When FSH is given by injection, this physiological signaling abolished. We have to substitute our own feedback mechanism by recording t ovary's response to the injections and, if necessary, varying how or if we gi further injections of FSH. We learn how the ovary is responding to the injec tions by measuring and remeasuring the amount of estrogen in the blood wi **serum estradiols** and by visualizing the number and size of the ovarian follicl with **transvaginal ultrasounds**. There are two reasons why such ovarian mor toring is necessary: to try to avoid dangerous degrees of stimulation that cou lead to OHSS; and so that hCG can be administered at the best time—with m ture follicles—so that we get healthy eggs.

Monitoring usually starts on the first day of a menstrual period, when v measure the levels of serum estradiol, **serum progesterone** and **serum LH**, to b sure that the bleeding truly represents a menstrual period, that it is the start a new cycle and not, say, an **ectopic pregnancy**, a **miscarriage** or **implantatic bleeding**. All three hormones should be low. During treatment cycles involvir a GnRH-agonist used according to the long protocol (see the box "The Lon Short and Ultrashort of GnRH-Agonists"), the physician may monitor th proper down-regulation of the pituitary gland with such tests over the course a week or more.

At Sydney IVF we typically repeat the serum estradiol after several days of stimulation with FSH to make sure that the dose of FSH is enough to achieve a response and is not causing a grossly excessive response. On about the eighth day of the cycle, we measure estradiol again and perform an ultrasound to see how many follicles are developing. Therefore, by day eight we know if a certain level of estrogen is coming from a number of follicles that need further growth before maturity or if that amount of estrogen is coming from just one or two follicles that are already mature.

From then until the follicles are close to two centimeters in diameter, we adopt a flexible approach in relation to the dosage of FSH, the duration of further stimulation and the timing of more estradiol measurements and ultrasounds. We generally expect follicles to become bigger in younger women than they will in women over 40.

If for some reason a GnRH-agonist has not been used, we need also to look for signs of the natural LH surge. This means more frequent blood tests, sometimes more than once a day, with measurements of serum progesterone, LH and estradiol. The last blood test is then taken at the time that hCG is given, usually in the evening. If this last test still shows progesterone and LH to be low, then we can be confident that ovulation will not be earlier than the expected 36 to 38 hours after hCG. If, on the other hand, they are high, then an educated guess needs to be made as to when the LH surge probably began. In practice it can often be assumed to have started in the early hours of the morning, which means timing the egg pickup for around midday—but there are exceptions. We also follow a very similar protocol in looking for the natural LH surge if we are conducting IVF with a natural, unstimulated cycle.

# Egg Pickup

The culmination of ovarian stimulation and monitoring is the egg pickup procedure—the aspiration of the fluid from immediately preovulatory follicles in which the eggs have detached themselves from the wall of the follicle and are surrounded by a mature cumulus (see Figure 3.6a). The egg pickup can be carried out directly during laparoscopy (see the next section on gamete intrafallopian transfer) or less directly through the side of the vagina, guided by transvaginal ultrasound, described in the section on in vitro fertilization (see also Figure 20.1). The eggs obtained can then be used immediately for gamete

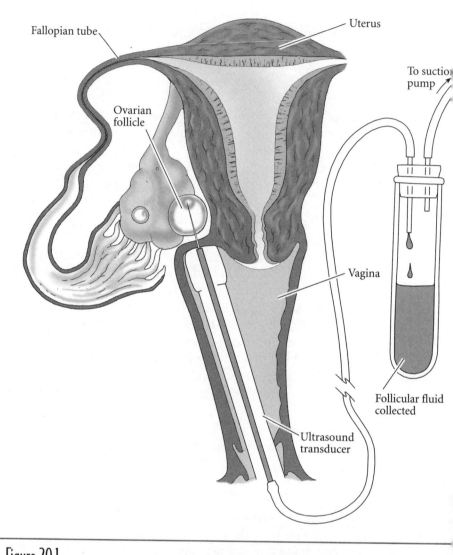

**Figure 20.1** Ultrasound-guided follicle aspiration for egg pickup through the vagina.

intrafallopian transfer, they can be fertilized in vitro for transfer a day or two later or for later transfer after freezing, they can be fertilized simply to gain information on sperm and egg function or they can be discarded.

# Gamete Intrafallopian Transfer

**Gametes** comprise sperm and eggs. Gamete intrafallopian transfer (GIFT) is the direct transference of sperm and eggs to the fallopian tube, where fertilization of eggs by sperm normally takes place. At least one of the tubes *must* be normal for this procedure.

## Laparoscopic GIFT

Although at Sydney IVF we have developed ways of carrying out GIFT by ultrasound (I discuss this further on), the established way of achieving access to the tubes with GIFT is by laparoscopy. Most people considering GIFT will have had a laparoscopy in the course of investigating their infertility (see Chapter 4).

In the process of laparoscopic GIFT, the eggs are collected from the follicles, either during the laparoscopy or immediately before by transvaginal ultrasound. We refer to this part of the procedure as **follicle aspiration** or, more colloquially, "egg pickup." The fluid we get from the follicles is kept at 37° Celsius (98.4° Fahrenheit) while the eggs are looked for and isolated by a scientist working in the operating room with a special enclosed microscope that protects the correct physical environment for the eggs. When the follicles have been emptied, the eggs and the prepared sperm are loaded into a transfer catheter, which is then passed through the open, **fimbrial end** of one or the other fallopian tube, to between two and six centimeters down the tube.

## Why Does GIFT Work?

GIFT increases the chance of pregnancy during the cycle of treatment in two ways. First, it makes sure that many sperm get into close proximity with the egg. Second, it increases by two or three times the number of eggs available to be fertilized in the treatment cycle. For GIFT to have a good chance of leading to pregnancy there are two special requirements. The first is that the sperm count needs to be high enough; after laboratory preparation, there should be more than 100,000 normal and motile sperm available for the transfer. The second special requirement for GIFT is ready access to a normal fallopian tube.

With ultrasound GIFT the eggs are collected the same way as with IVF, that is, by procedures through the vagina. For transfer, the gametes are loaded into a special two-part catheter developed by myself and Dr. Jock Anderson in 1987. This catheter system consists of an outer cannula that is passed through the cervix out into the corner of the cavity of the uterus (where the tube comes in), and an inner gamete cannula, which is then pushed several centimeters down the fallopian tube (see Figure 20.2).

In 1992 at Sydney IVF, the chance of pregnancy among women with comparable infertility having laparoscopic and the more recently developed ultrasound GIFT was about three to two in favor of laparoscopic GIFT. Therefore, this is the main reason that at Sydney IVF we still perform more laparoscopic GIFT procedures than ultrasound GIFT procedures. It is hard to move away from a familiar procedure that has a relatively good chance of working. In addition, even though no general anesthesia is involved in ultrasound GIFT, it does involve two separate procedures— the ultrasound-guided follicle aspiration for egg recovery and the passing of the catheter down one of the fallopian tubes. During laparoscopic GIFT, recovery of eggs and transfer of gametes into the tubes are usually carried out together.

There may be circumstances, however, when these new methods are more attractive, such as if a woman wants to avoid further laparoscopies and general anesthetics or if she has an intuitive notion that it is time to try something new. Before departing from establthods, however, a woman should discuss with her physician or the nursing staff at the assisted conception program what their latest experiences have been with the new methods.

## What Can Go Wrong with GIFT?

Apart from the risks of ovarian stimulation (see Chapter 11) and not getting pregnant in any particular cycle, there are three main hazards with GIFT. First there is the chance of a miscarriage (about 30 percent of pregnancies miscarried until the introduction of GnRH-agonist instead of clomiphene reduced the risk of miscarriage to about 15 percent). Second, there is the chance of a **multiple pregnancy**. It is also possible that the pregnancy will implant in the tube forming an ectopic pregnancy, a complication that has occurred in about 5 percent of clinical GIFT pregnancies at Sydney IVF, slightly higher than the risk after IVF with transfer of embryos to the uterus.

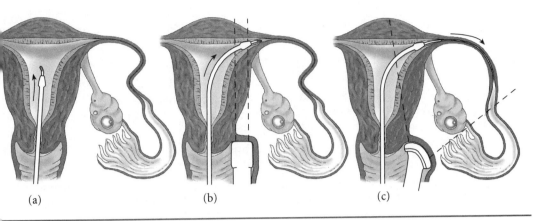

(a)                                (b)                                (c)

**Figure 20.2**  Ultrasound GIFT and ZIFT. The technique of ultrasound-guided catheterization of the fallopian tubes from the vagina, for gamete or embryo transfer to the tubes, as developed at Sydney IVF in 1987. The outer cannula is passed from the vagina, through the cervix, into the uterus (a). The cannula is directed into the angle where the tube joins the uterus (b). The fine inner catheter is passed out into the fallopian tube (c).

## What Is the Chance of Success?

The chance of a successful pregnancy with GIFT at Sydney IVF has averaged more than 30 percent per cycle since Sydney IVF started its laparoscopic GIFT program in 1986. In many months more than 40 percent of cycles have led to conception. Although such a success rate is considered to be very good—and many other centers achieve these results—it still means that at least as many people do not conceive as do conceive in any one cycle.

Although the key to success with GIFT may be to repeat it several times, it is informative to look in some detail at what sorts of factors have influenced the pregnancy rate with GIFT at Sydney IVF. The two main factors have been the man's sperm count and the woman's age, but we will consider some specific questions first.

Is the **duration of infertility** important? The length of time a couple has been infertile is not important if the woman is under the age of 39. Up to 1989, when we last did this analysis at Sydney IVF, of 11 women with 13 years of infertility or longer who had GIFT, four conceived in their first treatment cycle, and their pregnancies were normal.

What is the effect of a woman's age? A lot. Table B.1 in Appendix B shows the effect of age on the clinical pregnancy rate and on the pregnancy outcome after GIFT since Sydney IVF began in 1986. The probability of a clinically obvious pregnancy holds up well until about age 38, after which, unfortunately, t probability rate falls quickly. Even before age 38 there is an increase in t chance of a miscarriage with an increase in age.

Does the chance of pregnancy change with successive GIFT cycles? Amo women under 39, as shown in Table 2 in Appendix II, the chance of pregnan with GIFT has been highest for the first two cycles (especially the second cycl but the chance is still reasonable after that.

How many eggs should be transferred? To a large extent it is true that t more eggs transferred at GIFT the greater the chance of pregnancy. Unfc tunately, the hazard of multiple pregnancy also increases, with twins, triple quadruplets and so on representing quantum leaps in terms of unsatisfacto outcome and new opportunities for suffering. The problems of multiple pre nancy are those of prematurity and nonsurvival, an increased risk of birth d fects and the consummate difficulty in looking after three or more babies once, when they have all been safely delivered.

The Reproductive Technology Accreditation Committee of the Fertili Society of Australia produces guidelines that all Australian assisted conceptic units voluntarily agree to comply with. These guidelines limit the number eggs transferred to three, except in special, uncommon circumstances. T transfer of two eggs is recommended for many women and is usual at Sydn IVF for women under age 33 who are having GIFT and have been infertile f just two or three years. In the United States there is no such general policy place to limit the number of eggs transferred at once and different clinics di fer in their practices. Clinics that transfer more eggs or achieve slightly high pregnancy rates within one cycle of treatment require recourse more often **fetal reduction** to manage high-number multiple pregnancies. Clinics th limit the number of eggs transferred have recourse to freezing spare fertiliz eggs to provide further chances of pregnancy from the one round of ovaria stimulation.

## What Is the Effect of the Sperm Count?

The sperm count is critical for GIFT. For normal conception to take place, ju a few sperm are needed in the tube (probably fewer than 50 and perhaps few than 10; see Chapter 3), but these sperm in natural circumstances have bee highly selected for fitness during the journey up through the uterus. We fin that we need at least 100,000 motile, largely normal sperm for GIFT to have a optimal chance of success. We increase this number to 200,000 if a high pro portion of the sperm have abnormal shapes. This means that GIFT is only suitable for couples with normal sperm counts or sperm counts that are just moderately affected by oligospermia. As a form of assisted conception, however, GIFT is substantially more reliable—in terms of pregnancy rates and limiting the hazard of multiple pregnancy—than superovulation with intrauterine insemination.

# In Vitro Fertilization

In vitro fertilization (IVF) means the fertilization of eggs by sperm in the laboratory. The procedure is most obviously necessary when the fallopian tubes are blocked or absent, because the fallopian tube is where fertilization normally takes place. From the early successes of clinical IVF beginning in 1980, however, it was realized that IVF can help whenever there is doubt that fertilization is occurring. IVF was soon found to be equally effective for other diagnoses, including oligospermia (low sperm counts), the presence of sperm antibodies, endometriosis and unexplained infertility. IVF can also be successful when there are too few sperm available for GIFT.

# How Does IVF Work?

Like GIFT, IVF increases the chance of pregnancy during the cycle of treatment in two ways. First, it makes sure that many sperm get close to the egg—in the laboratory. Second, it increases the number of eggs available to be fertilized in the treatment cycle. The chance of something going wrong is generally too high with just one egg, although this kind of "natural cycle IVF" does have a place in young women with fallopian tube disease.

## Transvaginal Follicle Aspiration

After ovarian stimulation, the second special requirement for IVF is to get the eggs from the ovaries into the laboratory, where they can be fertilized. The

There are several reasons why fertilization may fail to take place in vitro:

• Sperm may fail to attach in great enough numbers to the egg's surrounding coat, the **zona pellucida**. This may occur because of insufficient numbers of healthy sperm or the presence of sperm antibodies. If a failure of sperm to attach to the zona is seen, future cycles should involve sperm microinjection.

• The recovered eggs have been deprived of follicle stimulating hormone. Sometimes, especially in so-called "good responders," the number of growing follicles is so high—and the rise of serum estrogen levels is so alarming—that a high risk of ovarian hyperstimulation syndrome (OHSS) is perceived, several days short of anticipated follicle maturity. One understandable response on the part of the physician is to considerably reduce the dose of FSH. If this reduced dose lasts more than a day or two there is the risk that all the follicles other than the largest will commence the process of **atresia**, critically deprived of support, offering (at egg pickup) oocytes that are no longer optimal or that might have become lost within the follicle.

• Ovulation itself may have been triggered (by injection of hCG) too soon or too late in the follicular phase for the particular follicle(s) concerned, resulting respectively in eggs that were substantially immature or substantially overmature at the time the hCG was given. It can be difficult to distinguish these states on the appearance of the recovered eggs in the laboratory or to distinguish them from the aged eggs described in the next paragraph.

• The recovered eggs, especially in a relatively "poor responder" with few follicles, may inherently fail to metabolize energy efficiently enough to carry them through **fertilization**, **cleavage**, **implantation** and formation of a healthy **fetus**. This is a manifestation of the effect of age in the woman and is thought possibly to be the result of increasingly faulty **mitochondria** in either the eggs or the granulosa cells (see the box " How Eggs Get Their 'Use-by' Date: Mishaps in the Mitochondria" in Chapter 7).

traditional way of aspirating the follicles and collecting the eggs was by lap aroscopy. (It was Dr. Patrick Steptoe's special expertise with laparoscopy in th late 1960s that led the Cambridge embryologist Dr. Robert Edwards to sugge to him the idea of collaborating to develop IVF in humans.) Nowadays we a most always do the egg pickup through the vagina, guided by ultrasound (see Figure 20.1), usually with just mild sedation and local anesthesia. In this way we developed Australia's first ambulatory care IVF program in 1986 at Royal Prince Alfred Hospital in Sydney.

Follicle aspiration for ultrasound GIFT or IVF is thus carried out during a vaginal examination while the patient is awake. The sedation is administered to take some of the anxiety out of the procedure. The ovaries will be scanned by ultrasound, as during the monitoring of ovarian stimulation programs. Local anesthetic will be inserted through the wall of the vagina around the ovaries, and the follicle or follicles will then be aspirated using a needle passed through the wall of the vagina beside the cervix, into the ovary. All that is generally felt during the procedure is some pressure on the ovary, followed by an ache that subsides. About one in 20 women experience considerable pain, however, so it is best to have the option available of general anesthesia. There is often a small amount of bleeding from the wall of the vagina. After the procedure the patient will spend a short time resting. Although the patient will not generally have been anesthetized, the use of sedation means arrangements should be made for someone to accompany the patient home.

# What Can Go Wrong with IVF?

A few things can go wrong with IVF. First, there is the hazard of ovarian hyperstimulation syndrome (see Chapter 11). Second, fertilization may fail, and the reason may lie with the sperm or with the egg.

Apart from not getting pregnant in any particular cycle, and apart from the hazards of multiple-ovulation induction (see Chapter 11), there are, as with GIFT, a number of hazards with IVF should pregnancy occur. First, there is the chance of a miscarriage or even an ectopic pregnancy; if the embryo drifts out of the uterine cavity into an abnormal tube it may not return to the uterus (see Chapter 14). Second, there is the chance of a multiple pregnancy; the risk of twins with three embryos transferred is about 20 percent and the risk of triplets about 5 percent. Third, there is the chance of **premature labor**; even with a single fetus the risk of going into labor early is increased, for reasons that are still obscure. An IVF pregnancy should always be regarded as at risk and the patient should be cared for by an obstetrician aware of its special nature (see Chapter 23).

# Fertilization by Sperm Microinjection

Sperm microinjection (SMI) is a method of in vitro fertilization that puts on
minimal demands on the number of sperm available and their motility. It is us
ful when there is an absence of fertilization with conventional IVF, either b
cause of problems with low sperm numbers or low sperm motility, or becau
of other barriers to the fertilization process, such as sperm antibodies.

## Where to Put the Sperm?

In conventional IVF, about 50,000 to 100,000 motile sperm are left in a sma
dish with the eggs. The eggs are surrounded by a glassy membrane called th
zona pellucida. Outside this there is a mucus-like layer that consists of cells d
rived from the follicle; this sticky layer is the cumulus, and its overall dimensio
give the **cumulus mass** a width about 10 times the diameter of the egg. It is the
layers that sperm need to get through to reach the egg with ordinary IVF. It
overcoming these layers that microinjection—manipulating the sperm at a m
croscopic level—or "micromanipulation" seeks to do (see Figure 20.3).

Before 1992 the sperm cell membrane was thought to have to merge wit
the egg cell membrane during microinjection. The sperm cells were injecte
through the zona pellucida, into the space immediately round the egg, th
**perivitelline space** (see Figure 20.3a)—a sperm microinjection technique calle
**subzonal insertion** (SUZI). Fertilization then took place normally. The bic
chemical process by which the egg cell takes the sperm head apart and reassem
bles its **chromosomes** (and hence its genes) happens in the normal way.

Until 1993 pregnancies from sperm microinjection around the world wei
relatively few. The first baby born was in Singapore in 1988. In 1990 there wei
two babies born in our program in Sydney and two in England, in an IVF pro
gram led by the British scientist Simon Fishel. In 1991 at Sydney IVF we ha
seven pregnancies from 59 cycles (12 percent), in 41 of which there was at lea
one embryo to transfer; there was also one pregnancy from a microinjected eg
that had been frozen, stored and thawed.

The situation has changed much for the better, with the advent in Belgiu
in 1992 of a sperm microinjection technique called **intracytoplasmic sperm i**
**jection** (ICSI, or sometimes **insertion**). In the ICSI procedure, a single sperm
injected all the way into the **cytoplasm** of the egg itself (see Figure 20.3b

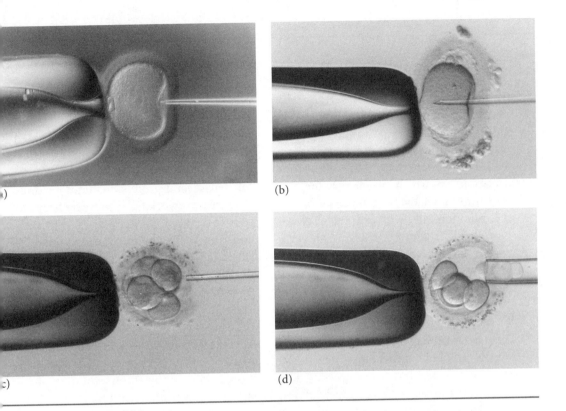

(b)

(d)

**Figure 20.3** Micromanipulation of eggs and pre-embryos. Sperm microinjection into the space around the egg (a) is called subzonal insertion, or SUZI. The technique has now been discarded. Sperm microinjection into the egg itself (b) is called intracytoplasmic sperm insertion, or ICSI. The zona pellucida around a pre-embryo is opened (c), either for assisted hatching or to enable pre-embryo microbiopsy. In a pre-embryo microbiopsy (d) one or two cells are taken from the pre-embryo to make a genetic diagnosis (referred to as preimplantational diagnosis). (Photos by Rosemarie Cullinan and Kylie de Boer, Sydney IVF.)

Success rates have more than tripled from sperm microinjection using ICSI at Sydney IVF and in many other programs. More than half the eggs we obtain will, with ICSI, be fertilized successfully, even with desperately low sperm counts. A quiet revolution in overcoming male-related infertility is going on around the world.

Only about 25 percent of the eggs we used to obtain at Sydney IVF would fertilize with sperm microinjection (SMI) using SUZI; not uncommonly, all eggs would fail to fertilize. For a practical chance of success we needed to get more than 10 eggs at the time of egg pickup, which meant that the wife needed to be relatively young. The barrier to fertilization rates with SMI by SUZI was the unpredictability of achieving an **acrosome reaction** for the sperm selected for injection (see Chapter 3), because without it the sperm cannot bind to the egg.

*You Would Prefer ICSI ...*

The need for the acrosome reaction, however, is probably unnecessary when the sperm is injected into the egg itself. The powerful disassembly machinery of the egg does not seem to be put off by acrosomes. Fertilization rates of mature eggs at Sydney IVF, with single sperm cells, including immature ones obtained from the testis itself, is now over 50 percent, an astonishing success story for intracytoplasmic sperm insertion. The final chapter on ICSI is still to be written. Many pregnancies have been achieved for the wives of men with blockages of the **epididymis** or the **vas deferens**—congenital blockages present from birth, infective blockages and blockages from vasectomy operations for sterilization—using sperm obtained from **microepididymal sperm aspiration** (MESA). The technique seems so powerful that several groups, including Sydney IVF, are now working at securing fertilization from men with severe oligospermia and even **azoospermia** by using immature sperm cells from the testis itself, a procedure known as **testicular sperm extraction** (TESE).

*...but Still Be Cautious*

In Chapter 9 we consider in detail the genetic conditions in men that might be passed on with these powerful ways of assisting conception, including **cystic fibrosis,** perhaps **congenital abnormalities** of the male genitalia and hereditary oligospermia. In addition, a small proportion of offspring may have an **aneuploidy** of the sex chromosomes.

More babies need to be born, and children followed through childhood, before we can be as secure with this form of IVF as we are now with IVF of the more established kind.

## How to Select the Sperm?

Experience has shown that the genetic makeup of sperm cells is not related to the sperm's motility. The presence of normal genes in the sperm cell seems to be more closely related to sperm shape than to sperm motility, although even with abnormal-looking sperm it seems the chromosomes are often still normal, but it is sperm motility that is most important for the sperm to get to the egg to fertilize it. The sperm cell for microinjection is therefore selected mainly on the basis of its normal shape and size. Some motility is also needed (it shows that the particular sperm is not dead).

# Embryo Transfer

With successful fertilization, the resulting pre-embryos can in principle be transferred the next day, when they are at the stage of a **zygote**, or later, while they are in stages of **cleavage**. There are three potential places to which the embryo can be transferred. The endometrial cavity is the commonest. Zygotes or day 2-cleaving embryos can be transferred to the fallopian tube (if it is not blocked). Later-cleaving embryos might one day be transferred directly into the endometrium itself, the "endometrial submucosa" (see Chapter 23).

## Uterine Transfer

When the eggs have been fertilized, we wait two to three days and then transfer up to three of the (cleaving) embryos back to the uterus. Such an **embryo transfer** is straightforward and painless. A fine plastic catheter that has been loaded with the embryos is passed through the cervix into the uterus. At Sydney IVF ultrasound is used to make sure that the embryo transfer catheter is positioned correctly in the endometrial cavity before the embryos are expelled.

## Zygote Intrafallopian Transfer

When IVF is to be used and at least one fallopian tube is normal, it might be an advantage to make use of the tube, even though the eggs have been fertilized in the laboratory. The reason is that fertilized eggs are normally in the tube for three days or so before traveling down to the uterus (see Chapter 3). During this time, therefore, eggs fertilized by IVF can be transferred to the tubes, either by laparoscopy or by an ultrasound-guided catheter (see the box "Ultrasound GIFT").

At Sydney IVF we have long favored GIFT and ZIFT when the fallopian tubes are normal. We still do. The medical directors of many very good IVF centers, however, are not convinced that GIFT, ZIFT, PROST, TEST and so on, even during laparoscopy rather than during ultrasound, increase the pregnancy rate overall in comparison with careful IVF and transfer of embryos direct to the uterus. They only offer IVF with direct transfer of embryos, two or three days later, through the cervix into the uterus. Their results can be very good indeed.

One recent study, published by Dr. Margo Fluker and colleagues from Vancouver, Canada, in the U.S. journal *Fertility and Sterility,* showed that direct uterine transfers were better, in these doctors' hands, than laparoscopic transfers to the tubes. My problem with this paper was not with their uterine transfer results, but with the extremely poor laparoscopic transfer results. I wonder if their embryos somehow had been jeopardized en route from the IVF lab to the operating room, or perhaps whether their transfers to the tube were as accurate as they could be. One reason that we at Sydney IVF continue to favor transfers to the tube when the tubes are normal, apart from our good results with it, is that transferring embryos deep into the tubes seems generally more secure than a catheter that has to negotiate the cervix. Ultimately, what is important is for your physician and your IVF center to do what brings about the best results for them—and thus for you.

The variations that are possible for transferring embryos go by a number of acronyms, including ZIFT (**zygote intrafallopian transfer**). Others know it as PROST (**pronuclear-stage transfer**) for transfers of fertilized eggs that have not yet divided and TEST (**tubal embryo-stage transfer**) for pre-embryos at the two-cell or four-cell stage. These procedures are only possible when the tubes are normal. They are more expensive to carry out than straightforward GIFT and IVF procedures but generally carry pregnancy rates similar to GIFT, even though IVF has been used to obtain the embryos. They are chosen instead of GIFT when sperm function is doubtful.

## What Is the Chance of Success with IVF?

The chance of pregnancy varies tremendously according to the clinical circumstances (see Appendix B). In addition to age, much depends on the sperm count

## Clinics with Unusually High IVF Pregnancy Rates

Some IVF centers consistently report high success rates with IVF—pregnancy rates well over 30 percent per cycle of treatment. These programs are obviously technically excellent. But before ranking such programs in their own, high echelon of achievement (and possibly paying a premium for their services), it can be instructive to take into account the policies the clinic follows with regard to a number of variables, one or more of which may turn out to be a disadvantage in your personal circumstances.

• Does the clinic offer GIFT? If not, a greater proportion of their IVF patients will have relatively fewer reproductive abnormalities, but this is not in itself a reason to not choose the clinic.

• Do they cancel a relatively high proportion of their IVF cycles? To keep their statistics looking good, cycles may be peremptorily canceled if, for example, estrogen levels show a limited rise in response to stimulation with FSH and fewer eggs are likely to be obtained than would be optimal (patients classified as "poor responders"). At Sydney IVF we never cancel a cycle unless at the request of the couple, because stimulation will not often turn out to be better a second time around. In 1992 the overall cancellation rate for assisted conception cycles at Sydney IVF was 3 percent.

• What is the average age of the women being treated? Results will be better if the average age is less than 35 years. The clinic may arbitrarily set a cutoff age.

• How many of the patients' cycles were first or second cycles? The average pregnancy rate at a good clinic will fall as more and more of their treatments are patients who have been treated before, perhaps somewhere else, without pregnancy, and who thus are increasingly likely to have low intrinsic fertility (this phenomenon of "self selection" for low fertility is described in Appendix A).

• How many embryos are transferred at once? Generally the greater the number, the greater the chance of pregnancy. Most European countries, as well as Australia, limit by voluntary rules or compulsory regulation the number of embryos transferred at any one time to two or three. In some programs in the United States and Asia, transferring up to six embryos at once is not uncommon. The transfer of high numbers of embryos decreases the **risk** of not getting pregnant in what, of course, can be a very expensive form of treatment, but it also increases the risk and aggravates the **hazard** of higher-number multiple pregnancy (see Chapter 9).

## Hydrosalpinx: Reintroducing a Villain

We met the hydrosalpinx in the box "Salpinx, Hydrosalpinx and Pyosalpinx" in Chapter 12. Whether present on one side or both sides, a hydrosalpinx spells trouble for getting pregnant— naturally or with IVF. The reason is complicated but important. A hydrosalpinx forms when a tube, damaged from **salpingitis**, becomes blocked at the outer, fimbrial end, close to ovary. Most hydrosalpinges, however, are not blocked at the inner, uterine end and remain in direct communication with the cavity of the uterus, the endometrial cavity. The **isthmus** of the hydrosalpinx is still open, as is the isthmus of a normal tube.

So what? Well, the problem starts when the follicles in the ovary start producing estradiol, either naturally or with ovarian stimulation. Estradiol from the ovaries causes the isthmus of the fallopian tube to become (temporarily) occluded (see Chapter 3). Meanwhile, estradiol stimulates the hydrosalpinx to fill up with even more watery fluid. Ovulation—or follicle aspiration for egg pickup—then takes place and the empty follicle starts to produce progesterone. Progesterone prepares the uterus for pregnancy in many ways. One of these ways, in normal circumstances, is to cause the isthmus to relax, admitting the pre-embryo, previously with its transport held up at the ampullary-isthmic junction, to the uterus, about three days after ovulation and fertil-ization (and the same time that is chosen in IVF programs to deliver IVF embryos to the uterus through the cervix).

The villainy occurs because it is this precise time, when embryos are floating free in the cavity of the uterus, waiting for the endometrium on each side to press down on it in anticipation of implantation, that the fluid from a hydrosalpinx comes splashing down through the endometrial cavity, inevitably posing a major threat to successful implantation. Pregnancy is lucky not to fail completely. Miscarriage is common among the implantations that survive the onslaught.

### What to Do About It?

At the least, the appearance of a previously unknown hydrosalpinx during ultrasound monitoring should mean emptying the hydrosalpinx at the same time (and in the same way) that the fluid is collected from the follicles to obtain the eggs. Then, a few days later, immediately before the embryos are transferred, if fluid is seen on ultrasound to have reaccumulated, the hydrosalpinx is aspirated again. We have seen pregnancy follow this sequence at Sydney IVF in a woman who had a number of previously unsuccessful IVF treatments. In the longer term, other options include removing the offending tube or tubes (**salpingectomy**), opening the tube with a microsurgical **salpingostomy**, or placing a clip on the isthmus (see Chapter 12).

and whether or not a high proportion of the eggs fertilize. We have had several pregnancies when only one embryo has been available for transfer, but we aim to transfer two or three embryos.

At Sydney IVF in 1988, the overall chance of clinical pregnancy with IVF and transfer of up to three embryos to the uterus varied in different months from 10 to 18 percent per cycle, and the statistics have not changed a great deal since. When there are four or more embryos to choose from for transfer in women under 39 years, the pregnancy rate is about 25 percent. Pregnancy rates for ZIFT have been higher, comparable to GIFT. Provided that the number of eggs is good and that they tend to fertilize, the key to success with IVF is to repeat it. It is best to give yourself more than just one or two chances for it to work.

Although IVF was developed to treat blocked tubes, there is one kind of abnormality of the tube that reduces considerably the chance of success with IVF. A significant number of such patients among an IVF clinic's clientele will hold down success rates considerably despite excellent laboratory practices (see the box "Hydrosalpinx: Reintroducing a Villain").

# Women Over 40

The chance of pregnancy, both in natural circumstances and with assisted conception techniques, falls rather quickly from the age of about 39. The chance of miscarriage also rises sharply among conceptions that do occur, and from the age of 42 more pregnancies miscarry than go to term, with natural conception or with assisted conception. The barrier to successful assisted conception is the nature of the woman's eggs. All of the eggs in the ovaries are formed before birth (see Chapter 3); after age 40 or older, many of the eggs will have abnormalities of the chromosomes or the mitochondria. The association between a pregnant woman's age and the risk of a fetal abnormality of the chromosomes, such as **Down's syndrome**, is well known. Although there are tests available to diagnose Down's syndrome in early pregnancy (**chorionic villus sampling** at about nine weeks or **amniocentesis** at about 15 weeks), remember that it is usual to transfer three eggs or embryos, so there is a risk that a pregnancy may be multiple, with one or more normal fetuses coexisting with an abnormal one. There is no satisfactory solution to this dilemma (one form of treatment, **fetal reduction**, is discussed briefly in the Glossary). Chapter 22 describes the use of embryo biopsy to make a diagnosis of trisomy 21 and other chromosomal abnormalities among pre-embryos while still in the laboratory.

Sydney IVF, like many clinics, has no arbitrary policies that include or exclude any age group from assisted conception technology. The actual probability of conceiving is best seen in the data on GIFT and IVF in Tables B.1 and B.2 Appendix B, which summarize the pregnancy experiences of women who co ceived with IVF and GIFT in the United States and Australia. It is ultimately t woman's decision, taking into account the medical advice she gets from her do tor. Although there may be peace of mind to be had from having tried IVF GIFT, there are reasons to be circumspect about embarking on assisted concep tion if you are a woman in her forties.

One novel way around the difficulties of older eggs—although easier sa than done—is to use eggs donated from a younger woman. Egg donation, well as embryo donation, sperm donation and surrogacy, are described in th Chapter 22.

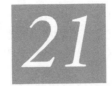

# 21

# Embryo Cryostorage

Professor Alan Trounson, working at the Centre for Early Human Deve opment at Monash University in Melbourne, started work in 1981 on stori animal embryos fertilized **in vitro** at extremely low temperatures (**cryostorag** He reported the first human pregnancy from a cooled, then stored, th warmed embryo in 1983. We know now that the risk of **miscarriage**, stillbir and birth defects is no higher with pregnancies established from transfer frozen-thawed embryos than is the case with transfer of fresh embryos. Embr "banking" is today indispensable in making reproductive technology as effecti as possible for infertile couples having **in vitro fertilization** (IVF).

# Freezing Embryos

Ordinarily, lowering the temperature of human tissues much below zero degree causes freezing. Ice crystals form and they damage structures within the cell The damage is irreparable. When thawed, the cells do not survive. Successf cryostorage of embryos has made use of "cryoprotectants," which are substanc

## Nature's Antifreeze

Many species of invertebrates—and, among the vertebrates, several species of frogs and at least one reptile—use dissolved substances of low molecular weight, such as glycerol and glucose, to survive repeated freezing and thawing of their natural, arctic habitats. We use similar chemicals in the laboratory to enable embryos to be cooled to extremely low temperatures and "cryostored."

Human embryos have been successfully vitrified and thawed, with resultant pregnancy, using three main cryoprotectants: dimethyl sulfoxide (DMSO), the substance first used by Dr. Trounson; 1,2-propanediol, which in most IVF centers has produced the best rates of embryo survival, and glycerol, which is nature's usual cryoprotectant in the invertebrate species, but which works for human embryos only at the more advanced stage of **blastocyst**. The pre-embryos are stored in liquid nitrogen.

that in high concentration cause solutions to become viscous and to solidify at low temperatures in such a way that ice formation does not take place (see the box "Nature's Antifreeze").

# Why Consider Cryostorage?

The main reason for cryostoring embryos is to reduce the need to stimulate the ovaries repeatedly, especially in young patients who produce large numbers of follicles and eggs in a conventional cycle of assisted conception. Usually an IVF or GIFT cycle will result in a number of apparently healthy pre-embryos in addition to the pre-embryos or eggs transferred in the particular cycle, which are then cryostored. If pregnancy occurs in the stimulated cycle, the embryos can be kept several years (or longer) for attempting a further pregnancy. If we predict a substantial risk of **ovarian hyperstimulation syndrome** (OHSS), then all embryos produced from an ovarian stimulation can be cryostored, with no further injections of **human chorionic gonadotropin** (hCG), and with no chance of more hCG from the pregnancy itself continuing to stimulate, possibly dangerously, the ovaries (see Chapter 11 for possible complications of ovarian stimulation).

# What Are the Dangers of Cryostorage?

Prior to the stage of transfer to the uterus, the pre-embryo's cells are "totipotent," in other words, each individual cell of the fertilized egg retains the same ability to develop into a complete embryo—a fetus with all its supporting membranes. Theoretically, therefore, if a four-cell pre-embryo is cooled and thawed, only one cell needs to survive for a normal embryo to result. Experience has shown that survival of cells is recognizable under the microscope. Pre-embryos with a high proportion (sometimes *all*, occasionally just *one*) of the cells visibly normal after thawing are selected for transfer to the uterus. Not all cells or pre-embryos survive cooling and warming. Information accumulated by the National Perinatal Statistics Unit in Australia has shown no harmful difference in the outcomes of IVF pregnancies after cryostorage of pre-

The National Health and Medical Research Council in Australia issued the following statement in 1983 (the sentiments are general and probably still hold up today): "Having accepted embryo freezing and thawing in principle, there is no time beyond which the maintenance of the embryo in the cryostored state becomes logically and unequivocally unethical. Yet, with time, the consequences are likely to become increasingly distasteful to the community. There will also be legal problems, such as questions of property, inheritance, and control over the use of and liability for loss of the embryos—any of which may increase with time. Arguments in favor of an agreed limitation thus become very strong. It would be undesirable for embryos to be stored beyond the time of reproductive need or competence of the female donor; embryos that have not been implanted should ordinarily be destroyed and discarded ten years after freezing, or earlier should the donor(s) wish it or circumstances compel it."

embryos, and this appears to be true even when some cells survive and others do not.

## Transferring Thawed Embryos

Thawed embryos can be transferred to the uterus either in a natural cycle (in which the midcycle **LH surge** is looked for and the embryos are transferred back three to four days afterward—to either the tubes or the uterus) or in a cycle in which we have complete control over the **endometrium** by the sequential administration of estrogen then **progesterone**. The chance of these cryostored embryos implanting successfully and leading to pregnancy is at least as good as it is with fresh, unfrozen embryos.

22

# Donation and Surrogacy

Our society loves children. We place a high premium on being a parent. But society is still ambivalent about creating families in ways that are not traditional. In Chapter 27, I question just how "traditional" today's nuclear family really is, but it only takes a generation or two of a certain kind of family structure to prevail in the community for people to regard it as being not just normal, but best.

People can understand and accept more easily those things that are familiar or they have experienced. And because most people have not had to face the crisis of infertility, and thus have little appreciation of the infertile couple's plight, they will not easily appreciate that children can, in fact, be brought up stable and healthy in a very wide variety of family structures. It is infertile couples, those without the luxury of having a choice, who are thus naturally in the vanguard in exploring the help—the "surrogacy"—others can provide by donating their sperm, eggs or embryos or their capacity to carry a pregnancy and have a baby for someone else.

To guide my way in this difficult moral and ethical field, I have lately found it most useful to consider how each and every person involved can *suffer*, and then how to make sure they are protected, rather than try to work from rather impersonal notions of people's rights and obligations.

# Sperm Donation

When a man's fertility fails because of a low sperm count, the personal consequences are complicated and sad. **Impotence** (usually temporary), loss of self-esteem and social withdrawal are common among husbands; anger, guilt and a wish to make amends are common among wives. More and more, the couple will turn to doctors who can use reproductive technology, such as **in vitro fertilization** (IVF) with **intracytoplasmic sperm insertion** (ICSI) before they accept **donor insemination** (DI). This technology is often at or past the limit of what is medically practicable and financially affordable.

## Secrecy

Of the several people involved in any case of DI, it is the infertile husband, more often than not, for whom maintaining secrecy is the most important. This is more so in some cultures than in others. For example, enlisting the help of a brother as sperm donor is an option generally rejected in favor of maintaining secrecy in the United States, where modern family structures are nuclear and insular. Among Indian Hindus, however, where more open and extended family networks persist, a brother's fraternal semen donation is an option often favored on genetic and cultural grounds. In Western societies, anonymous donor sperm banks have replaced acceptance of infertility, adoption, prudent adultery and divorce as the ways in which a woman might adjust to her partner's sterility.

The ostensible reason for sperm donors to be anonymous is the need to protect the social father, the recipient woman and the child from the embarrassment of acknowledging—and somehow having to include—the child's genetic father in their world. Many Western countries have now enacted laws whereby the social father, after a birth resulting from DI, is recorded as the legal and only father on the birth certificate.

But we as DI professionals also have a duty to sperm donors, many of whom in surveys have said they are willing to be approached by their DI offspring, even though their recruitment as donors has taken place with the expectation and promise of being anonymous.

## Genetic Paternity: Do We Tell the Child?

One of the lessons we have learned from the practice of adoption is that accidental discovery by an adolescent of his or her true genetic origins is too serious a hazard to allow even a small chance of happening inadvertently. Such a discovery means that the qualities most expected by a child of its parents, namely openness and truthfulness, will have been assumed mistakenly—a dreadful revelation, whatever the child's age. The same should be true of children from DI.

In time, a more sensitive and sensible approach to genetic parenting that eschews secrecy will probably prevail, but in the meantime, the first social experiment in removing secrecy from sperm donation has not been encouraging. Since 1985 legislation in Sweden has demanded openness concerning the identity of sperm donors to recipients. Despite predictions that donors would be frightened off by being known, it seems instead that men with different motives are volunteering to be sperm donors. The decline in DI in Sweden seems instead to be attributable more to the couple's wish for secrecy—abetted by traditional doctors—than to the donor's wish for secrecy. Dr. Mats Ahlgren, a colleague from Stockholm, Sweden, tells me that couples are advised by their doctors to travel to Denmark or Norway for the sake of donors remaining anonymous. But it is the husbands who probably feel most comforted by the

## What Sperm Donors Think

The apparent motives of sperm donors in donating their semen varies with the prevalent methods used in the community to recruit the donors. If donors are paid well (the United States is the one country where sperm donation is overtly commercial), most donors will at least seem to have donated for the money. Outside the United States, sperm donation has mainly been an altruistic activity, with reimbursement of costs common and only impoverished donors, such as students, thinking it is lucrative. Nevertheless, a small financial reimbursement seems to have a facilitatory effect, justifying or neutralizing an act that may seem otherwise a bit too self-consciously altruistic. The attitude donors have toward remaining anonymous to their unknown offspring may, in fact, not be very different between paid and altruistic donors.

The nonfinancial motives recorded among sperm donors include personal knowledge of and sympathy for infertile couples, and, especially among unmarried donors, a general desire to father a child or to pass on genes; sometimes donors are simply curious about their own fertility. Unless they are screened, sperm donors will include homosexual men. In France, where DI is coordinated nationally through the Federation Française des Centres d'Etudes et de Conservation du Sperme Humain (CECOS),

only men who are fathers are eligible to be sperm donors, a restriction that excludes well-motivated single men who want to be donors because they have no other hope of securing genetic descendants.

A curious phenomenon is alluded to by the results of one Australian study. Associate Professor Robyn Rowland of the Deakin University Department of Women's Studies, at an earlier stage of her career, found that the majority of donors who already had children were separated from their wives at the time they became sperm donors. From other sources we know that most marital separations in Australia are initiated by the wife, who more often than not receives custody of the children. It seems that in some way the men feel they are getting even. The French experience with married donors also mentions semen donation as "balm for a wounded ego." There may, therefore, be an element of compensation, spite or revenge for some sperm donors. In Dr. Rowland's study, a third of donors still living with a female partner had not told her and did not intend to do so. Otherwise, however, secrecy is not much of an issue for most sperm donors. Ken Daniels, a professor of social work at the University of Canterbury in Christchurch, reviewed donors in six New Zealand DI programs in the 1980s and found that 89 percent of donors had told other people of their involvement in sperm donation.

## What Sperm Donors Think (concluded)

Irrespective of the main motive for donating sperm, studies in all countries where sperm donation is accepted reveal that donors show great interest in providing useful information on their personal and professional characteristics—information beyond the physical features that form the usual basis for matching donor with intended social father. There is also a complementary interest among sperm recipients to know more than just the medical and physical features of the sperm donor. In our own DI program at Royal Prince Alfred Hospital in Sydney, we invite donors to write a paragraph or two to their anonymous offspring, a device that is more and more popular among donors and recipients alike.

The high level of curiosity donors show in the outcome of their donations is still not often rewarded by much information about what has happened. In 1975 Dr. R. Schoysman, of the Brugmann University Hospital in Brussels, Belgium, argued that "there is no reason whatsoever that he [the donor] should know the result," and that donors whose own children had tragically died would be "troubled by the fact that somewhere there is another child alive." I believe that the opposite might more often be true, that men may receive comfort or gratification from the knowledge.

Times have changed since 1975, but donors are still mostly told nothing, unless a **congenital abnormality** or an inherited disease appears among the offspring, information that can be medically important to the donor. Nowadays there is more and more support for retaining identifying information of donors, even if it is not used.

Curiously, in discussions of donors meeting "their child," it is usual to refer to the offspring in the singular, in parallel, presumably, with the experience of an adopted individual seeking out his or her parents. But five or six such children are not unusual for a sperm donor, in addition to his own natural ones. Whether or not they all will want to make contact with their genetic father is beside the point; just knowing that there are so many children about may itself be worrying. The student who goes through medical school selling his sperm repeatedly may come to regret the folly of his genetic excess.

We need to develop more respect for sperm donors. Such new respect should have one immediate consequence, namely to limit the number of pregnancies attributable to each donor, or at minimum we should be asking donors how many anonymous offspring they would be happy with. This principle is not new, but the reason for the limit has generally been to reduce the chance of inadvertent inbreeding (consanguinity) should any of the donor's children happen to marry.

Even if the chance, or **risk**, of inadvertently disclosing a DI child's true genetic paternity is small, the penalty, or **hazard**, is great. (For a discussion on the difference between risk and hazard, see the box "Risks and Hazards" in Chapter 9). Remember that today's DI children will be adults at a time when genetic testing for heritable vulnerability to disease may be common. The risk of accidental discovery can only increase.

Meanwhile, the anecdotal experience that social workers are gaining from meetings between genetic parents and their adopted-out offspring is shifting prevailing opinion away from the notion that behavior and personality are mainly determined culturally; more and more, they recognize the importance of genetic influences. This is a change from the emphasis placed on "nurture" over "nature" in most university courses in the social sciences up to the most recent of times. Such a move toward appreciating genetic determinants of behavior, more and more evident elsewhere, will increase the desire of DI recipients to know more about sperm donors. It should also sharpen our duty to inform the providers of sperm about the outcome of their donations.

anonymity. Inquiries made there by Dr. Daniels show that there is no shortage of donors happy to be identified.

## The DI Recipient

For the recipient couple, DI is a considerable challenge to the nature of their marriage. The infertile woman generally accepts the idea of DI faster than her husband, although in my medical practice I sometimes hear descriptions of disquiet by a patient about the thought of a stranger's sperm coursing through her body. The normal, social matter of choosing a genetic mate is effectively annulled; instead, with anonymous sperm banks, the reproductive choice passes to someone else.

For the infertile husband, the start of DI for his wife demands an acknowledgment of loss—a genetic dead end. The lasting importance of such a biological loss will depend on his ideas of social and genetic fatherhood, the supportive (or otherwise) attitude of his wife and friends and, probably least but

As embryo freezing programs have developed (see Chapter 21), fewer and fewer eggs obtained during IVF cycles are available for egg donation. Thus, egg donation is more and more likely to come from a donor who undergoes **ovarian stimulation** and **follicle aspiration** just for the donation, and who is usually known to (indeed is often very close to) the woman who receives the eggs.

This development, together with the risks of semen-mediated diseases and the general trend away from genetic secrecy, has caused patients and health care professionals, including doctors, to question why sperm donors should be anonymous, especially for patients from societies where extended family structures are common and where brothers as semen donors are morally preferable to strangers, and where we can recognize that more harm will come from sex between wife and husband's brother than from medically assisted insemination. Many people in Western societies are also realizing that loosening the idea of the nuclear family to allow a greater role for close relations and friends in forming functioning families is a sociological approach worth exploring.

### Pay for Attractive Sperm

There are commercial sperm banks in several countries, but only in the United States, with its strong national philosophy of pragmatism, is the sale of sperm for reproductive ends an industry. Doctors can order semen through the mail for their infertile patients matched to order by physical and other attributes. Prepared semen costs about $150 to $250 per 0.5 milliliter. In the United States, the presumption remains strong that buying sperm from a donor also buys off further duties toward the donor. Anonymity seems sacrosanct.

By 1980 a commercial sperm bank had been established where Nobel Prize winners could bequeath their talents widely, if they wished, by selling their semen. At least two sperm banks in California in 1992 specialized in the sale of sperm from gifted men. For example, at the Repository for Germinal Choice, described as a project of the Foundation for the Advancement of Man, approved applicants are given thorough descriptions of each available donor, from which they can make their selection. The price of the sperm depends on the donor's popularity.

nonetheless important, the compassionate approaches taken by the couple's health professionals—nurses, social workers and physicians.

All published studies on the outcome for children born of DI show that they develop physically and mentally as well as or better than their naturally con-

## Virgin Births and Lesbian Motherhood

Like celibate priests, devoted homosexuals and committed virgins have been pushed to the side in transmission of the human gene pool. Now, with **assisted insemination** and someone else's help in providing sperm, the last two of these three groups can bear genetic fruit without either purposefully transgressing their commitment or being blessed with divine intervention (DI Type II!).

Childlessness for an active heterosexual couple of reproductive age is a disability that calls for professional medical help. In his or her professional medical practice, a physician can and should be able to restrict professional obligations to treating medical infertility without venturing into areas of considerable social controversy or moral uneasiness and not be forced into procedures that are against his or her conscience. But assisted insemination itself needs no medical help; masturbation and injection of semen into the vagina allows conception to take place with neither intercourse nor an invoice for professional medical fees. Homosexuals, virgins and others can conceive in this way and have children without sex.

Homosexuals face resistance in the community if they want to become parents. We know that some male homosexuals wish to be sperm donors and many will, unless they are excluded for health reasons by special measures. Because of the risk of transmitting **HIV** infection by DI, many jurisdictions now require the same declaration of a safe "life-style" from prospective sperm donors as they do from blood donors, and homosexual men are in this way prohibited by law from becoming donors (at least when a physician is involved).

Still, the simplicity of self-insemination means that some women who seek pregnancy and children without ordinary sex will turn to homosexual men as sources of semen. As a biosocial phenomenon, it is inevitable. The compassionate doctor concerned about the risk of infection with donations of fresh semen might—if the law allows it—offer sperm banking to quarantine such dedicated semen while the donor

ceived peers. They are healthy, wanted and loved. Their parents, despite their emotional strain and psychological dramas, are less likely than average to separate and divorce.

The anonymous side of DI has been made possible and prevalent by the physical simplicity of getting semen from men. Programs of anonymous egg donation have, in contrast, been slow to develop, relying as they mostly have on spare eggs from women undergoing egg collection for IVF.

## Virgin Births and Lesbian Motherhood (concluded)

is tested serially for the AIDS virus with **serum HIV antibodies**.

Do medical professionals—or does society—have other duties to a virgin's or lesbian woman's desire to reproduce? We often advance the stable mother-father model for the psychological nurture of children, and we hear the refrain "the child's interests must come first" (as if we can anticipate how the child will grow up!). This model is held up as the disqualifying condition for virgins and lesbians. But nowadays it is a fractured model. Whether it is the resilience of children or the resourcefulness of single parents, today there are so many successful departures from the two-parent ideal that the argument that nothing be done to facilitate breaks from this standard is unrealistic and unsympathetic. Just what the difference might be with or without an adult male about the household, and whether it makes a difference if the child without a male role model in the family is a boy or a girl, needs more research.

Ultimately, however, it will be a matter for society to decide whether to apply public resources to such an extension of infertility to accommodate social childlessness; and it will be for individual doctors to accommodate or reject social childlessness as fitting in with their reproductive medical responsibility toward their patients.

The question remains open whether the loneliness of a child brought up by a virgin, with, in some cases, firm ideas of the repulsiveness of sex, can be overcome by his or her peers and education. Such fears may or may not turn out to be well founded.

I have written elsewhere (I admit with some support) about the biology of gay parenthood as a way of increasing the realization of human potential, but I suspect that there is still much to be learned in this area of sociology. Before pushing public policy one way or the other, it would be good to have more evidence on outcomes.

# Egg Donation

For some women, receiving donated eggs is the only way they will get pregnant. Egg donation is needed for women who have no eggs of their own (**primary ovarian failure**; see Chapter 10); for women who have eggs that are genetically unsuitable, such

Because the procedure for obtaining eggs for donation is usually difficult physically, one would expect the emotional compensation and the financial compensation to be greater than for sperm donation—and so it seems to be. A survey of 51 egg-donation programs by Dr. Mark Sauer and Dr. Richard Paulson in the United States showed that 30 of them, or about 60 percent, used only donors designated and introduced by the recipient couples themselves, implying that there was a personally identified sympathy for the infertility of a close relation on the part of the donors. The donors were usually sisters. In the programs that had commercial arrangements in which egg donors were paid, Sauer and Paulson found that the donor's compensation varied from $500 to $2,000 per follicle aspiration procedure. This price lies between that paid for a sperm donation ($50 to $100) and that paid for a surrogate carrying a pregnancy ($10,000 to $15,000).

Paying for eggs can also take a messier form—the discounting of the cost of IVF services for infertile patients who agree to make some of their eggs available for fertilization by a prospective recipient's husband. This practice necessarily puts a doctor in a position of conflicting interests. On the other hand, in at least one center in France, a majority of couples voluntarily and anonymously donate one egg if seven or more eggs are obtained at an IVF egg pickup and donate two eggs when there are more than 10. A study at Hammersmith Hospital in London found that more than 70 percent of women resting after their own embryo transfer would have agreed to donate eggs to infertile recipients, and 51 percent would have approved donation to single women. Women, even more than men, may be willing to be made known to their otherwise anonymous offspring, an observation that makes the 1991 recommendations of Great Britain's then IVF Interim Licensing Authority that egg donation should ordinarily be anonymous look awkward.

But in either case—anonymous or known—egg donors who are themselves infertile risk knowing that another woman may be pregnant while the donor herself remains infertile. This can be disturbing for the donor.

### Pregnancy After Menopause

Recently, considerable controversy came from the use of eggs from younger women, or even from female fetuses, to enable women to get pregnant whose own eggs were long gone. A commercial clinic in Rome, Italy, has since been behind women in their fifties and sixties getting pregnant and becoming mothers, and several U.S. clinics have followed suit. Governments elsewhere have been alarmed enough with this practice to legislate against it, generally using unfortunately simplistic, even arbitrary, logic.

## Commercial Eggs (concluded)

There are good biological grounds for being very cautious about using eggs from the ovaries of fetuses, or even from the ovaries of girls, quite apart from the immensely difficult, often tragic, personal and social circumstances that have led to the ovaries becoming available. In Chapter 3, I described how *all* the eggs in the ovaries are present well before birth and how the great majority of eggs are used up through the process of **atresia** before the first ovulatory menstrual cycle. We must hypothesize, in the absence of evidence to the contrary, that nature is ridding the ovaries of these eggs for a purpose, and that purpose may be that they are in some way defective. Until we know a lot more, many biologists believe we should not be thinking of bringing about pregnancies from such eggs.

Most of us will intuitively feel uncomfortable with the notion that women—particularly just rich women—can buy the opportunity to get pregnant at any stage of their lives. We can approach this issue, as has the popular press, from a number of angles, including the welfare of the intended child, social equity and so on. But the perspective that to me is the most clarifying has received scant attention, perhaps because it is at once more complicated and less emotional.

The key to me of the acceptability or otherwise of young eggs producing pregnancies for older women is to see the event from the perspective of the person who is going to provide the egg—the egg donor. Many of us are happy, in good circumstances, for a well-informed sister or friend of a woman with early menopause to go through an IVF cycle, including stimulation and follicle aspiration for egg pickup, out of affection and concern for the unfortunate woman. This can be an acceptable personal freedom to grant the donor, provided we can be sure that no undue or inappropriate coercion has occurred, and that she and the people important to her are properly informed and counseled—in other words, that they will not end up *suffering*. But can the same ever be true for a woman who is past her own normal menopause? More often than not, her friends will themselves be at or beyond the menopause, too, so for this purpose they will not be useful to her. Her relations, if they are to be young enough to be helpful this way, will most certainly be in some kind of dependent relationship and ought to be disqualified on these grounds (for sure, I would not be a party to a mother asking for egg donation from her daughter). Indeed, the only motive that remains viable is commercial—the payment of money to the donor by the recipient, directly or indirectly, with the doctor as the commissioning broker.

If these principles and existing laws remain firm, and if the matter is seen from the young donor's perspective, pregnancy for women after menopause will continue to be a nonissue for most of us.

as with certain X-chromosome-linked genetic diseases, or for women who ha
eggs that are simply inaccessible (a reason for egg donation in the 1980s b
nowadays almost unheard of because of the advent of transvaginal ultrasoun
for follicle aspiration). In addition, more and more older women, pr
menopausal or postmenopausal, are receiving donated eggs, as it is realized th
the limits to human fertility with age stem from aging of the eggs and not b
cause the uterus is older.

Egg donation, like sperm donation, can be motivated by sympathy for ir
fertile women, whether they are known to the donors or not, or by commerci
payments. Obtaining eggs, unlike sperm donation, is necessarily an intrusiv
operation, although the physical intrusion could just be part of another surg
cal procedure at which the eggs are obtained, and so be more or less incider
tal. Interestingly, most IVF programs involved with egg donation report ver
welcome, if not all that common, requests from healthy, normal women wh
are prepared to undergo an IVF cycle purely so they can donate eggs to an un
known recipient couple; although accounting for only about 10 percent or s
of egg donations, the recipients who benefit can usually be helped by no alter
native method.

There are other ways in which donating eggs is different from donatin
sperm. Whereas new laws have generally been needed to make sure that the so
cial father with DI is also the legal father, the connection between giving birt
and being the legal mother is *not* going to need special legislation. Thus, ther
are no special difficulties with ethical egg donation. But there are difficulties fo
that other most commercial, or most altruistic, of reproductive donations, ges
tational surrogacy.

# Surrogacy

For a woman to get pregnant and then give her embryo, and especially her baby
to an infertile couple is the pinnacle of reproductive generosity, or, in some case
to date, reproductive folly. There is evidence that female donors in general may
feel less ownership of their **gametes** and possibly their offspring than do male
donors. But I should add quickly that women generally have a greater wish than
men to know and to be known by the recipients and, especially when they par
with a baby, to *remain* known and in touch.

Another way of donating an embryo is for a woman to be inseminated with the semen of an infertile woman's husband. The embryo is then washed out of the uterus, just before implantation. The procedure carries medical as well as ethical hazards, including the possibility of pushing the embryo out into the tubes, resulting in an **ectopic pregnancy**. Ethics committees (see Chapter 26) outside the United States have generally not condoned such "womb flushing" for embryo donation. As IVF programs became prevalent in the United States during the 1980s, however, fewer and fewer clinical circumstances required womb flushing for treatment, so the method never became popular. A company that tried to commercialize the treatment—Fertility & Genetics Research, Inc., of Chicago—went broke. There are now no obvious circumstances where egg donation with IVF is not a better alternative for the prospective donor, ethically and medically.

## Embryo Donation and Receipt

We will consider first the situation in which embryos are donated after eggs have been fertilized in vitro, that is, a couple donates spare embryos after their own procreative needs have been met and there is no special physical risk for the woman. Such embryo donation seems to have happened around the world quite often, using (with permission) embryos placed in cryostorage after IVF that become surplus to the couple's own reproductive needs. From the point of view of both genetic parents, however, there are similarities to putting up a baby for adoption. The genetic parents' curiosity and possible wish to stay in touch are essentially unresearched as of 1997—we know very little about the actual outcomes. As with donation of sperm and eggs, recipients may expect more and more interest from embryo donors in being a part of their child's family; and, if the children are told or find out, they can also expect increasing interest from their children in knowing who their genetic parents are.

## Altruistic Surrogacy

It is not a new thing for a woman to conceive and give birth to a baby that she then gives away. (Some Australian Aboriginal communities practice the custom

as a treatment for infertility to this day.) If contact with the child is to be los
no doubt the giving was and is never easy. The custom by which an infertile wi
could "give" her maid to her husband for sexual intercourse and then claim th
child as her own is reported in the Book of Genesis.

Nowadays, however, the surrogate is likely to have been inseminated med
ically. The other modern difference is that it is only rather recently in our his
tory that Western society has developed the legal machinery that reinforces mar
riage and legitimacy of children. This legal framework has developed to th
point where there are now formidable legal obstacles to recognizing someone a
the mother other than the woman who gives birth.

Although altruistic surrogacy is not novel, and it needs no special repro
ductive technology, the surrogate runs the biological hazards of impregnatio
and pregnancy and the emotional hazards of giving up both the product of he
pregnancy and her genes, that is, both her genetic and gestational motherhoo
Throughout history the compensation for the surrogate has come from he
sense of generosity, added to by a continuing association with the child, even
at some distance. But in forecasting the outcome, it is worth recalling tha
Hagar, the surrogate in Genesis, looked with contempt on her infertile mistres
Sarai, who in turn dealt so harshly with Hagar that Hagar had to flee!

# Commercial Surrogacy

In commercial surrogacy, an infertile couple commissions a woman to have
baby for them, usually with the brokerage of a surrogacy agency, which typicall
retains about half of the fee paid. A legal, or hopefully legal, contract is signed
which to a great extent limits the right of the pregnant surrogate to make deci
sions for herself concerning medical and social matters while pregnant (such a
smoking), and, of course, the contract tries to compel her to give up the baby a
delivery. The United States is presently the one country in which the practice o
commercial surrogacy is accepted.

Today at least two forms of surrogacy need to be distinguished. In the first
and in 1997 becoming less common, assisted insemination is used for the surro
gate to get pregnant. The egg, in other words, is the surrogate's own. At the risl
of unfairly diminishing her generosity, she is, in effect, selling her egg first, leas
ing her body for the pregnancy second, and, third, giving up a baby who differs
from one more conventionally "her own" only by her not having chosen a mate
Genetically and biologically the baby is the surrogate's before and after she sells
it. Today this **genetic-plus-gestational surrogacy** is referred to as **traditional**

**surrogacy**. The first such surrogate to try to have her contract overturned in the U.S. courts and keep the baby was Mary Beth Whitehead. She was unsuccessful.

In the second form that surrogacy can take, the surrogate, or gestational carrier, receives an embryo fertilized in vitro using the egg and sperm from the infertile couple. Again perhaps unfairly diminishing her generosity, the surrogate sells the use of her body for its gestational function. This is **gestational surrogacy**. Unarguably the baby is genetically that of the commissioning parents. Unarguably, too, the surrogate mother is the gestational mother. The identity of the "biological" mother is now confused. Because there are few recent examples in society for not regarding the woman who gives birth to the baby as the natural mother, the law in most countries would define the surrogate as the legal mother, at least until the process of adoption transfers guardianship. Nevertheless, in the first such case in the United States in which the gestational mother attempted to have her contract overturned in the courts, the woman, Anna Johnson, like Mary Beth Whitehead before her, was unsuccessful. At the time of this judgment, which was later upheld on appeal, newspapers, if they can be accepted as a pointer to community attitudes, generally appeared content in their commentaries to regard the genetic parents as the biological parents.

## Medically Defendable Surrogacy

It is when the commissioning infertile woman has no uterus or when for some reason pregnancy would be exceptionally dangerous for her that surrogacy remains medically necessary for an infertile couple to secure genetic offspring. The commercial development of genetic-plus-gestational ("traditional") surrogacy in the United States in the 1970s was an alternative to IVF, before IVF became effective and available. In this respect it resembled the ill-fated commercialization in the United States of womb flushing to obtain embryos for sale. The developing practice of egg donation or sale, accompanied by IVF, should in the future diminish the medical need for this form of surrogacy to very low levels.

Several legislatures outside the United States have now started to respond to public opinion, which has consistently favored allowing altruistic surrogacy for valid medical reasons. This move recognizes that when a relative or close friend is agreeable to bearing an IVF baby for a woman without a uterus of her own she is being given the opportunity to be exceptionally generous. In carefully considered circumstances, there is the prospect of benefit for everyone involved—except paternalistic politicians who find the whole business too hot to handle. The legislation that is envisaged will make easier what is known as

The criticism that commercial surrogacy promotes the exploitation of women and infertile couples confuses the messenger (the surrogacy broker) with the message (the need of infertile couples and the readiness of third parties to fill the need). And the fear that commercial surrogacy leads to the "dehumanization of babies" is at odds with history. The interpretation we might give on a couple's commissioning a child from a surrogate when all else has failed is perfectly consistent with the historical trend toward ascribing more and more individual value to children. It is not the child but the autonomous surrogate herself who risks the experience of being "dehumanized"—a paid means to a lonely end. How can we estimate this hapless dehumanization, this suffering by the surrogate?

### The Pound of Flesh

One measure of exploitation in the selling of body parts—whether blood, gametes (sperm or eggs), embryos, babies or body organs—is the size of the broker's commission in relation to his or her efforts and, conversely, how much of the payment reaches the donor. In each case the people who commission the service are likely to be relatively wealthy, the person commissioned relatively poor. It is not clear in any of these cases that what an outsider might call exploitation is particularly important to the people who opt to be commissioned this way. In general, it can be difficult to devise ways of dealing with the problem of exploitation without seeming to want to lock people into poverty. It could be argued that society has an obligation to better the economic position of the potentially exploited to the point where they would not be tempted by the money or be coerced or forced through their personal situation to accept the role. But society has this obligation anyway, and such betterment might simply bring a higher price for the donation. Nonetheless, it was the rising price of wet-nursing that contributed to the decline in

"parental orders," in which a court can order, upon everyone's agreement, that child's birth certificate record the commissioning mother instead of the birt mother. The need for lengthy adoption procedures to complete the surroga arrangement can be overcome in this way.

Just how morally hazardous the practice of commercial surrogacy is, I ex pect, will continue to be revealed. There will be the occasional sad eventuality a baby born with an unexpected abnormality. More often, the hazards and th

## Exploitation and Autonomy (concluded)

popularity of that practice in England 300 years ago.

Society naturally aims to reduce the unfortunate circumstances in which people have little alternative than to sell a part of themselves. In the meantime, making the practice of surrogacy illegal is unlikely to work any better than illegality suppresses prostitution. Worse, it may make it more difficult to police those whose duty it should be to provide fair compensation.

Doing it voluntarily is an essential key to ethical donations of tissue and organs, whether the recipient is personally known to the donor or not and whether or not the donor is paid. But it is clear from the evident distress of Mary Beth Whitehead and Anna Johnson that bearing a child and giving it up, assuming there is no intention to deceive from the beginning, can be very difficult. An agreement to do so is not like other commercial contracts, any more, say, than was Shylock's pound of flesh in *The Merchant of Venice*.

The general unease that something so natural has become so unnatural—the clue to the dehumanizing side of surrogacy—lies not with reproductive technology but with the giving away of a child. It is this loss that is the source of the suffering, and it is the surrogate's suffering that is, or should be, a prime concern. The fact remains that forewarning, payment and notions of autonomy are poor compensation for loneliness and the loss of a baby. This sense of loss will happen often with the rigidity of predominantly commercial surrogacy, in which I predict that an ever-escalating price will need to be paid for privacy (to buy off the gestational mother), in comparison with the usually more flexible circumstances of a surrogacy agreement that from the beginning is more obviously altruistic and retains personal contact between parents, surrogate and child in an extended family. For this is a circumstance that, when carefully planned, has the capacity to achieve lasting personal benefit for everyone concerned.

suffering will, in commercial terms, be revealed by the high price that successful parents will need to pay to keep their privacy from the relinquishing surrogate. Commercial surrogacy will always be limited by the very real suffering the surrogate bears after her separation from the child.

23

# More Help
# on the Way

Progress in medicine is driven by imagination, innovation and research. In the last 20 years, reproductive medicine has depended on scientists, doctors and nurses demonstrating these qualities—a dependency that continues. This chapter looks at the developments in reproductive medicine being actively researched and examines what may be the technological keys to creating, amplifying, preserving or restoring a woman's control over her reproduction when there is infertility and when medical help is sought.

Also in this chapter I discuss storing unfertilized eggs for future reproduction (without having to fertilize them first); using immature eggs from natural cycles, or even from a resting stage, for IVF, avoiding the need for ovarian stimulation and finessing the postponement of reproduction achieved by storing unfertilized eggs; the promises and pitfalls of attempted gender selection, and making genetic diagnoses among embryos before they are transferred. The chapter closes with observations on present attempts to improve the effectiveness of embryo transfer directly into the lining of the uterus.

# Conserving Immature Eggs

Men faced with testis-threatening radiation therapy or drug treatment (for example, for treatment of cancer) can store their sperm cells for later use. All it takes is for a semen sample (or two or three) to reach a reproductive technology laboratory capable of freezing the prepared semen sample in a liquid nitrogen environment. In a procedure only slightly more complicated, such laboratories can also store early pre-embryos (fertilized eggs at the pronuclear stage or at an early stage of **cleavage**). In this case, however, the woman must first receive two weeks of stimulation of the ovaries to bring **follicles** to the point at which mature eggs can be obtained for their fertilization in vitro. Even if the woman has a partner willing to provide the sperm to fertilize her eggs, this wait before eggs can be obtained is often too long for her or her physician to postpone the start of the treatment.

## Unfertilized Egg Freezing

The holy grail in the field of preserving female reproductive potential is to reliably preserve eggs, first, without having to stimulate follicles to the point of ovulation, and, second, without having to fertilize the recovered eggs with sperm

## Poised to Spring

At the time of **ovulation**, the unfertilized egg is a tensioned spring waiting to be sprung. Unlike sperm cells (and fertilized eggs), recently ovulated eggs and eggs obtained from follicles just before ovulation in the ordinary course of IVF are tense with electrophysiological actions waiting to happen. When penetrated by a sperm, there is an electrical impulse that spreads quickly through the egg and initiates coating of the egg with mucus that stops more sperm from getting too close; it completes the second division of **meiosis**; it expels the second **polar body**, and it begins taking apart the sperm head that will change it into the male **pronucleus**, ready to merge with the female pronucleus—the process that ends in **syngamy** (see Chapter 3), by which 46 **chromosomes** are formed by the 23 from the sperm cell and the 23 from the egg cell.

This vulnerable electric state of the egg and the structures called "spindles" that hold the egg's chromosomes in the right place for completing meiosis and for **fertilization** are vulnerable to a fall in temperature. For example, ten minutes for an egg at ordinary lab temperature (say 21° Celsius or 70° Fahrenheit) instead of body temperature (37°C or 98.4°F) is enough to produce irrecoverable disruption to eggs in IVF programs. Melbourne embryologist Deborah Gook has had success with quickly freezing and thawing eggs to preserve these spindles, but many scientists believe the spindles are too delicate. The consequences of disrupting the spindles are producing chromosomal **aneuploidy** too serious for this procedure to be relied on and to become widely used.

before storage. The present emphasis for research is on freezing eggs well before ovulation—well before they acquire the delicate structure and machinery that enables them to receive a sperm cell and complete the process of fertilization (see the box "Poised to Spring" for details).

Resting eggs, in resting **primordial follicles**, may be the most stable of all to freeze. Some programs are freezing "slices" of ovaries, obtained by **biopsy** during **laparoscopy** (and usually packed with primordial follicles), for just this reason. But it is one matter to freeze the tissues, store them and thaw them. This we can do. Postponed for the moment is the question of how to bring the thawed, still-immature eggs to the point at which they can be fertilized. In principle, there are two ways we might try it—developing the follicle and its egg in the laboratory, which is called **in vitro maturation** (IVM) or simply

In experiments involving sheep and mice, Dr. Roger Gosden, working at the Department of Physiology and the Centre for Reproductive Biology in Edinburgh, and Dr. Jill Shaw, of the Centre for Early Human Development in Melbourne, have succeeded in removing pieces of ovary, cutting the tissue into slices two millimeters thick, freezing the slices and then transplanting the tissues back to the same animal some time after that animal—in the course of the experiment—had all other ovarian tissue removed. Ordinarily this should have been the end of ovarian function (and, of course, fertility) for these animals. In the majority of the animals the stored tissue, transferred either under the capsule of the kidney (a very vascular spot) or back to the region where the ovaries had been, was able to regrow and function normally, including ovulating. In some of the animals where the tissue was put back where the ovaries should have been, the animals were fertile.

The development of "ovarian slice freezing" promises the preservation of ovarian follicle function for women faced with a disease or treatment that threatens the survival of their ovaries, such as radiation treatment or chemotherapy for cancer or even **endometriosis**, if it is bad enough to threaten the ovaries. Preserving ovarian follicles at a young age might also become an option for women prescient enough to foresee a long career standing in the way of early pregnancy and family building. Although the numbers of follicles that survive the storage process is just a fraction of those removed, the experiments with sheep show that fertility can follow. With no other method in sight of overcoming the inexorable effects of aging on the ovaries' eggs (see the box "Mishaps in the Mitochondria: How Eggs Get Their 'Use-by' Date" in Chapter 6), banking a small amount of ovary might be a practical form of reproductive insurance.

transplanting the stored ovarian tissue with its primordial follicles intact back into the ovary itself (see the box "Saving Your Ovary for Later"). The principle such egg storage thus depends on is being confident that one or the other of these methods will sooner or later be perfected.

## Developing Eggs from Immature Tertiary Follicles

Take any egg out of its ovarian environment, separate it from its **follicle cells** and it will mature spontaneously. It will complete the first division of meiosis and theoretically at least, be ready to be fertilized. Researchers at Monash IVF in Melbourne have secured such fertilization using IVF techniques on eggs removed from **tertiary follicles** down to just a few millimeters in size. Two women have conceived and had babies from eggs obtained this way. Unlike the same procedure in cows, however, in which veterinary surgeons obtain pregnancy rates of over 60 percent using IVF with eggs from small tertiary follicles, the chance of women getting pregnant this way is still less than 2 percent. The smaller the follicle, the less likely it is that the egg will mature normally—and the more we have to learn about what is needed to get it to a normal, fertilizable stage.

Much more work needs to be done before human IVM from tertiary follicles becomes reliable, but the project is worthwhile and not just for reproductive insurance; it would also be good not to have to stimulate the ovaries for superovulation in assisted conception programs.

Meanwhile, even more work is needed before eggs from primordial follicles will be able to be used reliably after IVM. So far, a normal embryo with a successful birth has been achieved in just one mouse. A better option for primordial follicles after storage seems to be to put them straight back into the animal or person they came from and allow nature to develop the follicles (see the box "Saving Your Ovary for Later").

# Gender and Genetic Selection

As the London weekly magazine *The Economist* has stated: "People are generally free to choose how to bring up their children. If they want to choose their child's sex as well, why not?" The same could be said about choosing whether or not to try and suppress a familial trait considered harmful. And, in both cases, it is not as if people have not tried.

For centuries women and their husbands have visited witch doctors, astrologers and charlatans hoping to control that quintessential matter of chance, whether the next baby will be a boy or a girl. For probably much longer, perhaps since the origins of animal life generally, females have chosen consciously or unconsciously to mate with, and receive sperm from, males they perceive would enhance the fitness of their offspring. All that is really new is that today we are poised to use reproductive technologies that make these choices substantially more effective.

The following describes the present state of the technology that is needed to control gender and to screen embryos for genetic defects. When these technologies are developed to a point of practical usefulness, they *will* becom available, at least in some parts of the world, and people will pay money to see them out.

# From Hocus Pocus to Sperm Cell Sorting for Gender Selection

Since the discovery that the X chromosome is bigger than the Y chromosome scientists and others have tried to exploit the difference by aiming to separat the supposedly heavier X-bearing sperm (destined to form girls) from th supposedly lighter Y-bearing sperm (destined to form boys). To begin with, Y bearing sperm have long been thought to swim faster and thus get to the egg sooner. If you then conduct a race by abstaining from sex until the egg has been ovulated ("late sex"), you should increase the chance of having a boy. On th other hand, if you want a girl, this theory has it that you should have sex wel before ovulation, let the Y-bearing sports jocks run out of steam and the chance are that the slow but steady X-bearing sperm will be fittest by the time the egg appears in the fallopian tube ("early sex"). Landrum Shettles, a gynecologis from Alabama, popularized this principle in the 1970s, adding to the recipe a mildly alkaline vaginal douche (made by dissolving five grams of baking soda in half a liter of water) before intercourse for boy selection or adding a mildly acidic douche (20 milliliters of white vinegar in half a liter of water) before intercourse for girl selection.

Some fantastic results have been claimed for Shettles's method. For example, Dr. Cedric Vear, a family physician from rural New South Wales, reported in the *Medical Journal of Australia* in 1977 a perfect outcome among 10 consecutive couples. For some reason, he stressed the need to avoid frivolity, in order to, as he put it, "[impress] on both parties that the procedure is a scientific exercise and not an emotional or erotic skirmish." What a killjoy! What would he have thought of trying for a boy by holding off having sex until there is a full moon shining through the window then timing a climax to coincide with the crow of a rooster watching from the end of the bed? To be sure, Shettles did advise avoiding orgasm for conceiving a girl. Using the same Shettles methods, and publishing in the *MJA* in 1985, Dr. Barbara Simcock refuted Vear (and Shettles): among 73 women the success rate for choosing daughters was 50 percent; for choosing boys, she concluded that "the use of [a] modified Shettles's method appeared to decrease the delivery of a male child."

The enduring value of Dr. Shettles's work, demonstrated also by those who published both confirmatory and refutatory studies after him, is that, at least in Western countries, consistently more sex-selection-seeking people want girls than want boys. In Dr. Simcock's 1985 study in Sydney, 52 of the 73 couples wanted a girl, compared with just 21 who sought a boy. The same evidence of a preference for seeking females has been reported more recently from Ericsson-associated clinics.

No doubt this preference for girls over boys does not hold true in all parts of the world. In India and China, for example, there is ample evidence that boys are favored to such an extreme degree that abortion of female fetuses and even female infanticide are practiced to favor sons over daughters. Not just feminists are appalled by such brutality. Effective sperm selection would at the very least be preferable to abortion and infanticide, while the social changes come about that, with time, might put an end to what is plainly an extraordinary pressure in these countries to have sons instead of daughters.

More recently, attention has been focused on trying to separate X-bearing sperm from Y-bearing sperm in the laboratory, prior to assisted insemination. Most popular has been passing the sperm cells through a column of the human protein albumin, which was first reported in the British journal *Nature* in 1973 by R. H. Ericsson and others. Dr. Ericsson has since been associated with a number of clinics in the United States, Asia and Great Britain, at which it has been claimed that if couples use their albumin-based sperm cell separation techniques, they will conceive a child of the desired sex with more than the normal approximately 50 percent probability.

Ericsson's method reportedly produced enrichment of Y-bearing sperm. A number of investigators have explored this claim by testing the sperm obtained with a fluorescent dye that stains part of the Y chromosome, using a reliable technique called **fluorescent in situ hybridization** (FISH). Using FISH, investigators in laboratories from South Australia to Barcelona, Spain, have been unable to show significant enrichment for Y-bearing or for X-bearing sperm using albumin separation columns.

In 1989, the U.S. Patent Office granted a patent to the U.S. Department of Agriculture for the technique of sperm-cell sorting to concentrate X-bearing and Y-bearing sperm (in all mammalian species) by using a separation tech nique based on the different DNA content of these cells, and, using a technol ogy called flow cytometric sorting. Cell sorters based on flow cytometry are i wide use in medicine. Blood transfusion services, for example, use them to sep arate the different cells in donated human blood for specific transfusions of re cells (for anemia), white cells (for infections) or platelets (for bleeding).

Dr. Larry Johnson, working at the U.S. Department of Agriculture labora tories in Beltsville, Maryland, successfully adapted cell sorters to deal with th unusual flat shape of sperm cell heads. He stains the cells with a special, non toxic dye called a fluorochrome, which emits light when excited by ultraviole light from a laser. A sperm cell passing through the sorter is shot by the laser if a detector at right angles confirms that the sperm's flat surface is actually fac ing the laser, then a detector in line with the laser "reads" the intensity of emit ted light radiation. The sorter can be set to look for the slightly smaller amount of light a Y-bearing sperm emits or the slightly greater amount of emitted light of an X-bearing sperm. Either way, each sperm cell passing the test is then pushed electronically into a separate path leaving the cell sorter for collection and later use.

Dr. Johnson has used the fluorochrome-based cell-sorting method with sperm from a number of species, including rabbits, cattle and pigs. In addition to testing the resulting Y- or X-enriched sperm populations with FISH, the sex of offspring produced from inseminating the animals with these sperm fractions has been studied. Proportions of females ranged from 75 percent in pigs to 94 percent in rabbits when the cell sorter was set for enriching X-bearing sperm. Proportions of males when the cell sorter was set for enrich ing Y-bearing sperm ranged from 70 percent in pigs to 86 percent in rabbits.

Dr. Ed Fugger and Dr. Joseph Schulman, working at the Genetics & IVF Institute in Fairfax, Virginia, outside Washington D.C. , have successfully ap plied Dr. Johnson's method to human sperm. Writing in the journal *Human Reproduction* in 1993, Johnson, Fugger, Schulman and others reported an aver age of 82 percent X-bearing sperm and 75 percent Y-bearing sperm, depending on the setting of the machine for which type of sperm. Dr. Schulman has since reported the achievement of a human pregnancy of the wanted female gender for a couple who wished to avoid the risk of the genetic disease hemophilia in their next child (the gene for hemophilia being a recessive one found on the X chromosome, two of which in the baby stop expression of the disease), and tri als of sex selection for family balancing are under way using intrauterine in semination (IUI). Because of the rather slow nature of the cell-sorting process (each sperm has to be electronically tested one at a time and is then pushed to

## Serendipity with Sperm-Cell Sorting

Sperm-cell sorting is rather inefficient. Although the stream of sperm into the sorter is shaped as a rather flat ribbon, any sperm that does not present its flat face directly to the laser of the sorter will be rejected for not emitting a qualifying amount of light from the fluorescent dye bound to all its DNA. These sperm, even though they may contain the X or Y chromosome being looked for, and even though they might otherwise be completely normal, are dumped as junk sperm and not used. The difference in DNA content between X- and Y-bearing sperm is just 3 percent; the cell-sorting machines need to be kept in a fine state of tuning.

Any sperm, therefore, that reveals an amount of DNA outside this 3 percent tolerance will very likely be junked by the sorter, whether it is set for X or for Y. This means that a sperm with an abnormal amount of DNA for another reason, such as an extra chromosome or chromosome fragment or a missing piece of chromosome, will also be junked, potentially a wonderful means for selecting chromosomally normal sperm in IVF programs, whether gender is being selected or not. Indeed, sperm-cell sorting may turn out to be an essential tool in all IVF centers that use ICSI—if only to pick X-sperm to put an end to inherited male infertility!

one side or the other), the technology in 1997 is best suited for IVF, even ICSI, situations if there is any doubt about fertility for the couple. We thus have today the technology for changing the chance of a wanted girl from one in two to four in five, and for changing the chance of a wanted boy from one in two to one in four.

# Genetic Diagnosis in Embryos

Before cell-sorting technology was available to improve the chance of achieving female embryos, several British families at high risk of having children with hemophilia used IVF and biopsy of resultant pre-embryos to work out which were male and which were female. The rationale was (and is still) that genetic diseases inherited by sex-linked recessive inheritance will manifest in boys but

## Polar Body Analysis: Genetic Detective Work that Leaves the Embryo Alone

An abnormality in the number of chromosomes in a pre-embryo generally comes about because either the oocyte, or much less commonly the spermatozoon, brings to the fertilization one chromosome too many or one chromosome too few. Given that we will soon be able to be sure that the sperm's chromosome number is normal by cell sorting, it may be that we can also analyze the egg by a method that falls short of the relatively drastic step of taking out one or two cells from the pre-embryo.

The key may lie with the polar bodies, those products of meiosis by which the maturing egg rids itself of excess chromosomes. Remember (from Chapter 3) that the primary oocyte contains 92 chromosomes (we call these special chromosomes "chromatids") and that 46 of them go out with the first polar body, just before ovulation. If we analyze that polar body with FISH and see just one chromosome 21, for example, the odds are strong that the egg has held on to one of them,

and so will be destined to form a pre-embryo that has three of them—trisomy 21, or Down's syndrome. In a somewhat less likely situation, the egg may hold on to an extra chromosome 21 during the second meiotic division, which occurs with fertilization and which should expel 23 chromosomes. If the second polar body does not have a chromosome 21 on staining with FISH, again the odds will be strong that the pre-embryo will suffer from trisomy 21.

In 1996 it is still not possible to use FISH for all the chromosomes, partly because the fluorescent markers are not yet available for all chromosomes, partly because they are expensive and partly because there is a limit to how many different colors can be looked for meaningfully at once under the fluorescent microscope. We also need to know more about how long polar bodies remain intact and informative enough to give correct answers to the questions we would like to ask of them.

not in girls. The reason is that, being recessive, the abnormal gene will not be expressed (and therefore will not cause the disease) if there is a normal second gene (or **allele**) present among the chromosomes. For such genes on the X chromosome, one allele or gene is enough; the Y chromosome is too small to carry a complementary, savior gene. In addition to hemophilia, these sex-linked genetic diseases include Duchenne's muscular dystrophy (a wasting disease of the muscles) and Tay-Sach's disease (a degenerative disease of the brain and eyes).

By using the **polymerase chain reaction** (PCR) to amplify pieces of DNA known to be unique to the Y chromosome, researchers led by Dr. Alan Handyside at London's Hammersmith Hospital were able to distinguish male from female pre-embryos and to transfer just those that were female. The alternative for these families would have been to wait until pregnancy was established and then use either high resolution **transvaginal ultrasound** or conventional karyotyping of cells obtained by **chorionic villus sampling** (CVS) or **amniocentesis** to discover the sex of the fetus, aborting it if a male.

A number of IVF centers now have the capability of performing pre-embryo microbiopsy for preimplantational genetic diagnosis. Figure 20.3d in Chapter 20 shows such micromanipulation under way at Sydney IVF. For such chromosomal diagnoses as gender determination or discovering **trisomies** (including **Down's syndrome**, or **trisomy 21**, and **Klinefelter's syndrome**, which is 47,XXY) and monosomies (such as **Turner's syndrome**, 45,X), FISH is nowadays generally easier and more reliable for this purpose than PCR. For molecular diagnosis of specific abnormal genes, such as the gene for cystic fibrosis, PCR is the only method possible.

Although it is not likely that more than a tiny proportion of IVF eggs or embryos will be subjected to biopsy for genetic diagnosis any time soon, this is an important development for families affected by serious genetic diseases who have other reasons for considering IVF, in order to make diagnoses before embryos are transferred. Whether less serious genetic impairments will lead to such extreme technological intervention, only time will tell. A slippery slope into designer embryos? Well, if there *is* a slope, I would suggest that it is neither steep nor particularly slippery. As genetic knowledge and methods for diagnosis—and possible treatment—slowly accumulate, societies will have more time to debate these issues than prophets of impending Utopian doom would have us believe.

It is certain, however, that as sperm-cell sorting, intracytoplasmic sperm insertion and preimplantational diagnosis raise the value of individual embryos, not only will our expectations of (and our identification with) a single embryo grow, we will want to be surer than we can be in 1997 that an apparently normal pre-embryo that is transferred will in fact implant to form an embryo, a fetus and then a baby. Today, even in the best IVF programs, not more than about one in four or five transferred embryos implants successfully. It is possible that this will be improved by circumventing one or two of the possible barriers to implantation, namely the **zona pellucida** and/or the surface layer of the uterus's lining, the **endometrium**. After all, the implanted embryo is rid of its zona and sits snugly within the endometrium well before the menstrual period is missed (see Chapter 3).

# Direct Mucosal Embryo Transfer

If we can pick up sperm cells and place them within eggs, overcoming barrie to fertilization with sperm microinjection, why should we not pick up embry out of their zonas in the lab and, at the appropriate stage of visibly and gene ically tested normal development, place them in the uterus's lining?

Dr. Kasuma Kato, from Komatsu, Japan, has been successfully placing ea pre-embryos, still within the zona, into the endometrium by ultrasound-guide transfer through the wall of the vagina and through the wall of the uterus. Sydney IVF we have tried to duplicate these results but with little success. In a admittedly very difficult group of patients—with numerous prior unsuccessf embryo transfers—just two of 40 or so patients conceived. My colleague, Jo Anderson, who is very skilled at ultrasound (having introduced transvaginal u trasound scanning to Australia), has been to Japan to watch Dr. Kato, and Kato embryologist was with us in Sydney for some of the transfers. There was n doubt that the embryos were placed in the mucosal lining of the uterus and n in its cavity (as is the case with conventional transfers done through the cerv or with some transfers done by needle through the wall of the uterus). In oth words, the procedures technically went fine. The two pregnant patients bot miscarried.

There are two concerns with Dr. Kato's technique. First, no other IVF cen ters seem to have replicated his results. Second, it would make more sense to re move the zona pellucida around the embryos first, which means maintainir the embryos in culture longer, so that the **blastomeres**, the individual cells tha make up the pre-embryo, are capable of sticking together, which is a propert they do not display for a number of days after fertilization. Ideally, we woul bring the embryo to the stage at which it normally hatches through the zor pellucida, namely the stage of blastocyst, before doing the transfer.

## Assisted Hatching

Dr. Jacques Cohen, an embryologist until recently at Cornell University Hospita in New York City, has for several years championed a partial means of over coming the barriers to implantation. Having discovered that the zona pellucida of, especially, the eggs of older women can be thicker than usual and can seen (at least in culture) to resist the efforts of the blastocyst to hatch through i Cohen developed the technique he calls **assisted hatching**. He makes a sma opening in the zona using micromanipulation methods (see Figure 20.3c) similar to those used for sperm microinjection and for pre-embryo microbiopsy. The opening is big enough to allow easy passage through the zona once the pre-embryo expands, but it is small enough not to allow the blastomeres to drift out before they get sticky for each other.

Again, our experience at Sydney IVF has been mixed (and, judging from the published literature, so has the experience at other IVF centers), probably at least partly because of the temptation to restrict assisted hatching to the most difficult of IVF circumstances, when there can be other reasons why embryos are not doing well.

## Proper "Oomph" for Eggs and Embryos

In summary, there are still many reasons embryos do not do as well as we would like in the IVF lab and, after implantation, in a woman's body. In many cases there may be an inherent **embryopathy** present, acquired from the sperm or, more often, from the egg before fertilization. In some cases this embryopathy will be chromosomal. In many cases there is likely to be wear and tear of the egg's, and hence the embryo's, **mitochondria**. The situation is made more complicated by the likelihood that pre-embryos can be made up of cells that differ greatly in health, and they may well be struggling, first in vitro and then in vivo, to heal themselves by discarding blastomeres that are not up to it and replacing those that fragment with others that are stronger. In vitro culture conditions can make a critical difference for these embryos. Attitudes toward embryo research (see Chapter 27) in turn will make a critical difference to in vitro culture methods.

It makes sense to predict that the future will lie with eggs picked from their peers for their metabolic health; with eggs fertilized reliably by sperm sorted for their normality; with embryos cultured in the lab using techniques derived from a proper research-based appreciation of their nutritional needs; and with clinical techniques of embryo transfer to the endometrium that leave nothing to chance. Only then will infertility medicine—a woman's ability to get pregnant when medical help is needed—reach its full potential.

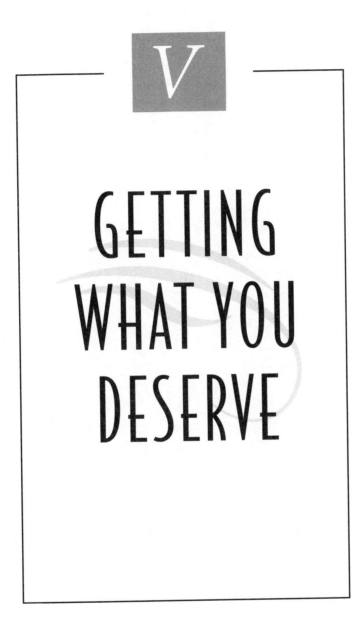

# V

# GETTING WHAT YOU DESERVE

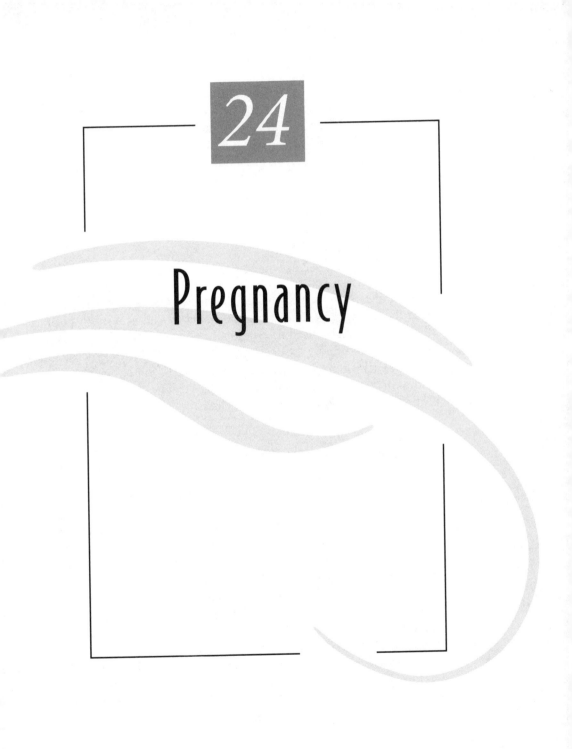

# 24

# Pregnancy

When that hoped-for moment happens—a **pregnancy test** is positive, abo
two weeks after the assisted conception procedure—the first response is em
tional: it's over! The time and effort and money has paid off. Infertility is
memory. But then you realize that it is not all over. There are still uncertaintie
Things can still go wrong. Even when things go right (and they do go right mo
often than not), there are new challenges.

# What Can Go Wrong ?

Bleeding after a confirmed pregnancy might mean a **miscarriage** or it migl
mean the presence of an **ectopic pregnancy**. It can also mean nothing at al
other than the slight bleeding within a normally pregnant uterus as new bloo
vessels form to support the developing fetus. Contact your gynecologist or you
IVF center (if you have had assisted conception). Do not do any vigorous activ
ity, and do not have sex until the bleeding subsides. An ultrasound will proba
bly be carried out sooner rather than later.

## Miscarriage, or Spontaneous Abortion

A pregnancy conceived but lost can cause more distress than unattained preg
nancy. The most common way for a pregnancy to be lost is through a miscar
riage, whether obvious clinically or subclinically. A **subclinical miscarriage** i
when the pregnancy test becomes positive but no **gestational sac** becomes visi
ble on **transvaginal ultrasound**; bleeding takes place sooner or later and can b
heavier than a normal period; no **curettage** is needed. On the other hand, a
"clinical miscarriage" is said to happen after an ultrasound shows an empty sac
in which an embryo may (for a while) or may not develop; in this case a curet
tage can sometimes be needed to empty the uterus and keep it in the best con
dition for another pregnancy attempt; sometimes it is advisable to have a **kary
otype**, or chromosome study, done on the miscarriage tissue in order to shec
light on why the miscarriage happened (see Chapter 7). The risk of miscarriage
is related both to the woman's age (see Table 7.1 in Chapter 7) and to the ab
normal reproductive circumstances of the conception (see the box "Miscar
riages and Infertility").

# Ectopic Pregnancy

An **ectopic pregnancy** is when the pregnancy develops in the fallopian tube instead of the uterus (see Chapter 14). This can happen after GIFT or after IVF (even though embryos are usually transferred to the uterus after IVF, they can migrate into the tube). An ectopic pregnancy cannot keep developing—sooner or later internal bleeding occurs. Its treatment is by an operation, sometimes involving a **laparotomy** (opening the abdomen with a horizontal cut at the pubic hair line), during which the tube will be opened for the pregnancy to be removed or, if damage is more substantial, the tube itself may need to be removed. Often, and especially with early diagnosis, an ectopic pregnancy can be treated during **laparoscopy**, and sometimes medical treatment with methotrexate is used.

# Hydatidiform Mole

Rarest of all the pregnancies that go wrong—assisted or not—are **hydatidiform moles**, abnormal from conception, usually without an embryo or fetus, and resembling a bunch of grapes when eventually expelled. The word "hydatid" means a little sac or fluid-filled vesicle. A "mole" in medicine can mean any blemish or faulty structure that is distinct from the normal tissue or organ surrounding it. Hydatidiform moles are benign tumors of the placenta (the afterbirth). The grape-like sacs represent swollen tongues of **trophoblast**, or placental tissue, which distends because there is no embryo or fetus present to put embryonic blood vessels into the trophoblast and to carry away the fluid the trophoblast absorbs, sponge-like, from the mother's circulation. The abnormal fertilization that gives rise to a hydatidiform mole is described in Chapter 3 in the box "Chromosomes and the Fate of Embryos."

Hydatidiform moles occur in less than about one in 1,200 pregnancies among European races; they can be much more frequent in some Asians (the frequency in Indonesia is said to be one in 100 pregnancies). In the United States, the incidence among African Americans is about half that in European Americans. The chance increases with the age of the woman (especially after age 40). There are reports of hydatidiform moles after infertility and its treatment, including assisted insemination, but it seems doubtful that there is a strong association with infertility or assisted conception that is independent of the woman's age. The risk after IVF is no more than would be expected by chance. Nowadays most hydatidiform moles are easily diagnosed early in

With engaging candor—and from an era (1952) that preceded the development of most effective methods for treating infertility—Dr. S. Bender, a British surgeon and gynecologist at the University of Liverpool, showed for the first time that the risk of miscarriage among infertile women is high. Of 313 first pregnancies among women with primary infertility (they had not been pregnant before), about 20 percent miscarried. This compares with a miscarriage risk of 12 to 15 percent among women with no infertility.

Miscarriages are thus more common after infertility than they are among pregnancies in women who have no trouble getting pregnant. In an article I published in the *American Journal of Obstetrics and Gynecology* in 1982, I analyzed most of the published articles on infertility and its treatment to that time. It became clear that both the reproductive abnormality behind the infertility and the new variables introduced by treatment could be responsible for this higher figure. Whereas the karyotype, or chromosome composition, of miscarriages that happen in the first three months (which is when most take place) is abnormal in 65 percent of cases or more (see Table 7.2 in Chapter 7), it is more likely to be normal in the circumstances of infertility and its treatment. In other words, there are reasons on top of the usual chromosomal mistakes at conception that can mar the environment for early embryos when fertility itself is reduced.

In my survey of infertility treatments to 1982, just three seemed to lower the risk of miscarriage to normal: ovulation induction with **bromocriptine** for **hyperprolactinemia** (see Chapter 10); operation for

pregnancy on transvaginal ultrasound, which confers a prolific pattern of echoes from the multiple fluid-filled sacs that compose the mole.

## Who's My Doctor?

Let us assume that your pregnancy avoids these last pitfalls. If you have been having assisted conception, you will have become used to the rather intense medical attention of the stimulation and the egg pickup. There is something of

**endometriosis** (see Chapter 16); and **donor insemination** for extremely low or zero sperm counts (see Chapter 22). In each of these conditions, should pregnancy have occurred naturally, the risk of miscarriage was considerably increased.

Most forms of **assisted conception** produce a rise in the risk of miscarriage over that expected in normal women. The risk of miscarriage after **gamete intrafallopian transfer** (GIFT) or **in vitro fertilization** (IVF) has been decreased by abandoning the use of **clomiphene**, which can have disadvantageous effects on the **endometrium** and hence on **implantation** of the embryo (see Chapter 10) in the **superovulation** regimen for stimulating the ovaries.

As it turns out, measuring the frequency of miscarriages—estimating the **abortion rate**—can be a much more sensitive way of gauging the correctness of a particular infertility treatment than measuring the **pregnancy rate** or even the **take-home-baby rate**! The reason is that there are too many variables that affect pregnancy rates and overall take-home-baby rates that have nothing to do with the treatment itself, especially the duration of the infertility and the age of the woman. Infertility clinics and assisted conception programs can present good figures by selecting carefully the patients whose results they report (see the box "Clinics with Unusually High IVF Pregnancy Rates" in Chapter 20), but they cannot easily do the same when reporting miscarriages as a proportion of the achieved pregnancies. The usefulness of using a low miscarriage rate as a signpost for good medical practice is not as well appreciated as it should be.

a letdown for the next two weeks while waiting for a period or a pregnancy test. If the pregnancy test is positive, it is still another two weeks before the transvaginal ultrasound can show if the pregnancy is in the right place (the uterus) and is healthy (of normal size for dates and with a beating fetal heart). During this time a patient might sense some loneliness: she is not ready yet to see an obstetrician for pregnancy care, and she senses that her infertility physician has done his or her job. But be reassured that, in fact, IVF clinics and infertility nurses love hearing from their pregnant patients, and your infertility physician certainly will be available for advice and to manage things if they go wrong. (Naturally, you will not be bothered by these considerations if your infertility doctor is also your obstetrician.)

But only time will tell if all is well. No one can further influence events any extent. In the great majority of cases the die has been cast at conception there is either a normal embryo or not—and only time will reveal which which. Nothing will rescue it if it is a "blighted ovum." Normal embryos are ge erally built to survive, but be sensible. Do not go on a ten-mile run or scuba di ing, but do not encase yourself in cotton wool either. Sex is fine unless there vaginal bleeding or painful spasms from the uterus; in these cases there is **threatened miscarriage** and sex with penetration or with orgasm can distu the pregnancy.

When *should* you get into touch with an obstetrician? The temptation ca be to see one as soon as possible. By all means phone as soon as seems sensib for an appointment eight to ten weeks from the date of the last period. It is di ficult to get an appointment with many obstetricians at short notice. But it is o ten better not to transfer to the care of an obstetrician until the pregnancy ha been confirmed as healthy. Instead, stay under the care of the gynecologist wh assisted with the conception for the time being. He or she may not be doing any thing special but knows what has happened so far and will be available if thing do not go right.

## With the Obstetrician

Your pregnancy, if you have had assisted conception, is not the same as that c everyone else. Do not let anyone tell you anything different. For a start, you wi probably be more used to sharing personal matters with your partner than witl friends and relations (see Chapter 25). For both of you, involving your friends relations and workmates in the pregnancy's progress will probably be less nat ural than it is for couples who got pregnant the straightforward way.

Second, you are going to be more anxious about your pregnancy. You alread know how unkind nature can be. This feeling will disappear but usually not un til the baby is born. Third, your pregnancy could be multiple, with extra risks o prematurity. After IVF, even for single fetuses, there is an extra risk of **prematur labor, small-for-dates** gestation and stillbirth. There is a small but real risk o **cervical incompetence**, a symptomless weakening of the cervix (see Chapter 7) which allows the pregnancy membranes to bulge through and then to break, al most always resulting in the loss of the pregnancy. This weakness may be related to the large number of gynecological procedures that have at various times been done for most people who have taken a long time to get pregnant.

## What Special Precautions Should My Obstetrician Take?

At Sydney IVF we recommend that all patients who are pregnant after assisted conception, whether the pregnancy is single or multiple, have vaginal examinations between the twelfth and twenty-eighth week of pregnancy to detect cervical incompetence early, or immediately if there is recent onset of back pain or vaginal discharge. If there is real evidence of cervical incompetence, then a protective stitch placed in the cervix (see Chapter 8) is essential treatment.

Even if there is no increased **risk** of things going wrong, the pregnancy may be practically irreplaceable, and the **hazard** of pregnancy loss is by its nature a greater one than for someone who has no trouble getting pregnant. An "at risk" approach to managing the pregnancy and the labor is appropriate for your obstetrician.

Finally, nature is not perfect and neither is medical care. The most painstaking attention cannot stop the unexpected from happening, and no amount of watchfulness will always mean a perfect outcome. But everyone should do their best, from the moment you first contact an infertility specialist or IVF center to when your baby goes home with you. If you think this is not happening, start asking questions.

## Should We Have Prenatal Diagnostic Tests?

There is no universally correct answer, because invasive tests always carry a small risk. Major malformations may be detectable on ultrasound after about 12 weeks. A formal malformation scan can be done on request at 19 weeks (just in time in Australia for an induced abortion to be allowable). Spina bifida, a serious **congenital abnormality** of the spinal cord, can be detected by blood tests (for **alpha fetoprotein**). Women over age 35 often have screening tests for **Down's syndrome**. This can be done by **chorionic villus sampling** (CVS) at about nine weeks from the start of the last period or by **amniocentesis** at 14 to 15 weeks. CVS has about a 1 to 2 percent chance of *causing* a miscarriage; the risk with an ultrasonically directed amniocentesis is less, but the pregnancy and therefore the emotional trauma of terminating it, if it is abnormal, are both more advanced. Whether you have a CVS or an amniocentesis, the procedu should be done by a gynecologist with a good deal of testing experience. Twi or triplets can often be tested separately, but deciding what to do should one normal and the other abnormal is an unenviable dilemma. Ordinarily, th are all aborted or all delivered, but **fetal reduction** can be available (see t Glossary).

# After the Delivery

The baby is born alive and she or he is well. Is this when the fun starts? Mayb Certainly life is not the same, especially with twins or triplets! Babies are d manding and the changes to your life are just beginning. Not everyone adjus readily. If the couple is older, it can be harder to accommodate the changes, e pecially after years of being together without children. Those who cope best a those who share their feelings and anxieties with their partner, health profe sionals and friends. Many IVF mothers have learned to organize their lives cope with repeated cycles of assisted conception; while they might be well pr pared in lots of ways, they may be less so in others. One important thing is keep in touch—with your partner and those who helped you—and be easy c the infertile couples you have gotten to know but who have not made it yet.

# Relief from
# Suffering

Infertility, its investigation and its treatment, has been referred to as an emo tional roller coaster. Optimism takes turns with despair. The cycle is worse assisted conception programs have been started, what with their expensiv promises and irregular, sometimes spectacular (sometimes multiple) successe Suffering comes not just from your childlessness; it threatens from every corn of your relationships with family, friends and acquaintances. It can even com from your treatment despite the best intentions of medical professionals. On th other hand, relief from suffering can come from changes, opportunities an good luck other than pregnancy. With advice and help your suffering may b contained and in time displaced by newer challenges and achievements.

# Family and Friends

As infertility develops it is profoundly isolating. In the beginning, as a coupl does not achieve pregnancy as quickly as expected, they might decide not to te anyone outside the relationship. You and your partner may even not reach th same conclusion about fertility at the same time. Then, as month follow month, and as ovulation and menstruation follow each other emptily, you clin together in mutual helplessness, often without seeking the support of those yo would normally confide in on less private matters—your workmates, friend and less immediate family.

On the other hand, it is a time when most couples' relationships strengthe and deep mutual commitment and empathy grow. I have been impressed, con sidering the level of stress involved, with how few infertile marriages come un stuck. But some undoubtedly do.

You will have debated whom to tell. In general, sex—and not getting preg nant in particular—is such a personal and private matter between the two o you that it might seem too painful to tell others. As time goes by, your sisters an friends conceive, but it gets harder and harder to share their joy. As their babie are born you might avoid family get-togethers and weekend barbecues witl your friends, then chide yourself for being so upset when you should be happ for them. The hardest times for you will probably be when close friends an nounce news of their pregnancy, then visiting the hospital after their baby' birth, attending the religious ceremonies, and so on. There are surely other ex amples you can tell me about.

Before awareness of your infertility reaches friends and relations, their re marks can be hurtful. You might be accused of being selfish, of not sharing you lives with children and of being self-indulgent and antisocial. You are too busy having a more private cultural and social time, building a big house, taking exotic cruises and vacations.

# Loss of Personal Power

It is common for a woman to question her feelings about her sexuality. She may feel that she is not a whole woman and be angry with her body, which does not seem to do anything right. She might sense a mystical but piercing punishment for a past abortion or a past child given up for adoption, a punishment for having intentionally put off having children to develop a career. This might be the time when either partner confesses to a past indiscretion (or two), adding a new twist to the suffering. Our minds can function in strange ways and sometimes a foreign, illogical thought about ourselves lodges there and refuses to leave, hurting us when we are at our most depressed and vulnerable. You might sometimes feel you are going mad, but such feelings are normal and counseling can help. Once such bogus imaginings are out in the open—in the safety of a counseling session—they have less power.

There is often a feeling of lack of control. Nowadays, with efficient contraception, having children for so many people seems such a careful and precise decision. So much care is taken with *not getting pregnant* that no one anticipates not being able to *get pregnant*. When infertility dawns it is a devastating shock. Anger that the ability to have children has been taken away can be overwhelming and sometimes frightening.

It seems that everywhere you go you are surrounded by pregnant women or new mothers. Senses of anger and unfairness overwhelm you. Other parents seem so callous, unsuited for the role and undeserving. The way they carelessly punish their child. You would never do that. If only someone would give you a baby. You can feel like taking one.

Two weeks of every four is spent in hope. Nature makes most people feel awful just before and during a menstrual period, the same period that reminds you that nothing is solved. It is a double whammy, a double kick in the teeth. Out come the cigarettes, perhaps, that you promise will be thrown out the moment there is a pregnancy. Or, more positively, you may say to yourself, "I must stay on an even keel, so I won't be disappointed if I'm not pregnant," or, "If I remain positive it will happen."

Not for Sensitive Souls: Pushed to Masturbate

An interesting but not unusual scene was painted by Dr. Aline Zoldbrod of Boston, speaking at the twelfth annual meeting of the Fertility Society of Australia in Sydney in 1993 on the subject "Men, Women and Infertility." The couple reach the infertility clinic, for the woman to be greeted with effusive salutations: "How are you? How are you bearing up? The blood tests have come through very well, and you will be pleased that the ultra-sound's showing a wonderful number of follicles. Please sit down and make yourself comfortable. We know you are having such a difficult time. We won't keep you a minute." Turning to the husband with the smile, the staff member says, "Here's your container for the sperm sample. The toilet's over there."

Exaggerated perhaps, but not too foreign. Ejaculation can be easier said than done. Some disheveled magazines are not necessarily the answer, especially when a need for a second sample—collected eggs patiently waiting in the IVF laboratory—follows hard on the heels of the first. At Sydney IVF, in addition to providing pristine, discrete cultural material in the private sperm-collecting rooms, we provide beer, Scotch and wine, to eliminate at least some of the angst and to dissolve some of the awesome sense of duty.

# Women and Men

Women and men, in general, differ in the way they respond to the strain of infertility. There is nothing too remarkable about being an exception to these generalizations, and too much should not be made of generalizations. In general, however, women are more likely to want to talk openly about their feelings, and their self-image is much more bound into the traditional role of bearing and nurturing children. Women are more likely to cry. Men have more opportunities to let off steam physically and mentally, by playing sports or by aggressive pursuit of business. More of their goals seem achievable. Talking a lot about the feelings infertility brings seems a waste of time for men, because it does not change the situation.

Dr. Ellen Freeman and her colleagues from the University of Pennsylvania evaluated 200 infertile couples and reported that more than 50 percent of infertile women regard infertility to be the most upsetting experience of their lives, causing at least as much suffering for them as divorce or the death of a close friend or family member. In contrast, the stress of infertility, or the suffering it causes, was rated as high by just 15 percent of men. Given that so many couples experience infertility, its threat to reproductive choice and reproductive future is probably *the* major cause of "psychological morbidity" (as the social scientists would call it), or **suffering** (as we will call it), among women in the community, and a lesser but still important one among men.

A destructive pattern can develop. As the realization of infertility sets in, a couple will talk openly and understand and accept each others' feelings. As time goes by, however, anger, depression and guilt tend to take over. The husband might grow tired of trying to support and console his wife and withdraw, feeling the situation is out of his control; there is helplessness and frustration. The wife might be bitter and resentful, especially of her husband's apparent other interests and protection from suffering. Before the fighting starts is an important time to seek help and fresh understanding through counseling. *Do* consider it. *Do not* be alone unnecessarily.

Women bear the brunt of tests and treatment, even when a low sperm count seems to be the reason. The subject of **donor insemination** (see Chapter 22) might enter the conversation. It might have been brought up before, to dismiss it, but it resurfaces. It might have been resisted in favor of highly complex **testicular sperm extraction** (TESE) and **intracytoplasmic sperm injection** (ICSI) procedures (see Chapter 20). Still, the subject comes up again. It is at this time that the male partner's feelings of inadequacy may first be thoroughly brought home—often acutely. Up to this point, many men will have escaped the full impact of infertility's power to blame, consciously or unconsciously deflecting it, partly to their partner, partly replacing it with other achievements. Not all marriages survive the realignment of power that can occur at this point.

# Goodbye Privacy

The medical world intrudes. We met this phenomenon—this series of phenomena—explicitly in Chapter 19. Sex is no longer a private matter. Everyone seems to get involved in it. How frequently? How frequent is frequent? Just for the heck of it—fending off embarrassment—you throw in a few extra intercourse ticks on the temperature chart. Friends and family believe they have a duty to make suggestions and give advice. In Chapter 19 we dismiss the notion

that you can have sex too often, the notion that it matters a scrap *how* you ha
it and the notion that orgasm for women is essential for conceiving. By no
however, more often than not, sex is a shared chore.

You might start avoiding sex because it is a reminder of your sufferir
What is the point of it if you cannot get pregnant? Men can resent having to pe
form on demand at the "right time of the month" with a partner who is past e
joying it. It is depressing, with seemingly no way out. But there are things y
can do to help.

## Living for the Present

Remember to use the time between IVF cycles to strengthen your relationshi
Make the most of the resources you have. It may be cold comfort, but you *are*
a better position to do things spontaneously than couples bound down by kic
You *do* have more money to spend than couples with children—or more tha
you will have once they arrive. It *is* interesting to go to the theater, see ne
movies, discover inexpensive restaurants, get to know wines and art and go awa
for weekends.

Plan your life. Decide ahead which months will be set aside for assiste
conception or infertility treatment, which months for pleasure. With a plan (
action that stretches for months ahead, you are less likely to feel the bump
month by disappointing month. Keep up the planning ahead, so that if it is di
turbed by a pregnancy, well, that's life! Meanwhile, consider plotting togethe
Defeat the calendar if need be to avoid particularly painful family reunion
Everyone is different, but scheming together is a positive way you can bolste
your relationship. At times it will have a touch of spice, of naughtiness and eve
humor.

Remember, you are not alone. Ten to 15 percent of couples take longer t
achieve a pregnancy than they think it should. Sometimes when you share you
diagnosis you find others in similar situations—their closets open, their chi
dren turn out to be adopted or their children turn out to have come from dono
insemination. There will be couples who have been trying longer than you hav

There are support groups formed by infertile couples and they can be a goo
send. They can help the loneliness and strike a note of fun. They stop you fro
protecting yourself against some realities that will otherwise foment and catc
up with you. Many of the larger ones, such as Resolve in the United States, pub
lish useful and entertaining newsletters, which is a minimum level of involve

## Champagne and Candles

Among the myths dispelled in Chapter 19 is the one that a moderate amount of alcohol might be harmful. Wine contains many natural antioxidants. Many people take the antioxidant vitamins A, C and E to try and improve fertility, especially sperm counts. All the medical evidence is showing that sensible amounts of wine, which includes enough to make you feel good, are conducive to good health. Never drink so much that it leaves a hangover, but a glass or two of wine can do wonders at a woman's midcycle!

If having sex "at the right time" has become a strain—part of the suffering instead of part of the solution—consider some private scheming based on knowing early in the day when there is to be an ovulation (with the urinary LH testing we talk about in Chapter 19). For a start, LH test-ing can give you both the confidence not to have sex more often than you both feel like, before and after ovulation. The only cooperation you need for this plan to work is that on just one night in the month you both agree that there is no going out with the boys or the girls, there are to be no business dinners both of you do not attend and neither of you bring work home—and that it may be at rather short notice.

Then, whether it is to be champagne, candles and your favorite food at home or an intimate restaurant that is on your short list and for which you had no problem getting a midweek last-minute reservation, you can both do much to revitalize numbed sexual appetites. You have taken control. You are having fun. And neither of you can do more—neither of you *need* do more—than you are doing.

ment that you can turn on and off just by picking up the newsletter to browse. Choose such a "consumer group" carefully; some smaller ones will have moved from the common experience of infertility to the common experience of children. It is human nature to parade your baby when it has taken so long. (The maternity gear they wear also often seems extravagant!)

Allow time for nurturing yourselves, time that is not work, not focused on fertility. Listen to a relaxation tape, go to an aerobics or yoga class, take a walk. When you are depressed these actions will seem a chore, but good comes from them, so be firm with yourself. Do not volunteer to take on additional commitments with work or family while you are having assisted conception, or at least during the months it is scheduled. You need time to cope with it properly, even though modern IVF centers, for the most part, will fit in with your working day better than you might think.

Lean on your counselor, your nurse, your physician. Never be afraid of as[k]ing questions (see Chapter 26 for more about your doctor). When everythi[ng] seems overwhelming, remember the most potent suffering comes when you a[re] thinking about a childless future; if you are not successfully living for the pre[s]ent, make some future plans. Recall how you got on top of it before, how y[ou] successfully fought off those feelings the last time. Allow your partner to grie[ve] the infertility in his or her own way. Do not expect the same feelings you hav[e]. Take advantage of quiet times to communicate—and not always about infert[il]ity. A walk around the neighborhood or going to a movie together can, at a m[o]ment's notice, be better than stewing and getting testy at home, even if it is rai[n]ing outside.

When a quarrel is substantial, abstinence will make the heart fond[er]. Nature's libidinous help will sooner or later be on the way! Keep an importa[nt] fact in focus—fertile marriages fail more often than infertile ones. For mo[st] couples, the shared experience of infertility has the power to bring you closer t[o]gether than having children.

Many of the ideas for this chapter, and their expression, came from Kerr[y] McGowan, infertility counselor at Royal Prince Alfred Hospital and Sydney IV[F]

26

# Your Physician's Duties

$A$ physician has a duty to do his or her best for patients—for an infert
couple—who ask for help. The General Medical Council in Great Britain, f
instance, insists that a patient has to be able to expect this of a physician wl
is consulted for any medical reason. In responding to this obligation, the phys
cian is accountable to the patient, to the physician's peers and to the gener
community.

This chapter will introduce you to the vocabulary and principles of ethic
conflicts, to informed consent to medical procedures and to values that need
be preserved in the relationship between you and your physician, perhaps as tl
going gets tough. Reading the boxes will give you a deeper philosophical basis-
more profound ammunition, if you need it—for exploring and taking part
differences of ethical opinion.

# Moral Dilemmas and Ethical Conflicts

In acknowledging a duty of care, a physician is obliged to put the patient's or tl
couple's interests ahead of other priorities, such as administration, profit or r
search. This may not always be completely practicable, but then the physicia
should tell the patient or couple about the particular conflict of interest, and tl
couple should have the opportunity of consulting another physician. For exam
ple, physicians who have administrative roles in public hospitals and see pa
tients professionally have a special duty to make sure that their patients a:
aware of constraints on resources affecting what treatment they can offer an
that they are accountable to managers as well as to their patients.

To some extent these conflicts affect the way every physician practices. B
how, in the case of a subsidized public hospital, should a physician do his or h
best for one patient who asks for more and more expensive assisted conceptio
treatment, knowing that to give in to such requests will straightaway disadvar
tage others? It is not easy. More generally, authorities, such as governments, ca
help in these ethical areas by making it clear how far society will fund such trea
ments or investigations and where the line will be drawn socially or medicall
An aggrieved patient or couple may blame an anonymous bureaucrat, but th
integrity of the physician-patient relationship is preserved by the physician di:
closing the limitations to the patient, and, if the patient wants it, arranging
second opinion with another physician.

Similarly, commercial considerations could tempt a physician to "oversei
vice" or to "underservice" (jargon for working too hard or too little), dependin

## Ethics: Moral Imperatives, Outcomes and Equity

There is no single set of ethical theories that is universally accepted. One way that thoughts can be ordered—and debate on matters of ethics disciplined—is by categorizing ethical considerations into three groups: fundamental beliefs involving duty, which are seen by adherents to be self-evident and not needing more basic proof (sometimes called **deontological ethics**); the belief that goodness or badness of consequences, whether actual, intended or predicted (sometimes called **teleological ethics**), is the basis for moral imperative, and belief in social utility, which extends the idea of the benefit of consequences from the individual to the whole of society (sometimes called **utilitarian ethics**). We will begin with this last idea.

Utilitarian ethics has been around in philosophical circles since the time of Jeremy Bentham (1748–1832), a British philosopher writing during the time of the Industrial Revolution. In its more refined form, Bentham's proposal was that ultimate good is that which promises or brings the greatest pleasure or benefit to the greatest number of people. Utilitarianism has since been more conspicuous in some societies than in others. Marxism, and the notion that the end justifies the means, brought notoriety to utilitarianism. In Western society, utilitarian ethical principles and debate are resurfacing, in the form of allocating finite, public resources among plural interests—in other words, ensuring **equity** in the community, or administrative fairness and **justice**.

Modern examples of mainly utilitarian debate include political ones on society's funding for IVF. The ethical debate in Australia that preceded public payment for IVF—like the debate that preceded payment for induced abortions and for public sponsoring of family planning associations—also drew on the other two categories of ethics. But it can be useful to make cost-benefit analyses in the utilitarian area independently, before confusing the cost-benefit issue with moral prejudice (that is, with deontological ethics) and with personal benefit or detriment

on whether the physician is paid fee-for-service (especially if the health-care or diagnostic facility is owned by that physician) or works within a system of global payment for a diagnosis-related group of medical services (as in a health maintenance organization for, or limiting their payments for, society's medical ills). Again, the patient or couple should be given the opportunity of consulting someone else after the physician makes the disclosure.

## Ethics: Moral Imperatives, Outcomes and Equity (continued)

(teleological ethics) before having to reconcile the three, which is like mixing apples with pears and with oranges.

Teleological ethical beliefs, or consideration of consequences, I regard here as relating not to society as a whole but to individuals, which in practice means the woman and her husband or reproductive partner. Consequential considerations are (or should be) objective—ones that can be identified, tested (if necessary experimentally) and then accepted or rejected. They should, at least potentially, be matters of fact and be verifiable or refutable through observation and experiment. For example, the proposition, "Sperm microinjection is unethical as a technique for IVF because there might be a high risk of producing babies with major deformities" becomes unacceptable as a teleological ethical argument if experience shows that the proposition is not true. This is not to say that consequential arguments can only rest on facts and not on fears; rather, consequential considerations need continually to take into account new **empirical** information as it becomes available. Because the data teleological considerations are based on can change with time, it is legitimate—indeed it is compulsory—for ethical conclusions based on consequences to be ever open to rethinking and to change. We might usefully call it "evidence-based ethics."

Deontological ethical beliefs are by their nature less flexible and less subject to experiment. Either they are innate or they are instilled in people as children through teaching and observation. The strength of a person's convictions or character implies that his or her deontological beliefs show substantial resistance to corruption by argument and observation. Incidentally, the similarity that the term "deontological" might have linguistically to "God-given" is a coincidence, although religious beliefs are encompassed by the term. The word's origin is Greek, meaning "that which is binding, a duty." Deontology is thus the philosophy of duty or moral obligation. Although deontological principles include ethical positions that appear to be God-

A third example of conflict of interest is when matters of conscience, especially the physician's own moral beliefs, clash with the patient's wishes. The physician's duty then is to disclose what is on his or her conscience and that such considerations are influencing the advice being given. It is not right, for example, for a physician working in a Catholic hospital to offer only **gamete-intrafallopian transfer** (GIFT) and not **in vitro fertilization** (IVF) for a couple with infertility because of tubal problems or a particularly low sperm count.

## Ethics: Moral Imperatives, Outcomes and Equity (concluded)

given or derived from scriptures, it equally includes a physician's fundamental compassion for, and belief that there is a fundamental duty to help, a couple distraught by their infertility.

Ethical debate soon spills over among these three categories, but the longer it takes for this mixing to start, generally the more sensible the particular debate will be. Consider, for example, the moral position that life is sacrosanct from the moment of conception and that IVF, because it creates surplus embryos that will be denied the chance to survive, therefore ought not to be pursued. (This is the position of many fundamentalist Christians.) Given that there are valid reasons for doubting the absolute truth of this position in principle, what is the best approach to contradicting this deontological position in practice? Is it the argument that the number of children that result from IVF outweighs the number of lost IVF embryos (a utilitarian argument)? Is it the argument that nature also wastes embryos in natural circumstances, so the lost embryos are

of no consequence (a teleological argument)? Or is it the argument that infertility causes so much and such intense human suffering that one has a compelling duty to invoke the only treatment that works (a deontological argument)?

Individuals intuitively consider all three aspects in reaching a conclusion for action or for a decision. It is not uncommon, for example, for a couple who have moral difficulties with embryos in vitro or in cryostorage to recruit financial constraints and health fears from ovarian stimulation to help them decide that enough is enough.

If the ethical question is serious enough in the community, a more formal accommodation will ultimately need to be sought that crosses the three sets of ethical categories. In its rawest form, such an accommodation in a plural society may consist of a vote on the matter, as occurred in Great Britain in 1990, when both houses of Parliament voted with two-thirds majorities to approve IVF and embryo research.

When IVF or donor insemination (either of which may be medically better) can readily be obtained somewhere else, your physician should make it very clear how he or she is constrained by personal or local institutional views of morality. For sure, in some cases, the patient or the couple might share the physician's particular view that it is immoral to create embryos and then not transfer all of them to the uterus. The point is that the discussion should be an open one, not one pushed paternalistically by the physician.

I propose that when there are unresolved differences of ethical opinion, provided the law is not broken, the responsibility for making ethical and moral decisions should rest with the people who most need to live with the consequence of the decision. Unfortunately, not everyone agrees with this notion. Society still has many people who want to influence or to make decisions for others (typically they then walk away to another case, to make someone else's decision, instead of staying to sort out the personal consequences). We still see this on the private matter of abortion. We still see it in questions of embryo research (see Chapter 27).

# Informed Consent

In circumstances that are nearly always uncertain, the physician and the couple need to work together closely to establish the ethical premises and the trust that are needed to make good medical decisions. Patients generally do not like to risk losing the goodwill of their physician. This is a point that should work alike to the advantage of the infertile couple and the physician. The physician ought to be in a position to share uncertainty regarding the outcome of treatment with the couple. They should form what the American physician Thomas Guthei and others, writing in the *New England Journal of Medicine* in 1984, called the "therapeutic alliance." It is not so much the notion of a patient's so-called **autonomy** (see the box "Autonomy and Respect for Persons") but respect for each patient that should lead the physician to ensure that patients are presented with the advantages and disadvantages of alternative plans for treatment. In making decisions that will affect them, the couple are invited to take as much responsibility as suits their circumstances as they see them. This is where the purpose and value lie in obtaining **informed consent** for medical treatment.

In a recent case before the High Court in Australia, a young woman lost the sight of her single good eye after an essentially elective operation on her diseased other one (*Whittacker v. Rogers*). The risk of such a complication taking place was extremely remote, but the penalty she (and her physician) paid was disastrous; she had not been told of this known hazard even though, the court agreed, she had asked the right question. The court affirmed the view that the information given in the process of consenting to medical treatment, at least in Australia, must be tailored to the patient's inquiries in a given medical circumstance and must not just be a reiteration of a list of probable or possible complications. Different countries might interpret the legal requirements of

## Autonomy and Respect for Persons

A person's autonomy, as a philosophical concept, derives from the systems of ethics developed by the German philosopher Immanuel Kant (1724–1804). Kant is important to moral philosophers because he proposed that innate human choice is the only proper subject matter of morals (and, incidentally, that all else in ethical judgments is regarded as a subclass of **value judgments** and hence loaded with the ethical system of the pronouncer—but more of this later). For Kant, in other words, morality was an autonomous matter—the self-determination of the will.

In the age of enlightenment, autonomy came to mean personal freedom. Now, in the late twentieth century, there is a call for every decision that affects a person to be made by that person. (If more than one person is affected by that decision then ideally they take part in making the decision.) On the face of it, autonomy is a good thing, provided at least that one person's autonomy does not infringe upon that of another.

In clinical medicine, patient autonomy becomes identifiable—and problematic—when ethical justification for decisions on medical care is based merely on the patient's informed consent. In the extreme case, the patient decides and the physician complies. The decision is the patient's to make and then the outcome of her or his decision becomes legally irrelevant. In such an extreme situation, informed consent becomes a mask for uncertainty, responsibility for which is transferred from the physician to the patient. This transfer is ultimately unfair if insisted on by the physician and unwise if insisted on by the patient, because the physician has been trained to have the knowledge the patient or the couple are seeking.

Thus, autonomy is a goal rarely completely reached in medicine, and sometimes it is completely lacking. There is an inherent imbalance of power in all encounters between professional and lay people, between physicians and their patients (or, in the extreme autonomy model, "clients"). This after all is why the client seeks the advice of a professional. In other areas of medicine, a sick or incompetent patient quickly loses autonomy and wants the professional to do his or her best on their behalf. This can also be the situation with infertility treatment, but it should not be assumed by the physician.

**Professionalism** can be described as the responsible practice of professional power. It implies involving the patient in making decisions where a choice exists and in explaining the situation if there seems to be little choice. **Paternalism**, on the other hand, can be defined as the irresponsible practice of professional power, where the patient is kept in the dark or is pushed into accepting the proposed treatment. Professionalism, by shunning paternalism, advances respect for persons and leads to a sensible and balanced sharing of uncertainty.

informed consent differently, but the judgment in this Australian case illustrate an important obligation. When offering treatment for infertility the physician i obliged to inform the couple of the consequences in as much detail as the cou ple want to hear. Printed information can help, to be sure, but the physician must first anticipate a need for the most relevant information and, should curi osity be slight, deliver it regardless (there is basic information everyone mus have), and second, continue responding to it for as long as curiosity persists. I time constrains this at one professional consultation then another opportunity needs to be made.

Thus, it is the patient who should decide how far discussion should go be fore reaching a decision on medical treatment. A physician should resist relying on only a signed consent form "for protection." All-encompassing forms for consenting to medical procedures seek to place too much weight on the patient Such a form—and such a polarized professional relationship—is good for nei ther the physician nor the patient, who is meant in this way to be dumped with responsibility for what eventually happens.

Taking responsibility is a two-way thing. Patients also need to take respon sibility for what happens. Do not expect your physician to second-guess you. If you want to know more before starting an IVF treatment cycle, for example, af ter reading the information brochures and signing the consent forms the IVF center provides, it is your responsibility to postpone starting if you do not feel ready. You have a right to know the chance of success, an estimate based on var ious assumptions and generalizations. But when you do start, it is your respon sibility to share with your physician the inevitable uncertainty concerning the outcome that is a part of any medical treatment.

# Responsibility in Infertility Research

There is probably no area in medicine where research and clinical practice are less distinct than in reproductive medicine and the use of reproductive technol ogy. This state of affairs has meant babies for infertile couples who otherwise would have outgrown their opportunities. For them the rapidity of research be coming practice has been a blessing. For others who have been less successful, there is often a sense of bewilderment and resentment, when expensive, un comfortable or even possibly dangerous maneuvers have failed to secure suc-

## The Helsinki Declaration, 1964

The Helsinki Declaration on the rights of humans in the field of medical experimentation states:

• A fundamental distinction needs to be made between medical research in which the aim is essentially diagnostic or therapeutic for a patient, and medical research in which the essential object is purely scientific.

• The responsibility for the human subject needs to rest with the medically qualified person involved and that it should never rest on the subject of the research, even though the subject has given his or her consent.

• Every biomedical research project involving human subjects should be preceded by careful assessment of predictable risks in comparison with foreseeable benefits to the subject or to others; and that concern for the interests of the subject must always prevail over the interests of science and society.

• The design and performance of each experimental procedure should be clearly formulated in an experimental protocol, which should be transmitted to a specially appointed independent committee for consideration, comment and guidance.

The Helsinki Declaration goes on to say that, in principle, medical research can be combined with professional medical practice:

• The doctor can combine medical research with professional care, the objective being the acquisition of new medical knowledge, only to the extent that medical research is justified by its potential diagnostic or therapeutic value for the patient.

• In any medical study, every patient—including those of a control group, if any—should be assured of the best proven diagnostic and therapeutic method.

• The refusal of the patient to participate in a study must never interfere with the doctor-patient relationship.

cessful pregnancy, and especially when there has been a lingering atmosphere of experiment.

The widely accepted current minimum code of conduct for clinical research experimentation is the Declaration of Helsinki of 1964 (in turn derived from the Nuremberg Code of 1947, and amended in 1975 and 1983), which established that, to be ethical, medical research must be meaningful, scientifically based, medically supervised, consented to only after evaluation of risks, confidential and truthfully reported.

More and more, ethical aspects of medical practice, as distinct from ethical aspects of research protocols, are presented to IECs for opinion. In the United States many institutions have set up rapid-response "ethics committees," distinct from their research review boards, to which controversial medical decisions can be referred, sometimes by individuals who have detected undue paternalism in clinical decisions made by colleagues. The danger is that ethical responsibility for the decision through such referral becomes remote and diffuse, with diminished rather than improved **accountability** for the outcomes. Nonetheless, ethics committees of both kinds can usefully help an individual researcher or practitioner share a moral burden by providing a forum for formal ethical consideration when that researcher or practitioner has doubts.

Institutional ethics committees have not yet evolved fully. Some shortcomings are quirky, others are pervasive. To start with, no committee will be better than the members that compose it, and the committee will depend particularly on the experience, intelligence and compassion of the person in the chair and the example he or she sets to the committee's other members.

A more general shortcoming of ethics committees finds its root in the following Helsinki principle: "In the treatment of the sick person, the doctor must be free to use a new diagnostic and therapeutic measure, if in his or her judgment it offers hope of saving life, re-establishing health or alleviating suffering." In other words, there is nothing much to constrain a physician from introducing new treatments outside formal clinical trials, and a very large number of surgical and medical innovations involving operations and the use of therapeutic devices (indeed most therapeutic medicine outside drug trials, including surgical operations on the fetus) have been introduced this way. By no means have all IVF centers involved their ethics committees when introducing new (for them) treatment modalities that may or may not have worked well in other programs.

The irony for the physician is that if he or she wishes to try a new treatment or operation, there is presently no need to refer the matter to an ethics committee, unless the practitioner wants to evaluate the new treatment or operation in a controlled or randomized study of its efficacy. This inconsistency imposes a major practical disadvantage to constructing proper evaluations of new treatments by individual practitioners and within institutions. The point, in practice, is so finely drawn that, for example, an IVF center's laboratory policy decision to use one culture medium for perhaps two months before switching to another for comparison is likely to escape the attention of the IRB, whereas a better-designed, simultaneous, randomly allocated comparison of culture media comes under full and critical external scrutiny.

Committees that review research protocols within institutions before they are put into effect have been established in most Western countries. Generally they are called **institutional review boards** (IRBs) in the United States and **institutional ethics committees** (IECs) in other countries. IRBs and IECs should be set up by all institutions that carry out a significant amount of research. They need to include lay men and women as members, and often there are members with legal and ethical (sometimes theological) experience. Their membership might include specialist physicians and scientists, who are meant to rule a research protocol unethical if it is not scientifically sound. In some institutions the moral and scientific roles in judging a research proposal to be ethical are devolved to two committees, which then meet to make joint decisions. IRBs and IECs are bound by the Helsinki Declaration.

IRBs and IECs cannot override laws and government regulations, but they can impose narrower constraints, which they often do, depending on the nature of the institution. For example, hospitals run by religious orders commonly limit the reproductive research they allow. Consciously or not, IECs and IRBs draw on moral, consequential and equity or resource-allocation considerations before they approve, improve or reject a research proposal. Members use their own ethical values as they seek to put themselves in the place of the research subjects, in order to protect them without unduly standing in the way of medical progress.

Increasingly, IRBs and IECs are being brought together in different countries within a framework of national ethical policy, sometimes by a government-appointed "super ethics committee," to which global or community-wide matters of ethical policy can be referred. In Australia, for example, a protocol was submitted to an IEC that involved flushing preimplantational embryos from the uterus of embryo donors impregnated by assisted insemination (see the box "Womb Flushing" in Chapter 22). The then-novel ethical hazards caused the IEC to refer it to the Medical Research Ethics Committee of Australia's National Health and Medical Research Council, which published a paper discussing the ethical difficulties, with a recommendation that studies of this sort not proceed. The same national ethics committee was responsible for formulating general guidelines for the ethical conduct of research involving in vitro fertilization and research involving the human fetus.

National ethics committees thus build from a starting point enunciated in the Helsinki Declaration to produce more country-specific sets of values, over which IRBs and IECs can add their own institution-specific values. Thus, there is a "ratchet function" through which, from Helsinki to the institution, ethical considerations can be tightened but not loosened.

# Ethical Principles in Practice

Whether infertility treatment is accepted medical practice or whether it is me[?]ical research can therefore be a vexing question. It is often not possible to ma[?] the distinction. What is there to guide the physician and the patient?

## Compassion

Treatment, whether established or relatively pioneering, should always be deli[?]ered with compassion, whatever the level of autonomy or privacy the patient [?] couple choose at that stage of their relationship with their physician. The pr[?] dent physician (or nurse or psychologist or social worker) will detect the level [?] willingness to share feelings and emotions the patient or couple have and w[?] respond to it. Complete physicians will make known their capacity for deep[?] feelings such as empathy (see the box "From Mercy to Empathy"). But the[?] deeper shared feelings are delivered by the physician to the patient at the p[?]

### From Mercy to Empathy

The words "sympathy," "compassion" and "empathy" have replaced biblical expressions of "mercy" and "pity" for giving meaning to important social feelings people show their fellows, falling deliberately short of the more psychologically invasive, sometimes sexually invasive, emotion of "love."

"Empathy," despite its Greek appearance, is not an ancient word. It was coined in 1912 to translate the German psychiatric term *Einfühlung,* or "feeling as one with," which is a rather risky degree of psychotherapeutic identification a physician, specifically a psychiatrist, can aim for with his or her patient. In modern usage, empathy probably more often represents *Mitgefühl,* feeling "with" someone, overlapping the word "compassion," which dates from 1625 in English usage. But in either usage, something deeper is meant than "sympathy," the German for which is *Sympathie.* Empathy does not need to characterize a health professional's relationship with each patient or client. This is neither practical nor is it always welcome. Rather, the potential for it is signaled in one way or another and it is a reserve to draw on when the occasion calls for it. Compassion, however, should be as obvious and as steady as bedrock.

tient's option—only if the patient wants to share them; they are not necessarily appropriate to every professional situation. In this way a patient's privacy can be protected without standing in the way of good medicine.

As new options for treating infertility become available, there are other principles and values that are important for patients, physicians and other health professionals, researchers, ethics committees and governments to consider. This is especially so when duties, obligations and rights of different people come into conflict.

# Duties, Obligations and Rights

"The rights of the child should be paramount" is a statement presently popular in our society among social moralists when trying to consider such complex situations as surrogacy (see Chapter 22). It stems from Article 3 of the United Nations Convention on the Rights of Children. Unlike Article 3, however, the statement is often used to refer to children who have not yet been born and even to children not yet conceived. Such a statement promises a shortcut to ethical wisdom, a quick way out of many moral entanglements that affect the family and the infertile couple in society. But there are limits to its context and its power to illuminate moral and ethical values.

Duties and rights are different perspectives of the same relationship. In a sense, they work from opposite directions. One person's right is meaningless without someone else's duty or obligation. For example, the argument in a democracy that everyone has a right to vote really means that governments are obliged to provide accessible polling stations and to count votes honestly and accurately; if you choose to stay at home on election day, no one has a duty to bring you the voting booth, so your right to vote has lost its meaning.

If a moral duty is perceived widely enough it gets to be seen as a right by the recipient—a right that may then spread to others in similar positions, producing a need to redefine the duties or obligations of others in an attempt to make everything seem fair and equitable. Incompatibilities or conflicts can arise between, for example, a physician's duty to the wife and to the husband (although it is rare in practice); perhaps more often, there is conflict between the physician's sense of duty and the rights that the couple have to secure the best medical advice and personal respect they consider should be offered. If you as a patient think that your rights are at variance with a physician's perceptions of his or her duties or obligations, then justice is best brought about by openness. You should be given the opportunity of seeking a second opinion, and if conflicting expectations persist you should take it.

There are instances when society, in seeking to accommodate rights, relies not just on physicians' self-motivated duties but adds to these duties by imposing obligations. In most countries, compulsory notification to public health authorities of certain infectious diseases, such as hepatitis C and **AIDS**, are examples of such an extrinsic obligation. Reporting of birth defects is another.

Ethical duties can conflict in many ways in medicine, particularly in reproductive medicine, because more than one client (or patient or autonomous person) is so commonly involved. Consider, for example, a sperm donor's desire for news of his progeny versus the desire of the couple that received the sperm for privacy. In this example different societies have imposed different obligations by regulation or law. In Sweden the donor is protected; in the United States the donor signs away all such rights. If society does not make obligations plain by regulation or law, a lot of thoughtfulness and compassion is needed to reach an equitable solution. Ethical "through-ways" or "shortcuts" that insist on wisdom through one-eyed focusing on moral duties or obligations—such as obligations to children not yet conceived overriding the wishes of the prospective parents seeking reproductive help—can be a bullying form of paternalism, given that such regulation of ordinary reproduction would not be acceptable.

## Doing Good, Telling the Truth and Achieving Justice

The moral force behind the notions of rights and duties in the relationship between physician and patient or an infertile couple arrives through a series of bioethical principles that have much general appeal and value. Again, however, these principles can conflict, so that a balance, sometimes controversial, needs to be struck. Balance may best be attempted within categories of considerations (see the box "Ethics: Moral Imperatives, Consequences and Equity"), before their strengths and weaknesses are compared across the categories to produce some sort of compromise in society in the form of public or professional policy. In a pluralist society, ethical tension will generally be least if these values are based on consequences rather than on shared moral perceptions of duty, except when such moral positions are virtually universal.

There is a widely recognized moral compulsion to tell the **truth**. Most agree that, as an ethical principle, truth should not be dispensed with simply for expediency, although occasionally for an individual the consequence or "end" (comfort) may justify unusual means (that is, withholding the truth). Integrity demands that truth not be dismissed for short-term gains alone. If, for a special reason, the truth is not told, the prudent physician will share the real truth and the responsibility for the untruth with others, such as the patient's husband or wife. I should add quickly that while this question might arise in dealing with terminal illnesses, the dilemma is not common among infertile couples; the trust they have in each other (see Chapter 25) should not be split. Nonetheless, it may be appropriate and kind to spare a 15-year-old from knowledge of all the consequences of **congenital absence of the uterus** (see Chapter 18) or **primary ovarian failure** (see Chapter 10) at first, while being more frank with her parents. Integrity as a value means more than always telling the literal truth and keeping promises; it calls for a consistency of approach that encourages faith in the judgment of a physician, nurse, psychologist or social worker.

The principle of **nonmaleficence**, or not doing harm, was made popular by the Hippocratic Oath, which says, "first, do no harm." As an ethical principle it often has a strong moral, sometimes religious, basis. "Thou shalt not kill" is an ancient expression of nonmaleficence. (Members of the Jainist religion in India take it to an extreme by breathing through a handkerchief, to avoid the accidental killing of flying insects, and by stepping carefully, so not to tread on ants.) When taken to override other ethical principles within the physician-patient relationship, nonmaleficence is a prescription for doing nothing. In modern, powerful medical practice the risk of doing harm is frequently accepted, and the same is often true in reproductive medicine.

**Beneficence** is the principle of doing good. Because to do powerful good may risk doing harm, or maleficence, the two principles often conflict. In medicine nowadays beneficence is the more widely observed principle, because it is recognized that greater ultimate harm can come from avoiding the risk of immediate harm. Instead, benefits are maximized while harms are minimized. Multiple ovulation induction for assisted conception is a good example. As an ethical principle, beneficence is determined largely by evidence, by the study of consequences for other individuals.

As the Oxford moral philosopher R. M. Hare has pointed out, no serious addressing of beneficence in the political process can avoid questions of equity. And controversy arises quickly in the political sphere if it means that our duties to some individuals (that is, these individuals' rights) are diminished for a greater good. Nonmaleficence then may properly become the basic moral obligation to everyone, irrespective of how lucky or unlucky is their station in society.

Justice, as a principle, means giving every person his or her due. **Distributive justice** is the distribution among members of our society those benefits (rights) and burdens (obligations) due them. The basis of distributive justice is the notion of fairness, the criteria for which involve equity and need. Debate over what is fair is the very substance of our political process.

# Threatened Values

Nowadays there is a considerable call in Western countries for what has come t
be called "evidence-based medicine" (as if it were something new). The moder
concept of evidence-based medicine is essentially an attempt to ration medica
treatments—or at least to ration publicly funded medical treatments—to thos
that have unequivocally been shown to benefit the condition being treated. Th
ethical practice of medicine has always demanded that the physician plac
highly the ethical values of **integrity**, **responsibility** and **accountability** in hi
or her individual relationship with patients and the community. This has natu
rally meant employing treatments for disease or suffering for which there i
good evidence of efficacy. But in keeping with the philosophy expressed in th
Helsinki Declaration (see the box "Ethics and Ethics Committees"), such med
ical practice has often paid scant regard to the financial cost of innovative treat
ment, at least when the cost has been borne by third parties. An increasing fo
cus on outcomes in medical practice generally—and in reproductive medicin
particularly—will be seen more and more in the next few years as those who
foot the bills call the shots.

**Assisted reproductive technology** has provided the excuse for the rapi
erosion of the rights of reproductive physicians and patients by governments in
many countries at a rate much faster than in other medical specialities, but spe
cialties nonetheless susceptible to cost restraint through evidence-based finan
cial pressures. It is not hard to see why. First, there is very little limit to the num
ber of people who are candidates for assisted conception in some form or other
public funding of it can clearly come under great demand without some form
of rationing. Second, there is the technology itself and its arousal of distrust; dis
trust of science is not far from the surface in today's societies no matter how
much we seem to take science and technology for granted. Many physicians in
advertently abet reproductive medicine's susceptibility to this degradation by
themselves referring to the service they deliver as reproductive "technology," im
plying that the technology is an end in itself rather than (as in other fields of
medicine) just an aid to practicing exact medicine. Third, we are concerned here
with an area of moral plurality of opinion. What are embryos? When do they
have autonomy? When does life begin? These are questions that have been hi
jacked by moral conservatives and fundamentalists with agendas that tangle IVF
up with the abortion debate.

The consequence is that society's trust in physicians, and often patients'
trust in their physicians, is under a threat greater than seen in any other area of
medicine. Several governments have imposed or are trying to impose on their

Equity has not been well served at the moral or social frontiers of reproductive medicine. Many governments have, with scant regard for the opinions of their infertile patients, banned embryo research on the basis of moral assumptions and banned gestational surrogacy on the basis of what is meant to be best for the family—but in each case patronizing their citizens for doubtful cause.

A **fetus** is utterly dependent on its mother. A **pre-embryo** in vitro is utterly dependent on the act of transfer into fallopian tube or uterus. Clearly neither the pre-viable fetus nor an embryo has autonomy, but it is popular to extend the notion of autonomy to them, in the form of their potential for autonomy in the future. A newborn child is also dependent on its mother, but respect for its potential autonomy is so widespread that society confers it with some of the rights of an adult. This is achieved in practice by promoting the **duties** of others and enforcing the **obligations** of others toward ensuring its well-being.

Producing pre-embryos for IVF or for research, then destroying those that are not transferred, will be equated with homicide by people who believe innately and intuitively that life starts at conception. For these people, producing pre-embryos that will not or might not be transferred to a woman in receptive circumstances is therefore morally unaccept-

able. This is what, for example, Cardinal Basil Hume, the Roman Catholic Archbishop of Westminster, England, said at the height of the IVF controversy in the 1980s, and it is what many other ordinarily moral people still believe.

On the other hand there is the belief (again usually innate) that humanness develops not instantly but in a sequence, a quick sequence, of **fertilization**, **syngamy**, **cleavage** and **implantation**, followed seamlessly by embryonic development, neural responsiveness, movement and development of the senses. The moral position that obliges increasing protection of these stages accommodates IVF. It allows research on human embryos in special circumstances, contraception that operates after fertilization and abortion in other special circumstances without calling it homicide or infanticide. This is what Dr. John Habgood, the Anglican Archbishop of York, said at the height of the IVF controversy, and it is what many other ordinarily moral people still believe.

Reconciling the two positions in the 1980s (and to date in the 1990s) has proved to be impossible. A spiritual observer on another planet might scratch his or her head and marvel at the energy that keeps such a trivial difference alive (trivial, at least, in comparison with the brutality, homicide and genocide that are still common over some parts of the globe). The moral gulf persists. Reconciliation is a fantasy. Arguments are won, drawn or lost by passion, noise, numbers and—generally to no one's advantage—by legislation.

Great Britain probably leads the world today in embryo research, in purposefully studying pre-embryos in culture to determine their metabolism and nutritional needs. This is partly the result of legislation enacted in 1990, the first time plural differences on the status of the embryo were reconciled by a parliament or congress to the apparent advantage of the infertile, when both the House of Lords and the House of Commons voted (with two-thirds majorities) to approve, in principle, embryo research for the advancement of knowledge. The price Britain's infertile couples have had to pay, however, is substantial. The Human Fertilisation and Embryo Authority, set up by the same act of Parliament that approved embryo research, levies an additional £40 (about $65) on the cost of every IVF treatment cycle conducted in Great Britain. The government of Victoria, Australia, is now preparing to introduce a similar tax.

### Brave New Canada ?

Canada's Royal Commission on New Reproductive Technologies reported in November 1993 as follows: "The Supreme Court has decided that the peace, order, and good government power can be invoked in support of federal legislative ac-tion. We are firmly of the belief that new technologies, as defined in our mandate, meet the criteria established by the Supreme Court, so that federal intervention . . . is constitutionally justified.

"More than any other aspect of health-related technology or service, the research and application of new reproductive technologies have significance beyond the individuals directly involved. Given rapidly expanding knowledge and rapid dissemination of technologies, immediate intervention and concerted leadership are required at the national level . . . citizens in provinces with insufficient regulation may suffer harm.

"The Royal Commission on New Reproductive Technologies recommends that the federal government establish an independent National Reproductive Technologies Commission charged with the primary responsibility of ensuring that new reproductive technologies are developed and applied in the national public interest."

Canada's Royal Commission on New Reproductive Technologies 1993 report inadvertently—but chillingly—recalls Aldous Huxley's Brave New World (1932): "A squat grey building of only thirty-four stories. Over the main entrance the words, CENTRAL LONDON HATCHERY AND CONDITIONING CENTRE, and, in a shield, the World State's motto, COMMUNITY, IDENTITY, STABILITY." In Huxley's brave new world, central governmental control of reproduction is advocated on the basis of what in the Royal Commission's words of maintaining the "peace, order and good government power" can be paraphrased to be Huxley's "community, identity, stability."

Margaret Atwood's 1986 novel *The Handmaid's Tale* concerns curtailment of random reproduction by a Christian fundamentalist government bent on efficiently repopulating a genetically devastated Republic of Gilead, inhabitants of which are largely sterile after a nuclear war; there is no high technology involved, just pervasive central government control of sex and getting pregnant. This novel might in some ways be a paradigm for modern Canada. The women in Gilead are no longer in control of their bodies. What is considered best for them is decided by others. As Atwood puts it, in the liberal days of anarchy, people had the freedom *to* have sex and to reproduce; in Gilead they are given the freedom *from* having to make difficult social choices for themselves.

The Royal Commission—all six members of which were women—decided with ironic paternalism that they know best what is in the "true interests" of Canada's women undergoing infertility treatment. In a closely argued, but in my opinion falsely premised, document, access to reproductive medical services—"reproduc-

tive technology" in the words of the commissioners—would at once be restricted yet universally available. Upon establishment of the "independent" (read exclusive of physicians trained in reproductive medicine) National Reproductive Technologies Commission, all Canadians with a medically defined need would have access to reproductive technology such as IVF (including anonymously donated sperm, eggs and embryos), whatever their married status or gender orientation. Private clinics would be banned.

At provincial clinics treatment would be allowed only for medical conditions where evidence-based certainty of efficacy is deemed by the commissioners to be satisfactory. Thus, IVF (and assisted conception generally) is to be available for disease of the **fallopian tubes** (see Chapter 12) but not for **oligospermia** (see Chapter 9) or for **endometriosis** (see Chapter 14), let alone for **relative infertility** of mixed cause or **unexplained infertility** (see Chapter 6), irrespective of **duration of infertility** (see Appendix A). On the other hand, and according to the commissioners, a woman—in her own true interests—would be prohibited from voluntarily donating her eggs or embryos to another woman she knows, voluntarily undergoing an egg retrieval procedure for her sister or best friend and making use of her remaining frozen embryos should her husband die before she considers her family complete (although she could, provided she has blocked tubes, qualify for new embryos produced from anonymously donated semen).

These prohibitions—these "freedoms from," as Margaret Atwood might put it—are founded not on evidence-based trials of personal good or personal harm done (social trials which in principle are as doable as medical trials) but on what the commissioners believe to be Canadian women's interests (or if not their own true interest, then "the national interest"). The price of Canada's Royal Commission and its two-volume report was in excess of Can$27 million—more than a dollar for every man, woman and child living in Canada—leaving more than a few Canadians with little stomach for what a permanent National Reproductive Technologies Commission would cost Canada and its infertile people.

infertile citizens the guardianship of statutory bodies that will regulate what can or cannot be done to them, what *may* and *may not* be done (under penaltie such as fines and imprisonment of physicians) and, of course, curbing wha *might* innovatively be done. Whether composed of men or women—or with scrupulous attention to gender neutrality and every interest group known to politics—these statutory "authorities" impose their priorities paternalistically on patients and their physicians and, to add injury to the insult, fund their own existence through a levy on patients' cycles of assisted conception treatment. No evidence has ever been systematically adduced—that is, evidence beyond that of mere anecdote—that patients want this protection or that it benefits them in any way. These authorities do not restrict themselves to ensuring high standards of medical practice; there are heaps of accrediting bodies that can do this much cheaper than government authorities. They are there to limit what takes place in the name of public opinion (rarely actually sought and, when known, usually ignored, as in the case of altruistic surrogacy in Australia) and in the name of what is presented as the community's moral values (or what a noisy group of people think they should be). Would that today's insistence on evidence-based medicine be joined by evidence-based ethics and evidence-based social policies!

I conclude this chapter by quoting Reverend Gordon Dunstan, professor emeritus of moral and social theology at the University of London and a writer within the theological tradition of the Church of England: "People who, as patients, experience a sensitive appreciation of human worth and dignity in their own relationships with their physicians will the more readily credit medical [people] with respect for human worth and dignity in the embryo, and trust them accordingly."

Embryo research in the United States, in Australia and, when Dr. Dunstan was writing in 1986, in Great Britain, became problematical in the late 1970s and early 1980s and not just because of the rather global fashion of not trusting science or physicians. Rather, it came about because the rapidity of developments, and some public carelessness and inarticulateness among the physicians concerned, enabled certain moral fundamentalists to succeed in confusing many people about whose humanness needs protecting in IVF laboratories. The resulting difficulties in conducting embryo research, and in properly exploring the social innovations that reproductive medicine can bring to our notion of the family, are the subject of the next chapter.

# Embryo
# Research and
# Society

Fertilize an egg in vitro. Look at the **pre-embryo** that develops over the ne four days. Then do not eventually transfer it back to a woman's reproduct tract (the **uterus** or the **fallopian tubes**). To some critics of reproductive tec nology, this is embryo research. Whether deliberate or not, a pre-embryo ( the box "Revision: What Is a Pre-Embryo?") is being created, one that will r end up back in someone's body. Do such embryos *have* to be created? If so, do it make much difference what happens in the laboratory over the few days th spend there before they are discarded?

This chapter examines the controversy over embryo research that has he in vitro fertilization (IVF) techniques back over the last 15 years, why objectio to embryo research should fade—and *will* fade soon and why "test-tube babie do not mean the same thing for society that Aldous Huxley is often meant have prophesied in his book *Brave New World* back in 1932.

So-called spare embryos (or, strictly, spare pre-embryos) are produced the ordinary course of IVF practice for two reasons. First, unless you have sp cial moral objections, it is usual to try to fertilize all the eggs obtained at yo **egg pickup**. This lessens the chance of having no embryos to transfer if some fa and gives the opportunity to store embryos for transfer later without operati

## Revision: What Is a Pre-Embryo?

Doctors and scientists involved with IVF have come to regret simply calling all fertilized eggs "embryos." It has led some people to think that embryo research (more accurately pre-embryo research) means keeping little fetuses in the laboratory for experimentation. What actually happens in nature (and for the first few days in the lab) is described fully in Chapter 3, but I will summarize it here.

The fertilized egg remains as a single cell for almost 24 hours; it then divides into two cells, four cells, and so on until, after about four days of growth (the maximum, incidentally, we can reliably achieve in the lab), it becomes a ball of 16 or 32 cells (a **morula**) and then—if all goes according to plan—it hollows out to form a **blastocyst**; it is at this stage that it normally is in the uterus. It is not until several days later (about a week after fertilization) that the first few cells in the middle of the blastocyst take on the earliest features of what will become, after implantation, the embryo, and later the fetus. The other cells—in fact *most* of the cells that make up this pre-embryo—develop into the afterbirth and the membranes that surround the fetus in the uterus.

to get another egg. In short, fertilizing all available eggs minimizes the need to stimulate the ovaries repeatedly; for most people, it is common sense.

The second reason spare embryos come about is that there is harm in transferring all embryos to the uterus or to the tubes if there are more than two or three available to transfer. The higher-number multiple pregnancy that results if more than three embryos implant and develop is likely to end in miscarriage before the fetuses are viable. This loss is in no one's interest—not that of the patient, the physician, the community (which shares the expense) or the fetuses. But to limit the number of eggs to be fertilized to the maximum that can be transferred—generally three—is to seriously handicap the logistics of IVF. The spare embryos that result are therefore usually discarded or stored (see Chapter 21). Sometimes a couple may ask that they be donated to another infertile couple.

# Why Do We Need Embryo Research ?

In the early days of IVF, before 1978 when the first IVF baby was born, there was little chance that the eggs fertilized in vitro would develop into babies. In this sense, the IVF practices of the 1980s could not have been worked out without embryo research in the 1970s. We believe that IVF techniques in the 1990s and into the next century will only be better than those of today if we can continue to learn more about the early events after fertilization, not just by growing in culture for several days those embryos that are additional to the ones transferred, but (when conditions allow it and when providers of eggs and sperm approve) by fertilizing eggs for the special purpose of scientific investigation. Let us be clear about it—this *is* deliberate experimentation with embryos. Just how big a moral question is it?

In most IVF cycles there are embryos (no one knows if they are normal or not) that will not be used; they will be discarded. How morally awkward is it then to look at them ("observational research") or to study the effects of different culture medium on their capacity to keep growing a few days ("interventional research")? How morally awkward is it to fertilize eggs in different circumstances so that we can work out how they will grow best? How morally awkward is it to make sure that a promising but still unproven fertilizing method or diagnostic embryo test does not damage embryos before we try the method out in clinical practice?

Few people who have experienced infertility have a moral problem with the issue of embryo research, but in the community the difference of opinion

## Ethical Embryo Research: An Example

At Sydney IVF in 1989 we used the National Health and Medical Research Council research guidelines to make sure eggs fertilized by sperm microinjection were genetically normal before we produced pregnancies for couples with desperately low sperm counts. In the neighboring state of Victoria, for moral cum political reasons this research had been stopped. To the benefit of our patients (and, later, patients everywhere), Professor Alan Trounson, at the time the head of the Centre for Early Human Development at Monash University in Victoria and scientific director at Sydney IVF, arranged for the scientists skilled in the required embryology and genetics techniques (learned with Victorian mice!) to spend two special weeks in Sydney. During those weeks, each of 16 couples, all previously unsuccessful with IVF due to extremely low sperm counts, volunteered to have an IVF cycle in which they knew there would be no embryos to give them an immediate chance of pregnancy. The reason was that every one of the embryos would have its **chromosomes** looked at, which, although providing information, would mean the embryos would be destroyed. Each couple stood to benefit if the technique being tested could be shown to be safe, at least as far as the chromosomes were capable of showing this safety.

Before we started the study, we submitted a research protocol for approval by the institutional ethics committee (IEC) at Royal Prince Alfred Hospital, which has ethical jurisdiction over all Sydney IVF's clinical and research activities.

The results of the study showed that more embryos after sperm microinjection (SMI)—the technique then was **subzonal insertion**, or SUZI (see Chapter 20)—had

concerning embryo creation is still widespread. Because there is no sign of a consensus developing, at Sydney IVF, for example, we believe that it is *your* moral belief that should prevail for your eggs, your sperm and your embryos. The principle we follow when we get consent for IVF treatment or for research on embryos is that it is the moral perspective of those who provide the embryo that is overridingly important.

In Australia, the National Health and Medical Research Council (NHMRC) has, in principle, approved research studies on embryos or pre-embryos up to the stage of implantation, that is, up to about a week after fertilization. Nevertheless, all special studies involving pre-embryos also need to be approved by an **institutional ethics committee** (see Chapter 26). In the Australian state of

## Ethical Embryo Research: An Example (concluded)

a normal chromosomal **karyotype** than after conventional IVF (part of the authorized **control group**) and more than other researchers had reported for embryos conceived normally. SMI, in other words, if anything, improved the chromosome situation for the average embryo.

As these outstanding results were prepared for publication in the European journal *Human Reproduction,* the IEC at Royal Prince Alfred Hospital approved stage two of the studies to go ahead, namely the application of SUZI directly for the benefit of our infertile patients. Within the year probably the world's second and third babies were born from this new technique. (Dr. Simon Fishel in Great Britain secured pregnancies from SUZI at about the same time, but without prior genetic studies.)

Ironically, yet gratifyingly, this interstate expedition by people who were Australia's best IVF researchers led directly to an amendment to the **Infertility (Medical Procedures) Act** in Victoria to allow research up to **syngamy**; previously, research had effectively been banned on eggs from the moment of penetration by sperm.

Nonetheless, in 1992 IVF researchers in Victoria were still pushed to go straight to human clinical trials of intracytoplasmic sperm injection (ICSI), the microinjection technique that has now replaced SUZI, without *any* prior genetic tests of embryos produced this way. This direct step to medical practice, without making use of safety tests on embryos that were easily available, was considered in Victoria to be more ethical than embryo research. Such reprehensible, bureaucratic, paternalistic moralism is beyond comprehension for most infertile couples.

Victoria, where most of the early Australian innovations in IVF, such as **embryo freezing** and **sperm microinjection**, took place, permission has, since 1984, also been needed from the Victorian government's **Standing Review and Advisory Committee**, a committee that has never given permission for meaningful embryo research beyond the stage of syngamy. (Syngamy, as a moral milestone, is a peculiarly Victorian moral invention; it defines human life as starting with contact between the sperm's chromosomes and the egg's chromosomes, about 22 hours after the sperm enters the egg.) Clinical IVF research in Victoria was brought to an effective stop by a particularly paternalistic attitude of government toward its citizens. In Great Britain, on the other hand, several centers have permission from the **Human Fertilisation and Embryology**

**Authority** to conduct embryo research by fertilizing human eggs in vitro (wi
the permission of the "parents") and to study the metabolism of human em
bryos in vitro—what nutrients they need, when and how much.

# Whose Humanness Is in Jeopardy?

It was once a virtue not to make an issue of a matter without good cause. Toda
it seems issues are often kept alive for the sake of it. Embryo research has bee
popularly contentious. For people who maintain that human life, with all i
need for protection, is there from the moment of conception (or, with a twis
under the Victorian Act described above, from the moment of syngamy, or th
joining of the chromosomes), embryo research is like homicide. In effect, em
bryos are conferred with **rights** to match the **obligations** the state of Victori
enforced upon IVF researchers through legislation.

Almost twenty years after the world's first birth following conception i
vitro, back in 1978, we have learned little more than we knew then about the nu
tritional needs of fertilized human eggs and early embryos. Scientists and phys
cians have had to wait while others have developed moral, ethical and politica
positions to work out the future place of human embryo research. To be sure
the clinical applications of IVF-related reproductive technology have advanced
To the joy of their parents, many thousands of babies have been born wh
otherwise would not have been. But the chance of birth after an embryo's tw
or three days of development after fertilization in the lab has been kept low b
confusion over whose humanness needs protecting in the IVF laboratory. Th
two moral positions on the matter—that human life starts at conception with
duty or obligation to protect it from that moment or that life develops in stage
with a graded duty or obligation that unfolds according to the circumstances—
have proved to be fundamentally irreconcilable.

Embryo research will be beneficial for future infertile couples, as it will b
for future embryos in vitro or in vivo. But it is obvious that there are many peo
ple who feel their humanity and that of others is under threat from the idea o
culturing human embryos for scientific curiosity instead of their own individ
ual benefit. These feelings sometimes change, either when more information i
made available or when the dehumanizing experience of infertility happen
close to home.

In the meantime, it needs to be made widely known that what happens t
embryos in the laboratory does not dehumanize or brutalize those who carr

How can **autonomy** and notions of **rights** be conferred on embryos or pre-embryos while they are still undifferentiated cells, logically weeks or months from any possible inherent notion of independence? Let us leave aside inspirations such as the soul and when it might enter a body, because we have already seen how futile and unhelpful such philosophical maneuvering has been in illuminating the morality of embryo research. Instead, a fable about two mice might help.

### ... and the Tales of Mice

The first mouse in the fable was a field mouse, genetically an outbred mouse, a free-range mouse, but he and his large extended family lived on a farm, where they inhabited and populated a wheat silo. By prospering, father (later, grandfather) mouse caused the farmer who owned the wheat silo to reach the conclusion that he and his growing mouse family were vermin mice. The mice were then exterminated by the farmer in the ordinary course of farm business. The farmer's children hardly knew about it, but, being brought up on a farm, they would in any case have thought nothing of it. If pests, whether bugs, insects or mammals, get in the way of producing food efficiently and hygienically then, without fuss, they're gotten rid of. The second mouse was a genetically inbred white mouse, identical to hundreds of thousands of other mice—a battery mouse we might call it if it was lined up with others to test the safety of batches of drugs or perfumes. But this particular mouse had the temporary good fortune to find itself in its own cage, as a pet mouse, with a proud young owner. Being an interesting piece of property, the mouse was lent to another child for awhile. This second child tormented the mouse until it died, and then gave it back, with glazed eyes and a cold, stiffening body. Understandably, everyone concerned with this unforgettable experience was sad, perhaps a little brutalized.

What do these stories have in common and in what ways do they differ? And how do they help us come to grips with human embryo research? Both are stories of intentional rodenticide. Now, are the

out embryo research. As I explain in the box "The Moral Position of Embryos in Vitro ...," my experience with newcomers to embryo laboratories is that the opposite happens: IVF, embryo research and knowing the couples whose hopes are present in vitro, all increase one's awe of and respect for that which is human.

IVF and embryo experimentation are very human and caring experiences for those directly involved with them. This fact—it is an observable fact and not

## The Moral Position of Embryos in Vitro ... (concluded)

ethics of rodenticide immutable? Or are the moral circumstances of these two stories different? Truly, they are different. However inconsistent it is for mice, and however we might luxuriate philosophically in the wrongs of rodenticide as our memories of mouse traps and rat catchers falls further into sociological and town-planning history, morality for most of us—our response to the death of the mouse—will equate with how we perceive our own notions of humanity to have been affected by the tales of the mice.

Rodenticide, at first sight, might not have much to do with embryo research, but it gives an insight into notions of humanity and into notions of what is dehumanizing. The rights of these two mice turn out to be different because of the effect the different obligations we have to the two mice has on our sense of humanity.

In the early stages of the debate on the morality of embryo research, I remember that a parallel was drawn by some less than scrupulous debaters between embryo researchers and the Nazi doctors of World War II who sadistically experi-

mented on human beings. This analogy was drawn by people who thought that fertilized eggs were human life that needed the same protection as children and adults. Can anyone who has been inside an IVF laboratory function seriously make this analogy? At Sydney IVF and at all other IVF centers I have seen, each embryologist—most of whom are women—is meticulous about her or his concern for the patient. They are not cynical, contemptuous or callous. Not one I know has been brutalized by the experience of what happens in an IVF lab. Each of them has gained steadily and considerably in their respect for the couples they treat and in their respect for the reproductive and personal potential of the eggs, sperm and embryos that are in their care. (As a result it is our scientists at Sydney IVF who will confirm with patients the number of eggs or embryos to be transferred, who will sit with the patient during an egg pickup procedure if she wants the company and the comfort and who are happy to talk with the patient about how the laboratory procedures are going or have gone.)

just my opinion—can be verified by anyone who takes the opportunity to vis one of our IVF labs. This fact should, and in due course will, put an end doubts about their morality in a plural society.

I believe, therefore, that our society will eventually embrace deliberate, un abashed, responsible embryo and fetal research in vitro, not because of coger logic on its ethics or because the pope changes his mind, but because the in portance of such research for advancing human health will outlive those who believe they should, for one reason or another, oppose it.

# Beyond Embryo Research: Brave New World ?

The two most contentious issues in treating infertility—surrogacy and embryo research—have both now been discussed. Let me sum up their context in our society.

Since the late nineteenth century, there have been several medical and social waves of liberation for women. These waves have consisted of female emancipation (the vote for women), development of effective contraception, better hygiene, the conquest of infection with antibiotics, privacy and the option of divorce for marriages that no longer work. Sigmund Freud discouraged the inhibition of sexuality in child rearing earlier in this century. Since then the women's liberation movement, now feminism, has intensified the pressure for change.

The 1960s and 1970s—the two decades that followed the invention of the oral contraceptive pill—saw a rise in sexual permissiveness that was at last unshackled from a corresponding risk of unwanted pregnancy. Abortion received widespread sanction in the 1970s. Only in the 1980s did the specter of untreatable venereal diseases from viruses start to slow down the gathering popularity of premarital and extramarital sex.

Moral standards have always waxed and waned, but the developments of the twentieth century have brought to practical fruition trends that have been taking place for longer. These trends have included improving technology, improving health and longevity, more effective personal freedoms and, very conspicuously, a steady increase in the individual value placed upon children.

The present fortunate position is that the survival of children can be taken for granted from infancy to old age, that we have command of contraception and that we are on the verge of commanding conception—all of which means, or soon will mean, that reproduction, for the first time in our evolution, is truly a matter of choice. Children are now regarded, perhaps sometimes overly so, as society's most important members, with the popular claim that, in matters of reproduction, the well-being of the child is important above all else. The historian J. L. Stone, however, has demonstrated that today's family in Western societies, as a result of this cultural evolution, is self-centered, inwardly turned, emotionally bonded, sexually liberated, child-oriented and, too often, temporary. The

different, separate ambitions of parents detach them from the home and fr〈
their dependence on each other. The guilt they feel over depriving children
adequate family life is countered by concentrating too much on their childre
(too often on their one child's) personal achievements. Children, according
this model, are becoming isolated within the family. For their socialization th
depend not on their family but upon their peer groups.

Modern families, especially it seems in the United States and Scandinav
but in many other Western countries, are more loosely structured and less em
tionally and sexually cohesive than has been the case for centuries. In Chapt
22 I mentioned how infertility can prove to be a better cement for a marria
under strain than fertility. To the Indian social anthropologist Professor Praka
Reddy, accustomed to close relations within his own extended family, the mo〈
ern, sequestered, small European family of the type he studied in the Danish v
lage of Hvilsager lacks spirituality, overly emphasizes individualism and h〈
children brought up independent, alone and lonely. As a "type," this family h
an impermanence, a transience, that recalls the chaos of earlier centuri〈
Reproductive technology is not to blame for us reaching this point.

There is little reason to suppose that today's Western "nuclear" family mod
has a special claim to be the best or that today's typical Western family will 〈
more lasting than its predecessors. It has been called "ethnocentric" (overly r
garding our own ethnic culture to be best) to assume that this one form of t〈
family is crucial to the survival of a society. This is the context in which 〈
should examine gamete donation, embryo donation and surrogacy. Cultur〈
evolution, like biological evolution, works best if society, like nature, is ri〈
enough and confident enough to accommodate diversity. In this way, changi〈
circumstances bring adaptation or, more precisely, they bring triumph for wh〈
in retrospect are "preadaptations"—the luxury of diversity produces good r
sults down the track that are unforeseen at the time the diversity is allowed 〈
flower. With the twentieth-century nuclear family now fragile, we need to wide
our concept of the family, to extend the notion of parenthood, to broaden o〈
social options, to give people room to move in finding solutions to societ〉
stresses and strains and how to bring up well-balanced children.

Looking into a future with the technology for test-tube babies has broug〈
many writers to remember Aldous Huxley's *Brave New World*. It has broug〈
many of these writers to be afraid of sliding down a slippery slope into the m〈
chanical, oppressive world Huxley predicted for the future. "Sanity is a rare ph〈
nomenon in public life," Huxley wrote in a new preface to his book in 1946, ju
after World War II. Huxley believed that governments would favor stability 〈
society over truly responding to popular will; he also believed this would cau〈
powerful governments to become too bossy, too intrusive and too totalitaria〈

The reluctance of politicians everywhere to grapple sensibly with altruistic surrogacy is a good example of government preferring order to change.

The sinister feature of the future in Huxley's predictions was not what was possible with IVF and life in test tubes. Rather, it was the total control the centralized Utopian government had over people's lives. (To imagine the horrors that central government control can have over sex and reproduction without any resort to technology read or watch the video of Margaret Atwood's book *The Handmaid's Tale*.)

It is surely a government's proper job to foster tolerance and plural opinions in society. It is not its job, gratuitously and paternalistically, to make personal decisions for its citizens. Decisions on assisting conception, like decisions on contraception and abortion, should be private and well-informed ones, taken by the people affected, helped by their professional advisers in a community framework of tolerance.

By dealing explicitly with ethics, morality and suffering, as by explaining the physiology and medicine of infertility, I hope this book helps you to understand what is happening, to communicate with your physician and to articulate your cause, your case and your concerns.

# Appendix A

## The New Fertility and Infertility Math

The last fifteen years have seen the transformation of the physician's approach to infertility. The development of **in vitro fertilization** (IVF) has so improved our capacity to overcome this most distressing of disabilities that we have had to overhaul many of our working ideas on how infertility can come about. This is not because new causes have been discovered. Rather, we have come to appreciate how apparently minor disturbances can combine to cause a major disruption in reproduction even when tests show that there is no complete or absolute barrier to getting pregnant.

A consequence of this change of approach is the need to alter our way of explaining what is happening to you. No longer is it good enough to say, "The chance of getting pregnant after this operation is 60 percent." It begs questions such as: "Yes, but how long will I have to wait?" "Is that 60 percent in six months, a year or five years?" "What effect will my long periods (or my husband's sperm count, or my endometriosis, or my age) have on this chance?" "How will one or more cycles of IVF affect my chances of ending up with a baby?"

The first purpose of this appendix is to set out the arithmetic behind the new approach to appreciating fertility and infertility—an approach introduced in Chapter 1. The second purpose is to judge the place of various options for treatment when a couple decides the pregnancy has taken too long and the time remaining is getting short.

Before going on, it might be useful to reread Chapter 1. As I say there, at best—and sometimes, no doubt, at worst—getting pregnant is a matter of chance. The overall chance will depend first on what the chance is biologically meant to be when you have sex at the right time; and, second, it will depend on the number of months (or cycles of ovulation) you can keep trying, before you get too old or too fed up.

The statistic that describes this monthly chance is the "monthly probability of conception," known among population scientists as **fecundability** (abbreviated $f$), and it is the probability (the chance) of achieving pregnancy in one ovulation cycle. You can express fecundability as a percentage, say 20 percent, or a proportion, say 0.2—they mean the same thing. You may recall from Chapter 1 that the 20 percent figure represents normal average fecundability for a population of couples in their twenties when they first start trying to achieve a pregnancy. Fecundability is similar to a number of other terms that are used, including "monthly fecundity" (strictly speaking, the monthly probability of a live birth resulting from one cycle exposed to the possibility of pregnancy) and, more simply, **monthly fertility**. Like every statistic in biology, monthly fertility has a wide range of values in the population, as shown in Figure A.1, which also represents, with an ellipse at the left end of the graph (marked S), a group of couples with a monthly fertility chance of zero, meaning **complete infertility** (in other words, **sterility**, which affects maybe 2 or 3 percent of couples trying to get pregnant—couples who have a complete barrier to getting pregnant that will always need more than just time to overcome).

Sterility is abnormal—that is a statemer beyond argument (and diagnosing it is th subject of Chapter 5). **Relative infertili** (also called *subfertility*) is a different matte Population scientists—impersonal species tha they are—might define relative infertility a what the bottom 5 percent of the populatio has, corresponding with the bottom 5 percer of the area of Figure A.1 (under the graph an marked RI). Fixing the limits of relative infer tility within the normal range of monthly fer tility shown is quite arbitrary (see Chapter 1 You and I would probably put the cuto rather higher than 5 percent. We would, in stead, call the situation relative infertilit whenever you think trying for pregnancy ha gone on long enough and you go to see you

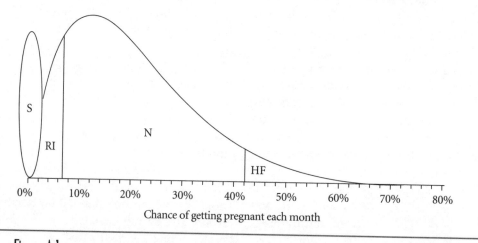

**Figure A.1**  Distribution of monthly fertility in the population. A graph showing the wide range of monthly fertility in a large group of young people. The average for the group is 20 percent. The ellipse at the left end of the graph (S) represents the 2 or 3 percent of couples who have zero chance of pregnancy—meaning complete infertility, or sterility. To define normal fertility (N), we can separate the lowest 5 percent and the highest 5 percent, leaving the middle 90 percent as "normal" (these cutoff points are arbitrary, however, and do not depend on any natural distinction). Couples in the "lower tail" of the distribution then have abnormally low fertility, or relative infertility (RI). Couples in the "upper tail" (equally abnormal, you could argue) have high fertility (HF).

ynecologist for tests and advice. Some people might say anything below average is enough to warrant having something done about it; gain your perception of how long it has taken nd how long you have are what is important, ut you might now be able to imagine the difficulty that arbitrarily defining infertility like his causes for some health care managers, politicians, radical feminists and others who are critical of expensive reproductive technology.

In statistics, incidentally, it is not just the bottom, say, 5 percent that is abnormal. Logically, the top 5 percent of a statistical distribution curve such as Figure A.1 is just as abnormal. It would correspond with abnormally "high fertility" (HF). This phenomenon (it is much less of a problem than it used to be before the days of effective contraception) is discussed in Chapter 1 under "High Fertility—A Disability?"

Tests for infertility can give us (and often do) results that are not conclusive. Pregnancy seems possible, but it has not happened yet. Sometimes the investigations are all normal; this is **unexplained infertility**. In practice, however, the distinction between infertility of known cause and unexplained infertility is much less important than it used to be. Although IVF was developed so that we could get around damaged fallopian tubes that were beyond repair—and undoubtedly this has transformed the treatment of sterility and serious infertility from this cause—it is in the modification of IVF to deal with relative infertility and unexplained infertility that the second, bigger transformation in treatment is taking place.

To understand relative infertility, and to understand when to use **assisted conception** maneuvers to try and overcome it, I make use of the special statistic of monthly fertility and show you how with time monthly fertility mounts up to what is called the **cumulative chance of pregnancy**. Take a first look at Figure A.2 for an introduction to this concept.

The classical causes of relative infertility are described in Chapter 7, but experience has shown that discovering a cause—and assessing the severity of a cause—is less important in determining monthly fertility (and hence the eventual chance of getting pregnant naturally as the months pass) than the **duration of infertility**. The other variable in determining the chance of achieving pregnancy naturally in circumstances of relative infertility is the time available for chance to have its way, or the **time left for conception**. There are some other points I need to cover before I place assisted conception in this context.

We can show in theory and in practice that the worse a diagnosed cause of infertility is, the better the chance of getting pregnant naturally will be after treatment, provided that the treatment corrects the problem properly and that the treatment does not, through side actions, interfere with any other aspects of reproductive functioning. Mild abnormalities discovered while investigating infertility, on the other hand, may turn out to be decoys, and attempts to treat them, especially if there is more than one, not only lures attention away from whatever the undiscovered "real" cause might be but risks introducing new disturbances that then take the distracting place of the original suspected abnormality or abnormalities. In medicine generally, physicians or surgeons are most likely to achieve beneficial outcomes when departures from normal are more than slight (see the box "Medicine's Perennial Paradox" in Chapter 1). Most of our

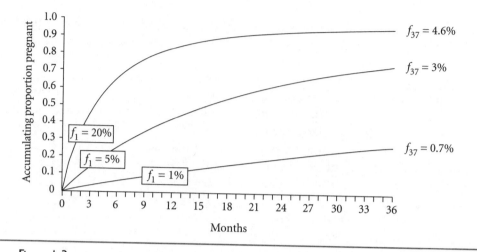

**Figure A.2** Accumulating chance of having gotten pregnant for three groups of women. The figures at the start of the graphs refer to their average monthly chance of getting pregnant in the first month (20%, 5%, or 1%). The figures at the tail ends of the graphs (4.6%, 3%, and 0.7%) represent the residual average monthly fertility of the women in each of the three groups still not pregnant after the three years, that is, for month number 37 ($f_{37}$).

treatments can have side effects, and these side effects are more likely to tip the balance unfavorably when the condition being treated is relatively trivial. This principle is particularly prominent in reproductive medicine and surgery.

You and your physician are especially likely to be frustrated in diagnosis and treatment when several abnormalities, possibly all individually mild, occur together. To demonstrate just how powerful such multiple problems can be in preventing pregnancy we need to understand the arithmetic of getting pregnant a bit better.

The now-standard medical way of judging the outcome of infertility treatment is called a "life curve." Figure A.2 shows three life curves: the cumulative, theoretical chance of *having become* pregnant during three years

of *trying* to get pregnant, based on the average monthly fertility values for the start of the three years that are given in the box labels for each graph. These values are averages, so as we progress along the particular life curve the average monthly fertility of the couples who have not gotten pregnant falls with each passing month, because it is more likely that those with above-average monthly fertility will conceive first. In constructing these graphs, I have assumed that all the known causes of sterility (complete infertility not resolvable by time alone) have been excluded by the usual tests, so that, at least theoretically, everyone would eventually get pregnant if time could just go on and on. The numbers on the right of Figure A.2 give the remaining average monthly fertility rate of those couples who are still not pregnant after he three years. Notice, incidentally, that in his way three years of no pregnancy diminishes expected monthly fertility from 20 percent per month to 4.6 percent per month, which is comparable to a decline that would be caused by introducing, at time zero, a disarrangement of anatomy or physiology that causes a 75 percent decrease in monthly fertility (that is, from 20 percent to 5 percent). Such is the power of "self-selection."

Let me put this plainly and boldly: **The longer the duration of the infertility has been, the lower the chance each month of getting pregnant will be—whatever the tests show.** One would think that this principle would now be so well known that, when infertility treatments are being compared in clinical studies, getting a **control group** who have spent the same time trying to get pregnant would be a necessity, but it is quite rare in the medical literature on treating infertility. Instead, study after published study still tries to compare one treatment with another or with no treatment among patients who have a certain "dose" of some deemed cause, such as a certain amount of endometriosis, a certain

reduction in sperm count and so on. This is fine in dramatically thorough causes of infertility; it particularly works with causes of sterility, but it does not work for mild causes.

It is not hard to imagine disturbances that cause the monthly chance of getting pregnant to fall in this way, that is, to about one-fourth of what it otherwise should be. Mild endometriosis, mild oligospermia, mild abnormalities of the cervix and mild peritubal adhesions are all good examples. In combination, however, these decreases have to be multiplied together (see Table A.1). In other words, whereas just one such abnormality is scarcely likely to come to the surface and result in infertility (pregnancy is delayed but it still happens inside an acceptable time), combinations can be disastrous, with monthly fertility chances that are more like those of intentional and effective contraception! This is also the reason why, when we investigate infertility, we see combinations of mild abnormalities rather more often than we should if we were sampling the whole population. As a result, oligospermia and endometriosis, for example, occur together more often among

| Table A.1 | Modeling the Effect of Multiple Minor Abnormalities on Monthly Fertility and Likely Time Needed to Get Pregnant | | | |
|---|---|---|---|---|
| Number of Factors | Average Fertility | % Pregnant in 2 Years | % Pregnant in 3 Years | Average Time Needed to Get Pregnant |
| 0 | 20 % | 93.6 % | 96.7 % | 3 months |
| 1 | 5 % | 63.8 % | 75.5 % | 2 years |
| 2 | 1 % | 20.7 % | 28.9 % | 7 years |
| 3 | 0.2 % | 4.7 % | 6.9 % | 40 years |

infertile couples than they would in a random sample of couples generally.

But the proper conclusion is not to forecast virtually untreatable infertility when we find such mixtures of disturbances. In reproductive medicine, it is often unreliable to correlate what we see in our tests with the real degree of disturbance. We cannot usually estimate, from the apparent or observed departure from normal that is disclosed by our investigations, just what the expected monthly fertility will be when a couple's fertility has never actually been put to the test. Many young women with endometriosis, for example, have come to see me because of pain but then get pregnant quite quickly when they try. Instead, I emphasize again the duration of infertility and the time remaining for conception as being the important guides for estimating the chance of a pregnancy happening, which is more important than working out the real or imagined, but capable of being labeled "diagnosis."

The technological interventions for assisting conception (see Chapters 20 to 22) share a capacity for increasing considerably the chance of getting pregnant in the month in which they are carried out. They achieve this by making much more likely the successful encounter of egg with sperm, resulting in fertilization, combined with multiplying the number of eggs or embryos in the reproductive tract. Their directness of approach to the problem means that very often, a whole series of diagnosed abnormalities can be got around in one maneuver. The same is true when there is no diagnosed abnormality. Depending on the circumstances, pregnancy rates of between 5 percent and 40 percent per cycle are achievable; for many instances of relative or unexplained infertility this represents up to a thirty-fold increase in monthly fertility. This then is how assisted conception finds its rightful place in relative infertility and unexplained infertility.

With assisted conception, pregnancy is thus still not certain, but the improvement seen over natural circumstances is considerable, and diagnosed causes of infertility, particularly if they appear to be mild, are less important than they used to be. I look at the results of treating infertility with assisted conception in Appendix B.

## Results of Assisted Conception

Several difficulties stand in the way of forecasting the chance of success with infertility treatment at any particular clinic. Whereas it true that not all clinics are equally good, in 1997 most well-established clinics are probably very comparable, at least technically. Not all clinics are experienced with all procedures, however, and a reasonable first step is to be sure that your clinic has firsthand knowledge of the particular procedure you need (or at least has an effective consultancy in place with an experienced embryologist and clinician), especially if you need an advanced procedure such as IVF with **intracytoplasmic sperm insertion** (ICSI), accompanied by **microepididymal sperm aspiration** (MESA) or **testicular sperm extraction** (TESE). Results from these advanced procedures should be no lower (and are often better) than IVF generally.

Once you are sure of a clinic's basic expertise, there are four factors that can readily outweigh real clinic-to-clinic differences. The first is the age of the female partner. The second is the number of previously unsuccessful assisted conception treatments she has undergone (generally the most fertile people conceive the quickest, wherever they go, so clinics particularly highly regarded can have a weighting of couples who have not been successful elsewhere, thus lowering their apparent overall success rates). The third factor is the clinic's policy on the number of eggs or embryos transferred in one cycle. The hazard of high multiple pregnancy restricts many clinics to the transfer of two or three eggs or embryos, with cryostorage of other normally fertilized eggs for comparatively simple additional opportunities later. Other clinics, especially in the United States, routinely transfer many more eggs or embryos and rely on **fetal reduction**, or selective feticide, to reduce higher-number multiple gestations to twins or singletons. The fourth factor is how prone the clinic is to cancel a cycle before proceeding with oocyte retrieval, or egg pickup.

Table B.1 compares **take-home baby rates** and **implantation rates** for the main different forms of assisted conception. National data for 1993 (the latest compiled data available) are provided from Australia (including a contribution from New Zealand) and the United States (with a contribution from Canada). In general, the age of women treated is in the low to middle thirties, with a considerable fraction (about 20 percent) in their late thirties or in their forties. **Gamete intrafallopian**

## Table B.1 Take-Home Baby Rates from GIFT and IVF: National Average Data from Australia and the United States, 1993

| | Australia | | | United States | | |
|---|---|---|---|---|---|---|
| | *Number performed* | *Live births* | *%* | *Number performed* | *Live births* | *%* |
| *GIFT* | | | | | | |
| Cancellations before egg pickup | | | 13% | | | 16 |
| Live births per egg pickup procedure | 3,663 | 761 | 21% | 4,202 | 1,182 | 28% |
| Live births per transfer procedure | 3,657 | 761 | 21% | 4,139 | 1,182 | 29% |
| Live births per embryo | | | 8% | | | n/a |
| *IVF, pre-embryos transferred to uterus* | | | | | | |
| Cancellations before egg pickup | | | 14% | | | 14% |
| Live births per egg pickup procedure | 6,638 | 565 | 9% | 27,443 | 5,103 | 19% |
| Live births per embryo transfer procedure | 5,549 | 565 | 10% | 24,410 | 5,103 | 21% |
| Live births per embryo | | | 4% | | | n/a |

**transfer** (GIFT) consistently produces a higher successful pregnancy rate than **in vitro fertilization** (IVF). For IVF, pregnancy rates are generally higher for transfers of pre-embryos to the fallopian tube (ZIFT or TEST) compared with transfers to the uterus. Results when eggs for IVF have been donated from younger to older women are better than for IVF in more conventional circumstances.

Table B.2 also indicates that the chance of a cycle of treatment producing one or more healthy babies might be greater in the United States than in Australia. A number of factors account for most or all of this difference, each attributable in part to the higher cost to the patient of assisted conception procedures in the United States compared with Australia, where universal government-sponsored medical in-

| | Australia | | | United States | | |
|---|---|---|---|---|---|---|
| | Number performed | Live births | % | Number performed | Live births | % |
| *GIFT and TEST: IVF, pre-embryos transferred to fallopian tube(s)* | | | | | | |
| Cancellations before egg pickup | | | 8% | | | 13% |
| Live births per egg pickup procedure | 541 | 67 | 12% | 1,557 | 380 | 24% |
| Live births per transfer procedure | 431 | 67 | 16% | 1,327 | 380 | 29% |
| Live births per embryo | | | 6% | | | n/a |
| *Frozen-thawed pre-embryo transfer* | | | | | | |
| Live births per embryo transfer procedure | 4,607 | 440 | 10% | 6,194 | 791 | 13% |
| *Pre-embryo transfers from donated oocytes* | | | | | | |
| Live births per embryo transfer procedure | 342 | 48 | 14% | 2,446 | 716 | 29% |
| Live births per embryo | | | 7% | | | n/a |

surance covers a significant part of the cost of up to six stimulated GIFT or IVF cycles. First, a much higher proportion of treatments in Australia are repeat cycles after previously unsuccessful ones. Second, the number of eggs or pre-embryos transferred per cycle of treatment is known to be significantly higher in the United States than in Australia, where a limit of three eggs or pre-embryos is enforced as national policy. This difference in transfer practices is reflected in the higher chance of having twins or a higher-number multiple pregnancy in the United States compared with Australia (see Table B.2 on the next page). Slightly fewer treatment cycles begun in Australia are cancelled before egg pickup. The importance of these and other variables on the results of individual clinics are explained further in Chapter 20.

**Table B.2**   Multiple Pregnancy Rates among Successful GIFT and IVF Pregnancies: National Average Data from Australia and the United States, 1993

|  | Australia | United Sta |
|---|---|---|
| *GIFT* | | |
| Single baby | 74% | 65% |
| Twins | 23% | 26% |
| Triplets | 3% | 7% |
| Quadruplets or higher | 0% | 1% |
| *IVF* | | |
| Single baby | 83% | 66% |
| Twins | 15% | 28% |
| Triplets | 2% | 5% |
| Quadruplets or higher | 0% | 0% |

# Glossary

Included here are all words and terms that appear in **boldface** in the text plus some extras. Words or terms that appear within the definitions in SMALL CAPS have their own entries in the Glossary.

**abnormal forms** an estimate of the percentage of sperm that have an abnormal shape of the head, midpiece or tail; part of the routine SPERM COUNT.

**abnormality** a departure from what is normal in a more or less exact medical sense. An abnormality can be *quantitative* (measurable with a number), *qualitative* (measurable but still apparent or obvious) or a matter of timing. Statistically, an abnormality is defined as signifying either a measurement or a yes-or-no quality that is outside what, for example, 90 or 95 or 99 percent of the population exhibits (*see also* STATISTICAL SIGNIFICANCE). "Abnormality" is a word without added value, unlike "defect," which has a negative connotation; thus, to avoid a gratuitous, negative effect it is preferable to say, for example, "birth abnormality" instead of "birth defect." *See also* ANOMALY.

**abortion** strictly, synonymous with "spontaneous abortion" or MISCARRIAGE. Loosely (and as used in this book), an induced abortion for early termination of pregnancy.

**abortion rate** the percentage chance that a pregnancy will end as a spontaneous abortion or MISCARRIAGE. The normal rate for clinically apparent miscarriages for young women is about 12 percent. The rate rises independently with age, the number of previous pregnancies and, especially, the number of previous miscarriages experienced. The rate is also higher with many causes of infertility when conception occurs with or without treatment.

**absolute infertility** STERILITY, or 100 percent infertility; also called COMPLETE INFERTILITY. See also RELATIVE INFERTILITY.

**absolute risk** your actual chance of having something or being affected by something. It does not usually mean "absolutely" in the sense of "100 percent," as in ABSOLUTE INFERTILITY. Usually given as a ratio, proportion or percentage: for example, the absolute risk of having at least some visible ENDOMETRIOSIS for women in their forties is about 20 in 100, or 20 percent; the chance or the risk of pregnancy each month for a normal young couple (normal FECUNDABILITY) is also about 20 percent, usually expressed as 0.2 (a proportion); the risk of a woman developing cancer of the ovaries by the time she reaches her seventies in North America, Europe or Australia is about 1 in 90, or about 1.1 percent. *See also* RELATIVE RISK.

**accountability** the sequel to responsibility, in which responsibility for the making of a decision continues to rest with the decision-maker as the effects or consequences from the decision unfold.

**acrosome** consider it the crash helmet of a mature sperm, present over the sperm head until the successful sperm binds to the coating of the egg known as the ZONA PELLUCIDA; imagine it to be like a balloon into which you push your fist (the fist being the sperm's head). *See also* ACROSOME REACTION.

**acrosome reaction** if the ACROSOME is a balloon-like crash helmet for the mature sperm, the acrosome reaction is the bursting of that balloon, releasing enzymes that digest a path for the capacitated, highly motile sperm to push through the ZONA PELLUCIDA into the PERIVITELLINE SPACE, where it can directly fertilize the egg.

**acute** medically, means sudden and quick; an acute inflammation is usually red, tender and may form pus. *See also* CHRONIC.

**acute salpingitis** *see* SALPINGITIS

**adenohypophysis** the glandular part of the PITUITARY GLAND, lying toward the front and thus also called the "anterior pituitary"; produces FOLLICLE STIMULATING HORMONE, LUTEINIZING HORMONE and PROLACTIN. Other hormones produced by the adenohypophysis include growth hormone, THYROID STIMULAT-ING HORMONE (TSH) and adrenocorticotrop hormone (ACTH). *See also* HYPOTHALAMUS.

**adenomyoma** *see* ADENOMYOSIS

**adenomyosis** an abnormal condition of th UTERUS in which glands from the ENDO METRIUM grow into the MYOMETRIUM, the mus cle of the wall of the uterus, causing local o general enlargement of the uterus, pain dur ing periods and perhaps heavier periods. A lo calized area of adenomyosis is called a "adenomyoma" and can be hard to distin guish from a FIBROID with TRANSVAGINA ULTRASOUND; unlike a fibroid, it is not easil removed by surgery because it is not clearl separable from surrounding tissue. There i no satisfactory long-term treatment; a HYS TERECTOMY can be done if symptoms are ba enough.

**adhesions** scar tissue, in particular betwee the SEROSA (surface lining) of abdominal o pelvic organs in the PERITONEAL CAVITY, tha can interfere with the access the FALLOPIAN TUBE has to the OVARY at OVULATION. Adhesion may be thin and transparent, like thin plasti wrap (sometimes called "filmy" or Grade 1) thicker and containing more scar tissue and blood vessels (Grade 2), or thick, dense and tough (Grade 3). Adhesions are caused by in fections, ENDOMETRIOSIS or a previous opera tion. Not all adhesions are important; it de pends on their location. *See also* INTRAUTERIN ADHESIONS.

**adrenal gland** a paired gland lying above each kidney, responsible for the essential hor mone cortisol and equally important with the ovaries in producing androgens in women. *See also* SERUM 17-HYDROXYPROGESTERONE.

FP *see* ALPHA FETOPROTEIN

I *see* ASSISTED INSEMINATION

ID (artificial insemination, donor; assisted nsemination, donor) *see* DONOR INSEMINATION

IDS (acquired immune deficiency syndrome) *see* HIV

IH *see* ASSISTED INSEMINATION, HUSBAND

lleles the many different forms that a particular GENE can take (and still function, for better or for worse, as a gene within that gene's job description). Genes come in pairs, one on each of the chromosomes that make up a chromosome pair. The two genes of the pair are not always the same. If your alleles are identical, you are HOMOZYGOUS for that gene; if they are not, you are HETEROZYGOUS. Abnormal alleles cause genetic disease or disability: if one allele is enough to cause abnormality, then the gene is dominant (DOMINANT INHERITANCE) and the abnormality is present in the heterozygous and the homozygous state; if two alleles are needed to cause abnormality; then the gene is recessive (RECESSIVE INHERITANCE), and the abnormality is present only in the homozygous state. Among alleles found on X chromosomes but not on Y chromosomes (which are smaller), a recessive gene will be unopposed in males (and thus will act as a dominant gene), whereas female carriers of the allele will be unaffected except in the extremely unlikely event that they inherit (or gain by mutation) a second abnormal allele; this mode of inheritance is called "sex-linked recessive inheritance."

alpha fetoprotein (AFP) a form of albumin (a protein in the blood) produced only by the fetus but that crosses the placenta and is thus detectable in the mother's blood, as well as being usefully measured in amniotic fluid by AMNIOCENTESIS; detectable in higher than usual concentration with certain "open" abnormalities involving the brain and spinal cord of the fetus (namely, anencephaly and spina bifida); present in lower than usual concentration in DOWN'S SYNDROME, or TRISOMY 21.

amenorrhea absent menstrual periods, usually because of absent ovulation (ANOVULATION) or because of absence of, destruction of or obstruction to the menstrual flow from the uterus, such as with INTRAUTERINE ADHESIONS (when it is known as ASHERMAN'S SYNDROME).

AMH *see* ANTI-MÜLLERIAN HORMONE

amniocentesis the sampling of the fluid from the amniotic or GESTATIONAL SAC. It can be performed, but with difficulty, from about 10 weeks of pregnancy but is more usually performed at about 14 weeks; cells from the FETUS can be set up in culture for a KARYOTYPE; for special diagnoses it can be examined more quickly by FLUORESCENT IN SITU HYBRIDIZATION (FISH) or by POLYMERASE CHAIN REACTION (PCR); other substances in the amniotic fluid, such as ALPHA FETOPROTEIN, can be measured to indicate whether the fetus is normal or not.

amniotic cavity *see* GESTATIONAL SAC

amniotic fluid the fluid in the amniotic cavity, or GESTATIONAL SAC; it is sampled during AMNIOCENTESIS.

ampulla the wide outer part of the FALLOPIAN TUBE, lying between the FIMBRIAL END and the narrow ISTHMUS.

ampullary-isthmic junction the point at which the wide AMPULLA of the FALLOPIAN TUBE meets the narrow ISTHMUS and the place where FERTILIZATION of the egg by a sperm cell normally takes place.

**ANA** *see* ANTINUCLEAR ANTIBODY

**androgens** male sex hormones, including TESTOSTERONE, the main androgen circulating in the blood in men and in women, and ANDROSTENEDIONE (which is weaker); produced in women more or less equally by the adrenal glands and the ovaries (in THECAL CELLS and hilus cells); produced in much greater quantity in men by the TESTES (testicles).

**androstenedione** a weak ANDROGEN produced in women by THECAL CELLS in the ovary and by the adrenal glands.

**aneuploid, aneuploidy** the gain or loss of one or more CHROMOSOMES, including TRISOMY (47 chromosomes) and MONOSOMY (45 chromosomes). *See also* POLYPLOID, POLYPLOIDY.

**ANF (antinuclear factor)** *see* ANTINUCLEAR ANTIBODY

**angular pregnancy** a pregnancy in which IMPLANTATION occurs in the "lateral angle" of the uterus—out to one side and very close to where the FALLOPIAN TUBES enter the uterus; MISCARRIAGE is common.

**anomaly** distinguishable from an ABNORMALITY in that the outcome of an anomaly may not lead to disease or disability. An anomalous kidney, for example, is in the wrong place but does its job perfectly well. The distinction between an anomaly and an abnormality, however, is loose and is not always observed.

**anorexia nervosa** "anorexia" means a profound loss of appetite, followed by loss of weight; "nervosa" means that there is a ner-

vous or mental basis for the state, in this cas a belief by the person affected, usually an ado lescent girl, and contrary to the perception c others, that she is overweight. She stops eat ing, and may induce vomiting or use laxative to keep the intestines empty and the stomacl flat. Menstrual periods stop because of th weight loss and underlying mental distur bance. Medical complications from induce vomiting and laxative abuse can be serious occasionally fatal. Treatment, which include psychological and psychiatric counseling, i difficult and not always completely accom plished; the younger the patient the better the chance of cure.

**anovulation** absence of OVULATION.

**anovulatory cycles** MENSTRUAL CYCLES cause by ovarian activity (or OVARIAN CYCLES) not ac companied by OVULATION; SERUM PROGES TERONE stays low, whereas some developmen of TERTIARY FOLLICLES and production o ESTRADIOL takes place. *See also* ANOVULATORY DYSFUNCTIONAL UTERINE BLEEDING.

**anovulatory dysfunctional uterine bleeding** irregular and generally heavy bleeding caused by ANOVULATORY CYCLES.

**anticardiolipin antibody** antibody made by the body's immune system that acts against components in the cell membrane. Looked for in the blood as a possible immune cause of RECURRENT MISCARRIAGES. *See also* LUPUS ANTICOAGULANT.

**anti-Müllerian hormone (AMH)** a hormone produced by the SERTOLI CELLS of the TESTES in a male EMBRYO to suppress the development of the MÜLLERIAN DUCTS.

**antinuclear antibody** (ANA); also **antinuclear factor** (ANF) antibody made by the ody's immune system that acts against com-onents in the NUCLEUS of the body's own cells, us sometimes producing an autoimmune isease. It is looked for in the blood as a screen-ng test for a possible immune cause of RE-URRENT MISCARRIAGES and for the potentially rious autoimmune disease systemic lupus rythematosis (*see also* LUPUS ANTICOAGULANT).

**nti-sperm antibodies**     same as SPERM NTIBODIES.

**ntral follicle**   a TERTIARY FOLLICLE.

**ntrum**   a fluid-filled space between the FOL-ICLE CELLS, the development of which marks he transformation of a SECONDARY FOLLICLE nto a TERTIARY FOLLICLE.

**RT**   *see* ASSISTED REPRODUCTIVE TECHNOLOGY

**rtificial insemination**   *see* ASSISTED INSEMI-ATION

**rtificial insemination, husband** (AIH)   *see* SSISTED INSEMINATION, HUSBAND

**aseptic necrosis of the femoral head**   liter-lly, noninfective death of the bone tissue of he top end of the thigh bone, where it forms he hip joint; a rare but serious complication from continued high dosages of cortisone-like drugs, including cortisone, prednisone and prednisolone, sometimes used for treating SPERM ANTIBODIES.

**Asherman's syndrome**   the combination of INTRAUTERINE ADHESIONS and AMENORRHEA.

**aspermia**   an absence of semen despite male orgasm. *See also* AZOOSPERMIA.

**assisted conception**   a group of medical treatments ranging from ASSISTED INSEMINA-TION to IN VITRO FERTILIZATION and its techni-cal variants, with the following common char-acteristics: increasing the chance of pregnancy each month, thus overcoming the medical disability of INFERTILITY; little or no spillover of therapeutic effect beyond the cycle or month in which treatment is invoked; and some form of procedural intervention, with sperm, eggs or embryos spending some time outside of the body.

**assisted hatching**   an IVF micromanipula-tion in which a small opening is made in the ZONA PELLUCIDA of the PRE-EMBRYO to help the BLASTOCYST emerge prior to IMPLANTATION.

**assisted insemination** (AI)   insemination, or injection of SEMEN or prepared SPERMATOZOA, into the vagina, cervix, uterus or fallopian tube, to aid fertility; a basic form of ASSISTED CONCEPTION. The husband's or male partner's sperm (AIH) or donated sperm (DI) can be used.

**assisted insemination, husband** (AIH)   AS-SISTED INSEMINATION in which the SEMEN from the husband or male partner is used.

**assisted reproductive technology** (ART) essentially synonymous with ASSISTED CONCEP-TION but tends to emphasize the technology instead of the medical help that uses the technology.

**asthenozoospermia**   *see* OLIGOSPERMIA

**atresia**   synonymous with ATROPHY, a process by which a tissue stops growing, loses its func-tion and degenerates. *See also* FOLLICULAR ATRESIA.

**atretic follicle**   a TERTIARY FOLLICLE that is no longer growing, no longer secreting estradiol and that no longer contains a healthy OOCYTE, or egg. *See also* FOLLICULAR ATRESIA.

**atrophy** literally, an absence of nutrition, but in particular the *result* of such lack in a tissue, which shrinks and loses its normal function. *See also* ENDOMETRIAL ATROPHY; FOLLICULAR ATRESIA.

**autonomy** an ethical principle in which value is given to maximizing an individual's contribution to the making of decisions that affect them; can be overdone by abrogating professional responsibility through misuse of the device of INFORMED CONSENT.

**autosome** a CHROMOSOME other than one of the SEX CHROMOSOMES (which are X or Y); numbered from 1 to 22.

**azoospermia** a complete absence of sperm (SPERMATOZOA) in the SEMEN caused either by an obstruction (usually in the EPIDIDYMIS or VAS DEFERENS) or by failure of sperm to form or to mature in the testis (called "maturation arrest"); detectable only by performing a SPERM COUNT, as semen looks the same whether it contains sperm or not. *See also* SPERMATOGENESIS.

**balanced chromosomal translocation** CHROMOSOMES occur in pairs in all cells except sperm and eggs; if part of one chromosome is found as part of a completely different chromosome it is translocated; for that person there is no net gain or loss of genetic material, so the translocation is balanced and there is no problem. But when that person makes eggs or sperm, some of these will have too much or too little genetic material. The same can be true for an embryo that results; the chromosomal translocation will then be unbalanced and the embryo will sooner or later be miscarried. *See also* CHROMOSOMAL CROSS-OVER and CHROMOSOMAL EMBRYOPATHY.

**basal body temperature** (BBT) **chart** a inexpensive way of detecting OVULATIC through the effect PROGESTERONE has on th HYPOTHALAMUS, increasing the body's tempe ature a few tenths of a degree; best recorde using a BBT thermometer (with a small scale than thermometers used to record fever or high temperatures) first thing in the morr ing before rising, and preferably in the vagin for accuracy. Day 1 of the chart is the fir morning when there is menstruation (a pe riod); commonly there is a dip in the temper ature just before the sustained rise that indi cates ovulation has occurred (a "biphasic chart); the chart typically records the days yo are menstruating, when you have sex an when you are aware of MUCUS or ovulatio pain. The BBT chart is best used to documen the presence and length of the LUTEAL PHASE especially if CLOMIPHENE is being used fo OVULATION INDUCTION, and for the timing o symptoms such as PREMENSTRUAL SPOTTING; i is not as good for predicting ovulation as LF testing in urine.

**BBT** *see* BASAL BODY TEMPERATURE CHART

**beneficence** the ethical value that come: from doing good. *See also* NONMALEFICENCI and SUFFERING.

**bicornuate uterus** a UTERINE ANOMALY in which the MÜLLERIAN DUCTS before birth do not join properly, creating a double uterus, in which each of the two sides receives just one fallopian tube and is smaller than a normal uterus.

**biochemical pregnancy** a somewhat insensitive term for when conception has occurred, producing a positive PREGNANCY TEST but no sign of a GESTATIONAL SAC on a TRANSVAGINAL

ULTRASOUND. *See also* SUBCLINICAL MISCAR-
RIAGE; MENSTRUAL MISCARRIAGE.

**biopsy** the taking of a small sample of tissue
for diagnosis under the microscope. Biopsies
of the ENDOMETRIUM can be done without
anesthesia, through the cervix (*see* PREMEN-
STRUAL BIOPSY); biopsies of the ovary or of the
lining of the peritoneal cavity (for example, to
detect subtle endometriosis) are done during
LAPAROSCOPY; a TESTICULAR BIOPSY is done to
determine why there is azoospermia. Using
microscopic techniques, even a PRE-EMBRYO
can be biopsied (*see* PRE-EMBRYO BIOPSY and
REIMPLANTATIONAL DIAGNOSIS).

**blastocyst** stage of development of the EM-
BRYO from the PRE-EMBRYO in which a fluid-
filled cavity forms in the formerly solid ball of
cells (the MORULA) about 5 days after FERTIL-
IZATION. For the first time, a distinction can be
made between a sheet of cells to one side,
which will form the embryo proper, and the
remaining, peripheral cells, which, after the
blastocyst "hatches" through the ZONA PELLU-
CIDA and undergoes IMPLANTATION, will form
the TROPHOBLAST.

**blastomeres** cells that compose the
BLASTOCYST.

**blighted ovum** an old-fashioned term for
an INEVITABLE MISCARRIAGE, meaning that the
OVUM (in its classical sense for professional
embryologists) has not developed normally
after FERTILIZATION, with only the supporting
tissues and no EMBRYO present. The term is de-
scriptive; it has no diagnostic value as to the
cause of the miscarriage.

**blood group and antibody screen** most
commonly done before an operation that can
cause significant loss of blood, especially if an
ectopic pregnancy is suspected, because a
blood transfusion might be needed; also done
for investigation of RECURRENT MISCARRIAGES,
when the rare but important antibody anti-
$T_jA$ needs to be excluded or detected.

**body mass index** (BMI) an estimate of a person's amount of fat calculated by dividing his
or her weight (expressed in kilograms) by the
square of the height (expressed in meters); normally between 20 and 25, although the upper
limit is higher with age. A BMI below 20 generally causes OLIGOMENORRHEA, then AMENOR-
RHEA, through ANOVULATION. A BMI much over
25 indicates obesity.

**bowel** the intestines; the small intestine
(small bowel) runs from the stomach to the
wider large intestine (large bowel), which
starts with the cecum, in the region of the appendix on the right side of the lower abdomen, ascends (ascending colon), turns left
(transverse colon), turns downward (de-
scending colon), becomes the sigmoid colon
(as it sweeps from side to side a bit), then the
rectum, before opening at the anus.

**breakthrough bleeding** bleeding, usually
light or "spotting," while on the birth control
pill or taking a PROGESTOGEN. It is common
and of no sinister importance in the first few
months of pill use but occurrence after many
months of satisfactory pill use can signal interference with the efficacy of the pill (a risk of
OVULATION and pregnancy) due to an inter-
current illness (involving, typically, diarrhea),
simultaneous taking of antibiotics, or taking
additional medications that speed up the pill's
metabolism; or it can signify coexisting pathology of the cervix or the uterus.

**bromocriptine** a drug that mimics dopamine, which inhibits production of PROLACTIN by the PITUITARY GLAND; used for the treatment of HYPERPROLACTINEMIA, with the tablets given by mouth unless they cause side effects, in which case the same tablets (but not the capsules) are used vaginally; made by Sandoz as Parlodel.

**buserilin** a GNRH-AGONIST made by Hoechst in Europe as Suprefact and administered as a nasal spray.

**CA125 antigen** a mucus-like protein produced in some circumstances by surface cells of tissues derived from the Müllerian ducts; its function is obscure but measurement as SERUM CA125 ANTIGEN can useful in diagnosing ADENOMYOSIS, ENDOMETRIOSIS and some cancers of the ovary.

**CAH** see CONGENITAL ADRENAL HYPERPLASIA

**canalization** see TUBAL CANALIZATION

**capacitation** an invisible change that mature sperm undergo to acquire accelerated movement and the ability to undergo the ACROSOME REACTION; brought about naturally when sperm swim up through the uterus and fallopian tubes, or brought about in the laboratory by spinning and washing the sperm through a series of solutions.

**CAT scan** a special form of X-ray taken with the person enveloped in the scanning apparatus, which builds up a particularly good image of any cross-section or series of cross-sections through the body, by the process of computerized axial tomography; particularly useful for investigation of the anatomy of the PITUITARY GLAND and HYPOTHALAMUS when a tumor is suspected and needs to be excluded. It is more widely available than an MRI SCAN which can give even clearer results.

**cautery** short for ELECTROCAUTERY.

**CAVD** see CONGENITAL ABSENCE OF THE VAS DEFERENTIA

**CBAVD** (CONGENITAL BILATERAL ABSENCE OF THE VAS DEFERENS) see CONGENITAL ABSENCE OF THE VASA DEFERENTIA

**cecum** see BOWEL

**cervical incompetence** weakness of the CERVIX of the uterus, usually because of previous operations but sometimes without prior injury, leading to MISCARRIAGE, typically in the second three months of pregnancy; diagnosed by examining the cervix during pregnancy, repeatedly if necessary; often causes no symptoms until the waters break (the pregnancy membranes bulge through the opening cervix), when it is usually too late to treat treated with a CERVICAL LIGATURE.

**cervical ligature** a suture placed circumferentially around the CERVIX to strengthen and support it for the treatment of CERVICAL INCOMPETENCE.

**cervical mucus** sticky secretion from the canal of the CERVIX, whose job it is to keep sperm out unless ovulation is about to take place, when the mucus becomes voluminous, watery, stretchable (SPINNBARKHEIT) and forms a crystalline ferning pattern when allowed to dry on a glass slide. See also CERVICITIS; KREMER TEST; INSLER SCORE; POSTCOITAL TEST.

**cervical mucus sperm antibodies** estimation of SPERM ANTIBODIES in the CERVICAL MUCUS; presence of these antibodies can cause

GATIVE TESTS of cervical mucus–sperm interction, including a negative POSTCOITAL TEST.

**rvical polyp** a POLYP of the canal of the RVIX; a cause of bleeding after sex (POST-ITAL BLEEDING) and sometimes accompaned by an ENDOMETRIAL POLYP, which can use INFERTILITY.

**rvical pregnancy** an ECTOPIC PREGNANCY cated in the wall of the CERVIX.

**rvicitis** inflammation of the CERVIX, usually cause of infection. Sperm might or might ot have trouble getting through the CERVICAL UCUS, which can be tested with a POSTCOITAL ST. Occasionally cervicitis can mean that ere is ENDOMETRITIS and SALPINGITIS.

**rvix** the neck of the UTERUS, lying between e body of the uterus (its FUNDUS) and the gina.

**lamydia** a germ, or infective agent, re-onsible for infection of and damage to the LLOPIAN TUBES. In men, chlamydial infection in cause nonspecific urethritis, with a tran-ent feeling of burning during the passing of rine or a yellow-colored discharge from the enis. In women, there can be a vaginal dis-harge or there can be mild or moderate ab-ominal pain from acute SALPINGITIS; it should e suspected whenever there is yellow-colored ucus in the CERVIX during the taking of a 'AP smear. There can be no symptoms in ei-her sex. The diagnosis is made by testing cell crapings from the canal of the cervix or from he urethra. As a germ, chlamydia is like a irus in some ways (it grows only inside cells) nd like a bacterium in others (it responds to ome antibiotics, especially tetracyclines and rythromycin). When diagnosed, both part-ers should be treated.

**chorionic gonadotropin** a GONADOTROPIN produced by the TROPHOBLAST of the PLACENTA that acts like LUTEINIZING HORMONE. *See also* HUMAN CHORIONIC GONADOTROPIN (hCG).

**chorionic villus (villi)** "tongues" of tissue of the placenta (TROPHOBLAST) that "lap" the mother's blood in the uterus, exchanging oxygen, nutrients and waste products between the fetus's blood vessels (in the villi) and the mother's blood; this tissue is sampled for genetic testing with CHORIONIC VILLUS SAMPLING.

**chorionic villus sampling** (CVS) a test done at about 9 weeks pregnancy at which, under ultrasound guidance, a catheter is passed through the cervix of the pregnant uterus to obtain a small sample of tissue from the PLACENTA (the afterbirth) for genetic testing, such as a KARYOTYPE.

**chromatid** *see* CHROMOSOMAL CROSS-OVER; MITOSIS

**chromosomal cross-over** ordinary cells of the body have 46 CHROMOSOMES in 23 pairs. The members of each pair do not necessarily contain the same GENES (which is why you can carry a gene for something RECESSIVE without being sick). During the cell divisions that produce the GERM CELLS (the process of meiosis), the 46 chromosomes first double to 92 before they end up with the 23 present in an egg or a sperm. Two of the four sibling chromosomes (chromatids) then randomly exchange bits of themselves in a cross-over. Nature jumbles up where the genes will go so that in the long run you do not always have to inherit two particular genes just because they are next to each other on a chromosome. Over the generations, there will sooner or later be a split between them during cross-over. Cross-over does not mean that genes can end up in any chromosome they like; unless translocated, they will remain in pairs (of ALLELES) within a particular pair of chromosomes. *See also* BALANCED CHROMOSOMAL TRANSLOCATION; LINKAGE ANALYSIS.

**chromosomal embryopathy**    when the embryo or fetus is abnormal because of a mistake in its CHROMOSOMES, with too much or too little genetic material. A cause of MISCARRIAGE.

**chromosome**    the mixture of a single long strand of genetic material (DNA) and supporting proteins. There are 46 chromosomes (23 pairs) in every normal human cell (other than the GERM CELLS). Each cell therefore contains all the genetic information needed to make a human being, but it is only in the first few days of the PRE-EMBRYO—if then—that all of a cell's DNA is accessible; once cells differentiate to have special purposes only the DNA they need remains unmasked. Chromosomes are located in the cell's NUCLEUS and come in pairs, so that each cell has two ALLELES of each GENE. *See also* CHROMOSOMAL CROSS-OVER.

**chronic**    medically, means slow to develop and lingering or long-lasting. *See also* ACUTE.

**chronic salpingitis**    *see* SALPINGITIS

**cilium (cilia)**    tiny hair-like projections on the surface of some cells, which are thus called "ciliated cells"; coordinated beating of the cilia move MUCUS and mucus-like substances (such as the CUMULUS MASS) on the surface of ciliated cells in the direction of the cilial beat.

**cleavage**    process by which a fertilized egg divides repeatedly over several days, forming for a time smaller and smaller cells; the process

begins at the stage of the ZYGOTE and en with a MORULA.

**Clomid**    *see* CLOMIPHENE

**clomiphene**    a drug that blocks the action ESTROGENS and so tricks the PITUITARY GLAN into thinking the ovary's FOLLICLES are n producing enough ESTRADIOL, so that natu FOLLICLE STIMULATING HORMONE production temporarily increased; the ovaries thereby a stimulated and follicles grow. Trade names a Clomid (Marion Merrell) and Serophe (Serono).

**coitus**    Latin for SEX.

**colon**    *see* BOWEL

**complete infertility**    absolute infertility (1( percent infertility), when there is no chance pregnancy happening without help, general because of no sperm, no ovulation or a con plete blockage to egg and sperm getting tc gether. *See also* STERILITY.

**complete miscarriage**    traditionally, any MI! CARRIAGE revealed to be complete upon car ful inspection of the expelled pregnancy tis sue, meaning that a uterine CURETTAGE wa not necessary to avoid the risk of retained tis sue causing more bleeding or infection. W can distinguish a complete from an INCOM PLETE MISCARRIAGE and whether or not cure tage should be done by use of a TRANSVAGINA ULTRASOUND, which is able to reveal retaine tissue.

**conception**    occurrence of pregnancy as indi cated by a positive PREGNANCY TEST that de tects HUMAN CHORIONIC GONADOTROPIN.

**conception rate**    the percentage of months o treatment cycles that result in CONCEPTION, in ding BIOCHEMICAL PREGNANCIES, ECTOPIC PREGNANCIES, MISCARRIAGES and all potentially able pregnancies (twins are not counted ice); less important for most purposes than e IMPLANTATION RATE, PREGNANCY RATE, viable egnancy rate and the TAKE-HOME-BABY RATE.

**nceptus** another word for EMBRYO or PRE-EMBRYO; literally, the "product of conception" d thus refers to any stage from the fertilized g (or ZYGOTE) to the FETUS.

**ngenital** an adjective meaning that something, especially an ABNORMALITY or ANOMALY, present from birth; the cause for such a condition can be hereditary (genetic) or an environmental factor operating before birth.

**ngenital abnormality** abnormal development of a body part during embryonic and fetal life, usually but not always apparent at irth. It can be inherited genetically or acquired by exposure to a physical or chemical sult, such as the action of a teratogen (a rug or other substance in the environment), uring development in the mother's uterus; w congenital abnormalities can be associated with a specific cause and an apparent ause might not be the true one.

**ngenital absence of the vasa deferentia** (CAVD) congenital absence of the two VASA EFERENTIA, which conduct sperm from the ESTES to the ejaculate; hence, a cause of obstructive AZOOSPERMIA; because the vas deferens on each side is usually affected, it is often alled "congenital bilateral absence of the vasa leferentia (CBAVD)." INFERTILITY is inevitable, ut can be overcome using IN VITRO FERTILIZATION with TESTICULAR SPERM EXTRACTION. The ause is usually the presence among the man's genes of one of the serious ALLELES for the ge-

netic disease CYSTIC FIBROSIS, which, having a RECESSIVE INHERITANCE pattern, results when there are two such alleles present; it can also come about when there are one or two of the less serious abnormal alleles for this condition. The more common of the abnormal alleles should therefore be screened for (using a specially set up POLYMERASE CHAIN REACTION on white blood cells). Should an abnormal allele be present ($\Delta$F508 is the most common seriously abnormal one), the woman should also be screened to predict the chance of cystic fibrosis occurring in the offspring.

**congenital adrenal hyperplasia** *see* SERUM 17-HYDROXYPROGESTERONE

**congenital anomaly** *see* CONGENITAL ABNORMALITY

**control group** when a research study or perhaps an experiment is done, the procedure, drug or process being tested or examined on the treatment group needs to be compared with a similar group that does not receive the treatment; this group is the control group, which can consist of, for example, people, embryos or research animals.

**corpus luteum (corpora lutea)** (Latin for "yellow body") the solid or cystic structure in the ovary after OVULATION; derived from the ovulating GRAAFIAN FOLLICLE; at first red and friable, as arteries and veins invade the collapsed follicle, before it matures into a little gland that is very efficient at producing PROGESTERONE, a hormone that is soluble in the fat, which gives the corpus luteum its yellow color. It provides its name to the second, or LUTEAL PHASE of the ovarian cycle, as well as to LUTEINIZING HORMONE, which causes the corpus luteum to be formed and sustains it until, in the event of pregnancy, it is supported instead by HUMAN CHORIONIC GONADOTROPIN.

**corpus luteum defect**    *see* LUTEAL PHASE DEFECT

**cryostorage**    storage at the very low temperature of liquid nitrogen of sperm, eggs or (very recently) unfertilized eggs in small amounts of ovarian tissue, after special preparation of these cells during cooling to replace much of the water they contain with a "cryoprotective" substance, such as dimethylsulfoxide, propanediol or glycerol. Storage is biologically safe for decades, but the existence of cryostorage "banks" (especially of embryos) has been a concern for some in society.

**cryptomenorrhea**    literally, "hidden menstruation"; apparent AMENORRHEA caused by an obstruction to the outflow of periodic bleeding from the uterus. Causes include an obstruction in the vagina, and typically there is periodic pain coinciding with the timing of the hidden menstrual flow.

**cryptorchidism**    literally (from the Greek), "hidden testicle," a condition in which there is incomplete descent of the testis or testes from the abdomen into the scrotum; synonymous with "undescended testis." *See also* ORCHIDOPEXY.

**CT scan**  *see* CAT SCAN

**culture medium (media)**    the fluid in which cells or tissues, including eggs, sperm and embryos, are grown; it consists of water, salts and nutrients. Different media have turned out best for different purposes. On the other hand, several different media seem to produce equal results for IN VITRO FERTILIZATION; traditional examples include Ham's F10, Whit-

tingham's T6 and Quinn's medium (said to based on "human tubal fluid," although in r ality very different from the fluid in the fa lopian tube).

**cumulative chance of pregnancy**    the acc mulating chance, month after month, of su cessfully getting pregnant. With a MONTH FERTILITY (a monthly chance of pregnancy, FECUNDABILITY) of, say, 20 percent, there is a 2 percent chance of pregnancy by the end of th first month, a 20 percent of 80 percent ( percent) chance of pregnancy *in* the secor month and so a (cumulative) 36 percer chance of pregnancy by the end of the secor month and so on. *See* Appendix A for detail

**cumulus mass**    a collection of specialize GRANULOSA CELLS surrounding the ovulatin egg in a sticky, mucus-like matrix; sticks to th fallopian tube's FIMBRIAL END after OVULATION

**curettage**    also called simply a "curette"or "D&C" (jargon for dilatation of the cervix an curettage of the uterus). When a curettage done to empty the uterus of normal or abnor mal pregnancy tissue, a special suction appa ratus is used and the operation is referred t as a "vacuum curettage." *See also* DILATION AN CURETTAGE.

**curette**    instrument for carrying ou CURETTAGE.

**CVS**  *see* CHORIONIC VILLUS SAMPLING

**cyproterone acetate**    a PROGESTOGEN that i particularly effective at blocking the effect o male sex hormones on the skin, thereby re ducing abnormal hair growth and acne Found singly in Androcur and in combina tion with an ESTROGEN in Diane-35, a formu lation used for oral contraception. Dangerou f taken in pregnancy, because it stops male fetuses from developing normal genital organs. Not available in the U.S.

**cystic fibrosis** a serious genetic disease with RECESSIVE INHERITANCE pattern characterized by a major disturbance of the body's mucus secretions, and thus a cause of incapacitating disease of the lungs. Important for infertility problems because the HETEROZYGOUS (carrier) state in men can manifest with AZOOSPERMIA due to CONGENITAL ABSENCE OF THE VASA DEFERENTIA, the infertility of which nowadays can be overcome with TESTICULAR SPERM EXTRACTION and IVF, thus risking inadvertent transmission. *See also* ΔF508.

**cytoplasm** the part of a cell that is not the nucleus (which contains the chromosomes); contained by the cell's plasma membrane and contains all the other cellular structures, including the MITOCHONDRIA. Genetic inheritance is mostly by way of the nucleus (with a contribution from mother and father); a small part is by way of the cytoplasm (with a contribution only from the mother). It is the cytoplasm of the egg (as a secondary OOCYTE) into which a sperm cell (SPERMATOZOON) is injected in the process of INTRACYTOPLASMIC SPERM INSERTION. *See also* MTDNA.

**D&C** *see* CURETTAGE; DILATION AND CURETTAGE

**danazol** a hormonal drug used for treating ENDOMETRIOSIS; related to male sex hormones (it is a weak androgen), it has occasional androgenic side effects, including weight gain and increased muscle bulk (it is an anabolic steroid), and facial hair; less commonly there can be deepening of the voice or enlargement of the clitoris. Manufactured by Sanofi Winthrop as Danocrine.

**Danocrine** *see* DANAZOL

**decapeptyl** a GNRH-AGONIST manufactured in Europe by Ipsen Biotech as triptorelin. Administered by a monthly injection.

**decidua** differentiated ENDOMETRIUM of pregnancy that is shed (like a deciduous tree sheds its leaves) as part of the afterbirth at childbirth or MISCARRIAGE; during pregnancy it has important hormonal functions. *See also* DECIDUAL CELLS.

**decidual cells** plump ENDOMETRIAL STROMAL cells, lying between the glands of the ENDOMETRIUM, formed under the prolonged influence of PROGESTERONE, especially with establishment of pregnancy; constitutes the DECIDUAL REACTION to form the DECIDUA of pregnancy and produce PROLACTIN (important for regulating water entering the AMNIOTIC CAVITY) and relaxin, which keeps the MYOMETRIUM quiet.

**decidual reaction** complete confluence of ENDOMETRIAL STROMAL cells lying between the endometrial glands, caused by prolonged (14 days or more) exposure to PROGESTERONE or a PROGESTOGEN; normally happens only with pregnancy. *See also* PREDECIDUAL REACTION.

**ΔF508** the most common ALLELE to result in CYSTIC FIBROSIS, when two ΔF508 alleles are present, or CONGENITAL ABSENCE OF THE VASA DEFERENTIA, when one ΔF508 allele is present in a man. A woman HETEROZYGOUS for this gene, with one ΔF508 allele will be a carrier for cystic fibrosis (and for CAVD) but will herself be otherwise normal.

**deontological ethics** in this book, a set of ethical beliefs in which principles and values are seen by adherents to be self-evident and not in need of more basic proof; the ethical principles are duty-binding, innately known and by nature resistant to change. *See also* TELEOLOGICAL ETHICS; UTILITARIAN ETHICS.

**deoxyribonucleic acid** *see* DNA

**depletion of eggs** the natural process in which the older a female fetus, girl or woman gets, the fewer the number of eggs left in the ovaries; the huge majority of eggs are lost because of ATRESIA, only a tiny fraction by OVULATION. When the eggs are more or less depleted there will be PRIMARY OVARIAN FAILURE and, in women who have had periods, MENOPAUSE will take place. INFERTILITY, however, usually precedes total egg depletion by up to 10 years. *See also* MITOCHONDRION.

**DHT** *see* DIHYDROTESTOSTERONE

**DI** *see* DONOR INSEMINATION

**diathermy** *see* ELECTROCAUTERY

**Diane-35** a formulation of the birth control pill that contains, as well as an ESTROGEN, the PROGESTOGEN known as CYPROTERONE ACETATE, which is particularly effective at blocking the effects of male hormones on the skin. Manufactured by Schering.

**dihydrotestosterone** (DHT) the most active male sex hormone or ANDROGEN; formed in target tissues from TESTOSTERONE, which is the main form of androgen circulating in the blood; testosterone must be converted to DHT before it can do its job.

**dilatation and curettage** (D&C) before CURETTAGE of the uterus, the cervix is dilated to admit the CURETTE.

**diploid, diploidy** the full, normal comple ment of CHROMOSOMES, numbering 46 (as 2 pairs). *See also* HAPLOID, HAPLOIDY.

**distributive justice** JUSTICE dispensed in th community to confer maximum value t those in need through the notions of fairnes and consistency.

**dizygotic twins** twins formed from two fer tilized eggs, or ZYGOTES; nonidentical twins.

**DNA** an abbreviation of deoxyribonuclei acid, a molecule made up of a variable se quence of units, the nature and order o which forms the genetic code. DNA is locate chiefly in the CHROMOSOMES, which form cell's NUCLEUS. A small amount of DNA (cod ing for fewer than 50 genes) is found in th MITOCHONDRIA. *See also* GENE; mtDNA.

**dominant follicle** the TERTIARY FOLLICLE, o GRAAFIAN FOLLICLE, that has the responsibilit for producing ESTRADIOL for the rest of tha particular OVARIAN CYCLE; picked out by th end of the first week of the FOLLICULAR PHAS of the normal ovarian cycle; its destruction whether accidental or intentional, means tha a new follicular phase must start, with OVULA TION two weeks later, whereas destruction o one of the tertiary follicles before one has be come dominant causes no interference with the timing of ovulation for that cycle.

**dominant inheritance** a pattern of inheri tance of a characteristic (such as brown eye color) or ABNORMALITY in which just one GENE or ALLELE is needed to confer the characteristic or abnormality, in contrast to RECESSIVE IN HERITANCE, which requires two abnormal genes. *See also* HETEROZYGOUS.

**onor insemination**   ASSISTED INSEMINATION n which SEMEN is used from a sperm donor who is not the husband.

**)own's syndrome**   or Mongolism, due to RISOMY 21. Chromosome 21 is the smallest of he autosomes (the nonsex chromosomes); risomies of the other autosomes tend to be ethal at an earlier stage of embryonic or fetal levelopment and are rarely seen as much.

**)UB**   *see* DYSFUNCTIONAL UTERINE BLEEDING

**luration of infertility**   one of the two most mportant variables (the other is TIME LEFT FOR CONCEPTION) that determine the chance of till getting pregnant naturally in RELATIVE IN-'ERTILITY, including unexplained infertility; he longer the duration of infertility, the maller the chance each month as time goes on; for details see Appendix A. *See also* 'ECUNDABILITY.

**luty**   a moral compulsion for ethical action hat is innate; the modern basis for DEONTO-LOGICAL ETHICS. *See also* SUFFERING.

**lysfunctional uterine bleeding**   (DUB) heavy bleeding from the UTERUS. *See also* ANOVULATORY DYSFUNCTIONAL BLEEDING; OVU-LATORY DYSFUNCTIONAL BLEEDING.

**lysmenorrhea**   painful menstruation; can be "primary," present in teenagers, generally in spasms around the start of the period, or "sec-ondary," developing only as a woman gets older and then typically lasting more than a day or so into the period, with prolonged aching as well as spasms. Primary dysmenor-rhea might or might not have medical impor-tance beyond the suffering the pain causes; normally it gets better as a woman reaches her twenties. Secondary dysmenorrhea is usually abnormal and can signify ENDOMETRIOSIS, FI-BROIDS, ADENOMYOSIS or PERITUBAL ADHESIONS.

**dyspareunia**   painful sexual intercourse that persists after the first few times or that devel-ops after months or years of painless sex.

**ectopic pregnancy**   a pregnancy IMPLANTED in an abnormal location, such as the FALLOPIAN TUBE, the CERVIX, the OVARY or the PERITONEAL CAVITY (abdomen).

**ectopic pregnancy rate**   the percentage of EC-TOPIC PREGNANCIES among total clinical preg-nancies (excluding BIOCHEMICAL PREGNAN-CIES). The rate is about 0.3 percent in normal women and is increased with abnormalities of the FALLOPIAN TUBES, ASSISTED CONCEPTION and other circumstances.

**efferent ducts**   fine passages in the RETE TESTIS conducting sperm cells from the tubules of the TESTIS to the EPIDIDYMIS.

**egg depletion**   *see* DEPLETION OF EGGS

**egg pickup**   *see* FOLLICLE ASPIRATION

**electrocautery**   use of a high voltage, high fre-quency electric current to coagulate or evapo-rate tissue during surgery; useful because it can be used during LAPAROSCOPY, particularly for stopping bleeding (by coagulation) and for treating ENDOMETRIOSIS (by evaporation).

**embryo**   a word used loosely to describe everything from a fertilized egg to a FETUS, in-cluding the PRE-EMBRYO. What is today called the embryo has for a long time been called the OVUM by professional embryologists.

**embryo biopsy**   *see* PRE-EMBRYO BIOPSY

**embryo transfer**   procedure by which the EMBRYO (age one to three days, and strictly a PRE-EMBRYO) is placed in the UTERUS or into the FALLOPIAN TUBE after IVF.

**embryopathy**   literally, pathology of the EMBRYO (or FETUS); can underlie a MISCARRIAGE.

**empirical**   an awkward adjective that can have contrary meanings in medicine. The word comes from the Greek for "experience." On the one hand, empirical medical practice is that which is based only on observation and experiment (praiseworthy); on the other, it can refer to medical practice that is based on very personal experience without taking scientific principles into account (not praiseworthy); at worst it refers to treatment that is chosen on no other basis than, "Let's see if it might work." In this book I use it in its first sense unless I draw attention to a contrary use of it by others.

**endocrinology**   the study of HORMONES.

**endometrial atrophy**   shrinkage of the ENDOMETRIUM through lack of support by, especially, the hormone ESTROGEN, or by the loss, through injury, of receptiveness to estrogen.

**endometrial biopsy**   *see* PREMENSTRUAL ENDOMETRIAL BIOPSY

**endometrial cavity**   the space inside the UTERUS lined by the ENDOMETRIUM.

**endometrial hyperplasia**   overgrowth of the ENDOMETRIUM, caused usually by prolonged action of ESTROGEN unopposed by PROGESTERONE (prolonged ANOVULATION), as is the case in, particularly, the POLYCYSTIC OVARY SYNDROME; potentially dangerous because it can eventually turn to cancer of the endometrium.

**endometrial polyp**   a POLYP of the ENDOMETRIUM, sometimes without symptoms, sometimes with abnormal bleeding, such as INTERMENSTRUAL BLEEDING, PREMENSTRUAL SPOTTING or heavy periods (MENORRHAGIA, OVULATORY DYSFUNCTIONAL BLEEDING); a cause of INFERTILITY and of failure of ASSISTED CONCEPTION to result in pregnancy; diagnosable with TRANSVAGINAL ULTRASOUND.

**endometrial stroma**   loose connecting-type tissue that lies between glands of the ENDOMETRIUM; contains STROMAL CELLS that by late LUTEAL PHASE (or SECRETORY PHASE) have responded to PROGESTERONE by becoming plump, confluent and sheet-like (the PREDECIDUAL REACTION), in preparation for pregnancy; with successful IMPLANTATION this stromal cell response is completed (the DECIDUAL REACTION) to form the DECIDUA.

**endometriosis**   a common condition in which tissue like the lining of the uterus, or ENDOMETRIUM, grows somewhere else, sometimes causing DYSMENORRHEA, PREMENSTRUAL SPOTTING, INFERTILITY, DYSPAREUNIA and OVULATORY DYSFUNCTIONAL UTERINE BLEEDING.

**endometritis**   inflammation of the lining of the uterus, or ENDOMETRIUM; can be ACUTE or CHRONIC.

**endometrium**   the lining of the UTERUS, which contains the endometrial glands and the ENDOMETRIAL STROMA. *See also* MYOMETRIUM.

**endorphins**   opium-like substances produced naturally in the brain that give a feeling of well-being. Production of endorphins is stimulated by many natural circumstances and by intense exercise (to which people can become

dicted); they are depressed in PREMENSTRUAL
NSION.

ididymal sperm aspiration    *see* MICRO-
OPIC EPIDIDYMAL SPERM ASPIRATION

ididymis    a finely coiled tubular structure
ing next to the testis in the scrotum, which
nnects the TESTIS to the VAS DEFERENS and
rough which sperm cells pass and gain in
aturity.

RT    *see* ESTROGEN REPLACEMENT THERAPY

tradiol    the most powerful natural ESTROGEN.

strogen    the general name for one of the two
rincipal female sex hormones (the other is
ROGESTERONE) responsible for stimulating
rowth of the female reproductive system (the
agina, the CERVIX, the UTERUS and the FALLO-
AN TUBES) and growth of the breasts; the
ain estrogen is ESTRADIOL, produced by the
eveloping FOLLICLE in the ovary, as well as by
e CORPUS LUTEUM, the PLACENTA and the
ody's fat tissues (through conversion from
ale sex hormones, or ANDROGENS, in the
lood); after menopause the main estrogen is
e weaker one, estrone, largely derived from
onversion of ANDROSTENEDIONE by the body's
t.

strogen replacement therapy (ERT)    the
herapeutic use of ESTROGEN to stop the effects
f MENOPAUSE after the ovaries have been re-
oved or have stopped functioning. If the
terus is still present, the hormone regimen
ust include at least 11 days of PROGESTOGEN
sage each month or there will be a risk of EN-
OMETRIAL HYPERPLASIA and cancer.

strone    a weak ESTROGEN, which needs to be
onverted (in target tissues such as the uterus)
to the strong estrogen ESTRADIOL before, as
a hormone, it causes an estrogen effect; the
main estrogen in blood after MENOPAUSE;
formed from estradiol when that hormone in
tablet (or oral) form is absorbed across the
intestines.

ethics    a set of principles and values that govern behavior to accord with a notion of
morality. *See also* BENEFICENCE; DEONTOLOGI-
CAL ETHICS; JUSTICE; NONMALEFICENCE; SUFFER-
ING; TELEOLOGICAL ETHICS; UTILITARIAN ETHICS.

ethics committee (Great Britain and
Australia)    a mandated committee of an institution (hence INSTITUTIONAL ETHICS COM-
MITTEE, or IEC) that conducts medical research. It meets regularly and is composed of
specialist and lay individuals who consider the
ethical implementation of protocols for research, according to the requirements of the
1975 Declaration of Helsinki on clinical research and human experimentation and any
other official determinations relevant to the
particular environment of the researchers. Its
purpose is to gauge and to minimize risks run
by the subjects of research; its decisions are
binding on researchers. In the United States
this committee is called an INSTITUTIONAL RE-
VIEW BOARD.

ethics committee (United States)    a socially
derived, multidisciplinary committee of a
hospital. It meets irregularly, often at short
notice, to help in the making of ethically difficult clinical decisions aimed at ascertaining
and preserving the patient's best interest.

ethinylestradiol    orally effective form of
ESTRADIOL that resists being converted to ES-
TRONE; generic name for Estigyn.

**extra-Y-chromosome syndrome**  a TRISOMY with a KARYOTYPE of 47,XYY, that is, a male with an extra Y chromosome; affected men tend to be tall. Surveys of penal institutions have indicated a higher than expected frequency, perhaps implying that affected men are at increased risk of being criminals.

**fallopian tube**  the hollow organ, about 10 to 12 centimeters long, that effectively joins the ovary to the uterus on each side; composed of the FIMBRIAL END, the AMPULLA, the ISTHMUS and the INTERSTITIAL SEGMENT.

**falloposcopy**  the procedure of looking inside the FALLOPIAN TUBE with a tiny (half a millimeter diameter) flexible, fiber-optic instrument from the direction of the uterus. *See also* SALPINGOSCOPY.

**fecundability**  technical term for the monthly chance of pregnancy, or MONTHLY FERTILITY, either for an individual (measured over time) or for a population (the number of conceptions occurring in one month). For any individual with UNEXPLAINED INFERTILITY and in milder cases of RELATIVE INFERTILITY, chiefly determined by the DURATION OF INFERTILITY; once calculated this way (see the details in Appendix A), an estimate of the chance of still getting pregnant naturally (as opposed to undergoing ASSISTED CONCEPTION) will chiefly be determined by the TIME LEFT FOR CONCEPTION. *See also* CUMULATIVE CHANGE OF PREGNANCY; NORMAL MONTHLY FERTILITY.

**fertilization**  entry of a sperm cell into an egg: their "marriage"; the egg is activated by this event, so that cortical granules are expelled that stop further sperm binding to the egg; the second division of MEIOSIS is completed, with expulsion of the second POLAR

BODY; and the machinery of the egg is starte[d] which will form PRONUCLEI of the male and f[e]male CHROMOSOMES prior to SYNGAMY.

**Fertinex**  highly purified METRODIN, with [no] residual LUTEINIZING HORMONE, thus equiv[a]lent in activity to RECOMBINANT FSH; calle[d] METRODIN HP outside the U.S. Made [by] Serono. *See also* SERUM ESTRADIOL.

**fetal reduction**  also called "selective abo[r]tion" and "selective feticide"; a controversi[al] and emotionally hazardous way of dealir[g] with a higher-number multiple pregnanc[y] (such as, especially, triplets, quadruplets [or] higher) because all the EMBRYOS or FETUSES a[re] at risk of being lost before viability; while ca[r]rying out TRANSVAGINAL ULTRASOUND, a leth[al] substance such as air or a solution of pota[s]sium is injected into the visibly beating hea[rt] of one or more of the embryos, thus reducir[g] the number of surviving embryos to two [or] one. Generally regarded as a more stressf[ul] procedure than even an induced ABORTION both for the person undergoing the operatio[n] and for the ultrasound doctor asked to do i[t]. Few people regard the availability of fetal r[e]duction to mean that the greatest care do[es] not need to be taken to avoid higher-numbe[r] multiple pregnancies in ASSISTED CONCEPTIO[N] programs. There is the HAZARD of loss of th[e] remaining fetuses from MISCARRIAGE, but th[e] RISK of this with an experienced ultrasoun[d] doctor is low.

**fetus**  an unborn baby, from the time the EM[-] BRYO is fully formed (from head to limbs[)] from about eight weeks from the LAST MEN[-] STRUAL PERIOD until delivery.

**fibroid**  also called a myoma, a benign "tu[-] mor" of the muscular wall of the uterus (MY[O-]

ETRIUM); it is more common with increasing age but can occur in women in their twenties; it can be single or multiple and can be located on the outside of the uterus (a
SUBSEROUS FIBROID), within the wall of the
uterus (an intramural fibroid) or protruding
into the cavity of the uterus (a SUBMUCOUS FI-
BROID). The closer it is (or they are) to the cavity, the more likely it is that a fibroid will disturb reproduction (either as MISCARRIAGES or
sometimes as INFERTILITY) and disturb menstrual bleeding. *See also* MYOMECTOMY.

**fimbria (fimbriae)**   *see* FIMBRIAL END

**fimbrial end**   also "fimbriated end," the open,
outside end of the FALLOPIAN TUBE in contact
with the surface of the ovary, from which it
picks up the ovulated egg from the ruptured
FOLLICLE; it is composed of delicate fimbriae,
finger-like projections of the tube lined by
cells with tiny hairs (CILIA), which beat toward
the inside of the tube, carrying the sticky CUM-
ULUS MASS into the AMPULLA before FERTILIZA-
TION; easily damaged by infection (SALPINGI-
TIS) or careless surgery, after which it can be
blocked, resulting in a HYDROSALPINX, or have
its correct movement inhibited by ADHESIONS.

**fimbriectomy**   an operation for STERILIZATION
or tubal ligation in which the FIMBRIAL END of
each FALLOPIAN TUBE is removed; it has a higher
failure rate than most other sterilization operations on the tubes and can result in a HYDRO-
SALPINX in later life, especially if ESTROGEN RE-
PLACEMENT THERAPY is used after menopause.
The operation to reverse it, SALPINGOSTOMY, is
much less often followed by pregnancy than
after other reversal operations.

**fimbriolysis**   MICROSURGERY of the fallopian
tube's FIMBRIAL END, involving careful dissec-

tion of fimbriae that have become stuck together from ADHESIONS; generally has a better
outcome than SALPINGOSTOMY, which must be
resorted to if the fimbriae are too damaged to
dissect.

**FISH**   *see* FLUORESCENT IN SITU HYBRIDIZATION

**fluorescent in situ hybridization** (FISH)   a
technique of genetic diagnosis in which a region of a CHROMOSOME is stained with a dye
that emits colored light when exposed to ultra-
violet light; a marker for chromosome 21 will
normally show two spots of light, whereas
three spots of light would indicate TRISOMY 21
(DOWN'S SYNDROME); useful because the technique is accurate with just one cell, making diagnosis possible in an IVF embryo before
transfer. *See also* PREIMPLANTATIONAL DIAGNOSIS.

**follicle**   normal structure in the OVARY that
contains the egg, or OOCYTE; all are formed as
PRIMORDIAL FOLLICLES 20 weeks before birth
and remain microscopic in size until growth
starts (FOLLICULOGENESIS), a few weeks before
the cycle in which the particular follicle will be
a candidate to ovulate; about 3 millimeters in
diameter at the start of a cycle, and about 2
centimeters in diameter when ready to ovulate; makes more and more ESTROGEN (particularly ESTRADIOL) as it grows; the number growing and their rate of growth can be monitored
by TRANSVAGINAL ULTRASOUND. *See also* ATRETIC
FOLLICLE; GRAAFIAN FOLLICLE; PRIMARY FOLLICLE;
SECONDARY FOLLICLE; TERTIARY FOLLICLE.

**follicle aspiration**   procedure for obtaining
eggs involving the passing of a needle into a
mature (or GRAAFIAN) FOLLICLE, either directly
during LAPAROSCOPY or via the vagina guided
by TRANSVAGINAL ULTRASOUND; known also as
"egg pickup" or "ovum pickup."

**follicle cells** cells of the FOLLICLE that surround the egg; an increase in number is what causes the follicle to grow; in TERTIARY FOLLICLES they are responsible for converting androgens from surrounding ovarian THECAL CELLS into ESTROGENS, particularly ESTRADIOL; a tertiary follicle's cells are also called "granulosa cells."

**follicle stimulating hormone** (FSH) the hormone, or GONADOTROPIN, produced by the PITUITARY GLAND that makes the TERTIARY FOLLICLE grow; obtained from human sources in a mixture with LUTEINIZING HORMONE (LH) as HUMAN MENOPAUSAL GONADOTROPIN (hMG), extracted from the urine of women who have been through MENOPAUSE (HUMEGON, METRODIN and PERGONAL); and HUMAN PITUITARY GONADOTROPIN (hPG), from human pituitary glands removed at autopsies (now obsolete). Pure FSH can be made synthetically with gene technology. *See also* RECOMBINANT FSH; SERUM FSH.

**follicular atresia** the process by which a PRIMARY FOLLICLE or TERTIARY FOLLICLE stops growing, leading to disappearance of its FOLLICLE CELLS and the OOCYTE, or egg, they contain; such a follicle is an ATRETIC FOLLICLE.

**follicular phase** the part of the ovary's monthly cycle before OVULATION, dominated by the presence of, first, a cohort of growing TERTIARY FOLLICLES, and then by the DOMINANT FOLLICLE, and the ESTRADIOL these follicles produce; normally around 14 days in length, but quite variable, being often much longer for the first few MENSTRUAL CYCLES after the first period (MENARCHE) and typically getting shorter in the months or years leading up to EGG DEPLETION and MENOPAUSE. Corresponds with the PROLIFERATIVE PHASE of the endometrial or menstrual cycle.

**folliculogenesis** strictly, the process by which FOLLICLES are first formed in immature ovaries, 20 weeks or so before a female fetus is born; in the woman, it means the growth of a PRIMORDIAL FOLLICLE into an early TERTIARY FOLLICLE, a transition that confers receptiveness of the follicle to FOLLICLE STIMULATING HORMONE (FSH); the stimulus for folliculogenesis and its timing for individual follicles remains a mystery.

**free androgen index** the ANDROGEN (TESTOSTERONE) in blood that is not bound to carrier proteins, so it is immediately available for action in the tissues; more likely to be increased in the POLYCYSTIC OVARY SYNDROME than SERUM TESTOSTERONE.

**FSH** *see* FOLLICLE STIMULATING HORMONE

**fundus** the body or main part of the UTERUS (leaving out the CERVIX), particularly its topmost part.

**galactorrhea** demonstrable milk production from the breasts other than while purposefully breast-feeding; caused by HYPERPROLACTINEMIA or, sometimes, by disease in the breast or wall of the chest.

**gamete intrafallopian transfer** (GIFT) procedure for assisting conception in which unfertilized eggs plus sperm (GAMETES) are transferred to the FALLOPIAN TUBE, so that FERTILIZATION occurs in the normal place, with several possible advantages: better, stronger and faster-growing embryos might result compared with those after IN VITRO FERTILIZATION; these embryos arguably reach the uterus at the right time after fertilization; and the

ach the uterus in an anatomically correct di-
ction. Some of these advantages, if they are
al, might also apply to the procedure of ZY-
TE INTRAFALLOPIAN TRANSFER (ZIFT).

**mete**   generic term for the mature GERM
LL, that is, an egg or a sperm.

**irtner's duct**   *see* MESONEPHRIC DUCT

**nder**   politically correct term for distin-
ishing the male from the female SEX.

**netic-plus-gestational surrogacy**   *see* TRA-
TIONAL SURROGACY

**rm cell**   the gender-neutral word for OVA
d SPERMATOZOA. *See also* HAPLOID.

**station**   pregnancy.

**stational sac**   a fluid-filled bag of mem-
anes in which the EMBRYO forms, visible on
ANSVAGINAL ULTRASOUND from about five
eeks from the LAST MENSTRUAL PERIOD; techni-
lly, the "amniotic cavity" (and later in preg-
ncy can be sampled with AMNIOCENTESIS).

**stational surrogacy**   surrogacy in which
e woman who is the SURROGATE (or gesta-
onal carrier) for the intended pregnancy re-
ives embryos from the commissioning in-
rtile couple, who have undergone IN VITRO
RTILIZATION; then, by becoming pregnant,
rries (or gestates) the pregnancy, she gives
rth and then gives up the baby to the baby's
enetic parents. In principle, the practice can
e done for altruistic or commercial reasons.

**IFT**   *see* GAMETE INTRAFALLOPIAN TRANSFER

**lucose tolerance test**   *see* PLASMA GLUCOSE

**nRH**   *see* GONADOTROPIN-RELEASING HORMONE

**nRH-agonist**   a GnRH-ANALOG that briefly
stimulates the PITUITARY GLAND to release FOL-
LICLE STIMULATING HORMONE (FSH) and
LUTEINIZING HORMONE (LH) but then quickly
puts a clamp on it, stopping these hormones
from competing with administered hormones
and, particularly in women, suppressing the
LH SURGE, which otherwise can spoil the timing of EGG PICKUP in an assisted conception
program (such as IVF or GIFT). Examples include BUSERELIN, GOSERELIN, LEUPROLIDE, NA-
FARELIN, and TRIPTORELIN.

**GnRH-analog**   synthetic hormones related
to the natural hormone GnRH, or GONADO-
TROPIN-RELEASING HORMONE. *See also* GnRH-
AGONIST; GnRH-ANTAGONIST.

**GnRH-antagonist**   a GnRH-ANALOG that immediately suppresses the pituitary gland from
releasing FOLLICLE STIMULATING HORMONE
(FSH) and LUTEINIZING HORMONE (LH); not
available commercially yet but likely to replace GnRH-AGONISTS for many gynecological
purposes (especially ASSISTED CONCEPTION)
when clinical trials are completed.

**gonad**   a gender-neutral word for the organ
that produces GERM CELLS. *See also* OVARY;
TESTIS.

**gonadotropin**   any hormone that switches on
the function of the GONADS. There are two
main families of gonadotropins: the gonadotropin that stimulates the growth of the
FOLLICLE, or FOLLICLE STIMULATING HORMONE
(FSH), and those that cause OVULATION from
the mature follicle and stimulate the CORPUS
LUTEUM that results to develop and to produce
PROGESTERONE, namely LUTEINIZING HORMONE
(LH) and HUMAN CHORIONIC GONADOTROPIN
(hCG); FSH will cause growing follicles to
produce the estrogen ESTRADIOL provided that
a small amount of LH (or hCG) is present;

FSH and LH are produced in the PITUITARY GLAND, whereas hCG comes from the PLACENTA in pregnancy. In men, FSH stimulates the SERTOLI CELLS of the TESTICULAR TUBULES, and hence drives SPERMATOGENESIS; LH and hCG stimulate the LEYDIG CELLS to produce TESTOSTERONE. *See also* the individual named hormones.

**gonadotropin-releasing hormone** a hormone produced by the HYPOTHALAMUS of the brain to regulate production of FOLLICLE STIMULATING HORMONE and particularly LUTEINIZING HORMONE. Can be administered to induce OVULATION when it is deficient, particularly in AMENORRHEA due to weight loss or excessive exercise, but it has to be given in small amounts directly into a vein, every 60 to 90 minutes for the two weeks of a normal FOLLICULAR PHASE (with an electronic syringe-driver), mimicking its natural pattern of secretion.

**Gonal F** RECOMBINANT FOLLICLE STIMULATING HORMONE manufactured by Serono.

**Goretex®** the nondissolvable product used in a special surgical specification as a barrier to the formation of ADHESIONS.

**goserelin** a GNRH-AGONIST manufactured by ICI as Zoladex and administered by monthly injection.

**Graafian follicle** a large, mature TERTIARY FOLLICLE that will respond to an adequate LH SURGE or injection of HUMAN CHORIONIC GONADOTROPIN (hCG) by undergoing OVULATION, releasing its egg; produces ESTRADIOL and, with exposure to LUTEINIZING HORMONE or hCG, PROGESTERONE; named after Reijnier de Graaf (1641–1673), the first person to see

and appreciate the importance of the ovari follicle.

**granulosa cells** FOLLICLE CELLS from a TE TIARY FOLLICLE.

**HA** *see* HYPOTHALAMIC ANOVULATION

**habitual abortion** a rather insensitive way saying RECURRENT MISCARRIAGES.

**haploid, haploidy** the state of a cell with CHROMOSOMES (half the normal DIPLOID chr mosome state), found normally only in sper cells and eggs as SECONDARY OOCYTES. *See a* MEIOSIS.

**hazard** an event, usually unwanted, som times in the sense of a penalty. Unlike RIS which has a number attached to it (it is QUAN TITATIVE), a hazard is "yes" or "no"—it is eith realized, or experienced, or it is not; althoug one hazard can be worse to experience tha another, you cannot put a figure on it (it QUALITATIVE).

**hCG** *see* HUMAN CHORIONIC GONADOTROPIN

**hermaphroditism** *see* INTERSEX

**heterotopic pregnancy** the coexistence of normal pregnancy in the uterus with an EC TOPIC PREGNANCY.

**heterozygous** the genetic state when th pair of GENES under consideration consists two ALLELES that are different. Disease or di ability can follow if one of the alleles is once seriously abnormal and dominant (s DOMINANT INHERITANCE) over the other allel *See also* HOMOZYGOUS.

**hirsutism** hair on the face, chest (betwee the breasts or around the nipples), abdome thighs that is getting worse, is worse than her family members or is worse than usual r one's race; more likely to be important edically if the menstrual periods are disrbed (if there is OLIGOMENORRHEA or AMENRRHEA). *See also* POLYCYSTIC OVARY SYNDROME.

**IV** human immune deficiency virus, the rus that causes acquired immune deficiency ndrome, or AIDS. Type 1 and type 2 viruses e recognized and both are usually tested for SERUM HIV ANTIBODIES.

**MG** *see* HUMAN MENOPAUSAL GONADOTROPIN

**omozygous** the genetic state when the pair f GENES under consideration consists of two LLELES that are the same. Disease or disability an follow if the alleles are seriously abnoral, a condition known as RECESSIVE INHERIANCE (an example is CYSTIC FIBROSIS). *See also* ETEROZYGOUS.

**ormone** a chemical substance, natural or not, vhich acts as a signal from one part of the body o another, via the bloodstream. The study of ormones is the science of endocrinology, and he hormone systems of the body are collecively known as the endocrine system.

**ormone replacement therapy** (HRT) *see* STROGEN REPLACEMENT THERAPY

**PG** *see* HUMAN PITUITARY GONADOTROPIN

**IRT** (hormone replacement therapy) *see* ESTROGEN REPLACEMENT THERAPY

**Huhner's test** *see* POSTCOITAL TEST

**human chorionic gonadotropin** (hCG) a GONADOTROPIN produced by the PLACENTA in pregnancy (specifically, it is produced by the TROPHOBLAST); the generic name for PREGNYL

and PROFASI, which are preparations of hCG obtained by extracting it from the urine of pregnant women; mimics the action of LUTEINIZING HORMONE, but has a very much longer duration of action (which has important advantages); given as an injection to stimulate OVULATION from a mature FOLLICLE 38 hours after the injection or to stimulate ongoing function of the CORPUS LUTEUM, particularly its production of PROGESTERONE. Typically given after a course of FOLLICLE STIMULATING HORMONE in ASSISTED CONCEPTION (GIFT and IVF) programs 36 hours before the expected time of FOLLICLE ASPIRATION, and then in further, smaller doses to support the corpus luteum (or corpora lutea) that follows; no cases of transmitted (infectious) disease have been recorded after its use. It is also the hormone of pregnancy that is measured in a PREGNANCY TEST.

**human menopausal gonadotropin** (hMG) a mixture of FOLLICLE STIMULATING HORMONE (FSH) and LUTEINIZING HORMONE (LH) extracted for therapeutic use from the urine of menopausal women (who normally produce these hormones in high concentration); marketed as HUMEGON (Organon) and PERGONAL (Serono). METRODIN (Serono) is hMG from which most LH has been removed. FERTINEX (or "Metrodin-HP") is Metrodin from which other urinary proteins also have been removed, resulting in FSH that acts like RECOMBINANT FSH. No cases of transmitted (infectious) disease have been recorded after the use of any of these preparations.

**human pituitary gonadotropin** (hPG) a mixture of FOLLICLE STIMULATING HORMONE (FSH) and LUTEINIZING HORMONE (LH) extracted directly from PITUITARY GLANDS obtained at autopsies; never used routinely in the United States, where HUMAN MENOPAUSAL GONADOTROPIN was used instead; not used anywhere in the world since 1986, when it was shown that CREUTZFELDT-JAKOB DISEASE (CJD), a deadly form of dementia, could be transmitted from its use due to contaminating and infected brain tissue; before 1986 it had been used mostly for OVULATION INDUCTION in women with AMENORRHEA, for which other hormones or drugs had not been effective, although sporadic instances of its use for IN VITRO FERTILIZATION are known outside the United States.

**human recombinant FSH**   *see* RECOMBINANT HUMAN FOLLICLE STIMULATING HORMONE

**Humegon**   mixture of HUMAN MENOPAUSAL GONADOTROPINS containing FOLLICLE STIMULATING HORMONE manufactured by Organon; virtually equivalent to PERGONAL.

**hydatidiform mole, complete**   a highly abnormal pregnancy resembling a bunch of grapes, and a result of FERTILIZATION of an egg by one or more sperm in which the egg's CHROMOSOMES are excluded from SYNGAMY. Instead syngamy involves either a single X-chromosome-bearing sperm (which first divides into two, giving a 46,XX hydatidiform mole) or two sperm, one X-bearing, one Y-bearing (giving a 46,XY hydatidiform mole). In either case, no embryo forms, just TROPHOBLAST, the CHORIONIC VILLI of which thus have no fetal blood vessels to take fluid away, causing the villi to swell and to look like a soggy bunch of grapes. The clinical manifestation is a uterus that is usually big for the gestational duration, often with vaginal bleeding.

The diagnosis is made by a characteristic appearance on TRANSVAGINAL ULTRASOUND. In small proportion of cases, a hydatidiform mole becomes invasive and malignant (cancerous), so after treatment by VACUUM CURETTAGE careful follow-up for 12 months with serial measurements of HUMAN CHORIONIC GONADOTROPIN is usually advised before another pregnancy is attempted.

**hydatidiform mole, partial**   *see* TRIPLOIDY

**hydrosalpinx**   blockage of the outer or FIMBRIAL END of the FALLOPIAN TUBE, resulting in its distension by watery contents.

**hyperplasia**   an abnormal increase in the number of cells seen in a sample of tissue. *See also* ENDOMETRIAL HYPERPLASIA.

**hyperprolactinemia**   an increase in SERUM PROLACTIN; may be accompanied by GALACTORRHEA.

**hypospadias**   a congenital abnormality in males in which the urethra does not reach the tip of the penis but opens near its base; the penis is usually short and curved, which can make sexual intercourse difficult, contributing to INFERTILITY.

**hypothalamic anovulation**   absence of OVULATION caused by insufficient GNRH drive from the HYPOTHALAMUS, so that the PITUITARY GLAND does not produce enough FOLLICLE STIMULATING HORMONE; usually accompanied by absent periods (AMENORRHEA).

**hypothalamic chronic anovulation**   *see* HYPOTHALAMIC ANOVULATION

**hypothalamus**   part of the brain lying immediately above and connected to the PITUITARY GLAND; responsible for producing GONADOTROPIN-RELEASING HORMONE, among other hor-

nones and substances (including the ENDOR-
HINS, dopamine and serotonin); in women
when conditioned to cyclical function by a
ack of exposure to male sex hormones before
pirth) it resonates with the OVARIAN CYCLE and
cooperates with the pituitary gland to cause
corresponding cyclical production of FOLLICLE
STIMULATING HORMONE and, particularly, a
:imely LH SURGE; responds to PROGESTERONE
py raising the body's temperature (*see* BASAL
BODY TEMPERATURE CHART).

**hysterectomy** a surgical operation at which
the UTERUS is removed, usually including the
CERVIX (hence a "total hysterectomy") but not
necessarily including the FALLOPIAN TUBES and
OVARIES.

**hysterosalpingogram** an X-ray of the ENDO-
METRIAL CAVITY and the internal outline of the
FALLOPIAN TUBES; performed by injecting a
fluid medium that blocks X-rays through the
cervix, so that it first fills the endometrial cavity and then flows out along the tubes, finally
casting shadows between the loops of intestine if the tubes are open. The test is uncomfortable, because of contractions of the
uterus, which can be partially overcome by
taking one of the same drugs that are used
to treat DYSMENORRHEA (such as an NSAID).
*See also* SELECTIVE SALPINGOGRAM.

**hysteroscopy** an examination of the ENDO-
METRIAL CAVITY of the UTERUS by a thin fiber-
optic instrument, similar to the instrument
used for LAPAROSCOPY; can be done in the
operating room under general anesthesia
(often in association with laparoscopy) or
with or without sedation in the physician's
office.

**ICSI** *see* INTRACYTOPLASMIC SPERM INSERTION

**IEC (institutional ethics committee)** *see* ETH-
ICS COMMITTEE

**IMB** *see* INTERMENSTRUAL BLEEDING

**immunobead tests** tests that look for human
antibodies attached to cells, especially antibodies attached to sperm cells (SPERM ANTI-
BODIES). The test involves tiny plastic beads
coated with antibodies to human antibodies;
if they are seen to attach to sperm cells then
the presence of antisperm antibodies on the
sperm cells is inferred by the observer.

**implantation** the process by which the embryo's TROPHOBLAST attaches to the mother's
ENDOMETRIUM and penetrates it, establishing
contact between the trophoblast's developing
CHORIONIC VILLI and the maternal blood. *See
also* BLASTOCYST.

**implantation bleeding** a small to moderate
amount of vaginal bleeding at the time implantation becomes established; can be confused with a menstrual period.

**implantation rate** the proportion of transferred embryos in an IN VITRO FERTILIZATION
procedure that produce a GESTATIONAL SAC
visible on TRANSVAGINAL ULTRASOUND. Unlike
for the CONCEPTION RATE and PREGNANCY
RATE, twins (with separate sacs) are counted
separately.

**impotence** inability to sustain an erection of
the penis and hence to ejaculate. Occasional
impotence is of no special psychological or
medical importance. Although persistent impotence is most often due to psychological
causes, medical tests are important.

**incomplete miscarriage** any MISCARRIAGE before all miscarriage tissue has been expelled.
Traditionally a uterine CURETTAGE was done

after a miscarriage, in the belief (often accurate) that there would still be some immature pregnancy tissue left in the uterus that could cause more bleeding and get infected. Nowadays we can distinguish an incomplete from a COMPLETE MISCARRIAGE (and whether or not a curettage should be done) with a TRANSVAGINAL ULTRASOUND, which is able to reveal retained tissue.

**induced abortion**   *see* ABORTION

**inevitable miscarriage**   traditionally, any bleeding from the vagina during early pregnancy with, on vaginal examination, opening of the cervix. Today, the diagnosis can be made much sooner (and distinguished from a THREATENED MISCARRIAGE) by not detecting a normal embryo on TRANSVAGINAL ULTRASOUND.

**infertility**   not getting pregnant as quickly as expected. *See also* SUFFERING.

**informed consent**   an administrative and legal device by which approval to proceed based on known or predicted consequences is obtained and recorded from a patient or from a volunteer for medical research, thus avoiding an accusation for what might otherwise be an assault. Just what "informed" means can be the subject of much legal and ethical wrangling. One modern interpretation is that it means as much as the person giving the consent demonstrates that he or she wants to know, although most doctors, ETHICS COMMITTEES, INSTITUTIONAL REVIEW BOARDS and courts underpin this with a minimum everyone consenting *should* be told about the procedure.

**Insler score**   a score (out of 12) for the quality of MUCUS in the cervix, gauged by scoring each of the following from 0 to 3: the cervix should be open; the volume of mucus should be good (although every woman will be different for both these parameters, they will be consistent in one woman from ovulation to ovulation); the mucus should be clear, watery and stretchy (SPINNBARKHEIT); and the mucus should produce a complete ferning pattern when it is allowed to dry on a microscope slide. The first two criteria vary at ovulation in different women (so anything above a score of 9 or 10 can be normal), but the same woman should achieve the same Insler score from one ovulation to the next. *See also* CERVICAL MUCUS.

**institutional ethics committee** (IEC)   *see* ETHICS COMMITTEE

**institutional review board** (IRB)   the U.S. equivalent of an institutional ETHICS COMMITTEE, set up to govern the ethical conduct of medical research.

**integrity**   a systematic ethical goal that preserves the values of TRUTH, ACCOUNTABILITY, equity and consistency.

**Interceed®**   a cloth manufactured by Johnson and Johnson and used for minimizing ADHESIONS in the PERITONEAL CAVITY after a surgical operation involving the FALLOPIAN TUBES or OVARIES. The material, woven from fibers of modified cellulose, are placed over abdominal surfaces, the serosa of which is likely to have been damaged, then dissolves in about a week or two into simple sugar molecules (which are absorbed by the body and metabolized); in the meantime, the cloth keeps the covered surfaces apart while the serosa reforms. Controlled trials have shown Interceed to be effective in preventing or reducing adhesions, but an adhesion-free result is not guaranteed. In my experience Interceed is exceptionally seful when dense adhesions resulting from previous operations are being treated.

**intermenstrual bleeding** (IMB)  bleeding between periods that are usually otherwise regular; if it happens while on the oral contraceptive pill it is called BREAKTHROUGH BLEEDING; if it happens over a few days before a period starts properly it is PREMENSTRUAL SPOTTING; if it happens after sex it is POSTCOITAL BLEEDING; these forms of IMB have different, usually important, causes.

**intersex** also called "hermaphroditism," a state of confusion regarding the assigning of gender, usually because of ambiguity of the genital organs at birth. There is male intersex if the KARYOTYPE is 46,XY, female intersex if it is 46,XX.

**interstitial segment**  the innermost part of the FALLOPIAN TUBE, passing through the wall of the UTERUS (the MYOMETRIUM) to join the ISTHMUS to the ENDOMETRIAL CAVITY.

**intracytoplasmic sperm insertion** (ICSI)  an IN VITRO FERTILIZATION technique involving sperm microinjection (SMI), in which one or more sperm are injected through the ZONA PELLUCIDA, across the PERIVITELLINE SPACE, through the vitelline membrane (the egg cell's membrane) and into the substance (or CYTO-PLASM) of the egg itself; has largely replaced subzonal sperm insertion (SUZI) because it is not a requirement for the sperm to have undergone the ACROSOME REACTION.

**intramural segment**  *see* INTERSTITIAL SEGMENT

**intrauterine adhesions**  ADHESIONS inside the ENDOMETRIAL CAVITY caused by prior infection (ENDOMETRITIS), especially if there has been a CURETTAGE during the period of infection. The circumstances in which this combination is most common are treatment for a MISSED ABOR-TION and treatment of a postpartum hemorrhage (bleeding a few weeks after the birth of a baby). *See also* ASHERMAN'S SYNDROME.

**intrauterine insemination** (IUI)  ASSISTED INSEMINATION into the uterus, either for DONOR INSEMINATION (DI) or with husband's semen (AIH). IUI can be carried out with a woman's natural cycles or with ovarian stimulation (SUPEROVULATION) using CLOMIPHENE or FOLLI-CLE STIMULATING HORMONE; a form of ASSISTED CONCEPTION.

**in vitro**  Latin for "in glass," meaning "in the laboratory."

**in vitro fertilization** (IVF)  FERTILIZATION of the egg by sperm in the laboratory; necessary if the FALLOPIAN TUBES are diseased or missing; useful if sperm fertilizing capacity is doubtful, because evidence of fertilization can be seen before the egg is transferred as an EMBRYO. *See also* ASSISTED CONCEPTION.

**in vitro maturation** (IVM)  maturation in the laboratory of the egg (as a PRIMARY OOCYTE) obtained from an immature TERTIARY FOLLICLE until it becomes a SECONDARY OOCYTE competent to be fertilized by sperm using in vitro fertilization. The smaller the follicle, the lower the proportion of eggs that mature successfully. ICSI can be used to increase the proportion of eggs that will fertilize, but the embryos on average do no better, and so no advantage is conferred by ICSI in this situation.

**in vitro penetration test**  one of several tests of the ability of sperm to penetrate cervical mucus at the time of ovulation or under the influence of estrogen. *See also* KREMER TEST; POSTCOITAL TEST.

**IRB**  *see* INSTITUTIONAL REVIEW BOARD

**irritable bowel syndrome**  also called "spastic colon syndrome," a distressing dysfunction of the intestines in which there is overactivity of the involuntary contractions of the intestines' muscular wall and increased pain signals coming from those contractions. Treatment is based on decreasing the contractions (with a diet high in fiber, sometimes with antispasmodic drugs) and attempting to reduce the action of the pain-carrying nerves, both by sedating them (this means general sedation so it is often not very acceptable) and by reeducating them to be less sensitive. Treatment is time consuming and, ultimately, not always satisfactory. The symptoms of the irritable bowel syndrome are often confused with those of ENDOMETRIOSIS; they are sometimes made worse with, and at the time of, PREMENSTRUAL TENSION. Typically (but not always), there is an alternating tendency toward diarrhea or constipation; sometimes there is nausea with the spasms.

**isthmus**  the narrow, inner part of the FALLOPIAN TUBE, about 3 to 4 centimeters long; lies between the AMPULLA and the INTERSTITIAL SEGMENT of the tube.

**IUD**  abbreviation either for "intrauterine death" (death of a FETUS, prefacing a stillbirth) or for "intrauterine (contraceptive) device," which is sometimes abbreviated IUCD.

**IUI**  *see* INTRAUTERINE INSEMINATION

**IVF**  *see* IN VITRO FERTILIZATION

**IVM**  *see* IN VITRO MATURATION

**justice**  the ethical value to be had in a community from conferring rights and obligations in a way that is fair and accords to other ethical values (NONMALEFICENCE, BENEFICENCE). *See also* DISTRIBUTIVE JUSTICE.

**Kallmann's syndrome**  CONGENITAL absenc of GONADOTROPIN-RELEASING HORMONE in th hypothalamus, together with a congenitall absent sense of smell, causing in women PRI MARY AMENORRHEA and ANOVULATION, and i men failure of puberty.

**karyotype**  a test that displays the CHROMO SOMES after relevant cells are grown in tissu culture; a normal female karyotype is desig nated 46,XX and a normal male karyotyp 46,XY.

**Klinefelter's syndrome**  a TRISOMY with a KARYOTYPE of 47,XXY; that is, a male with a extra X CHROMOSOME; a cause of AZOOSPERMIA

**Kremer test**  an in vitro (laboratory) test o the interaction between sperm and CERVICAL MUCUS, in which the mucus to be tested i drawn into two very fine glass tubes (another two tubes are filled with mucus that is known to be good) to give a four-way test between: husband's (or male partner's) sperm and wife's (or female partner's) mucus; husband's sperm and known good mucus; known good sperm with wife's mucus; and known good sperm with known good mucus. Because of the laboriousness of the test it is usual to administer ESTROGEN for at least a weak to the wife to ensure that the mucus is optimal.

**K-selection**  a reproductive strategy where survival of a species is optimized by placing a premium on individual survival despite fluctuations of the environment; favors large animals (and large animals favor this strategy); and favors animals that get pregnant more than once and the offspring of which require much postnatal care before sexual maturity is reached.

acing of pregnancy is important for survival mother and offspring and thus favors the olution of RELATIVE INFERTILITY. The opposite productive strategy to *r*-SELECTION.

**paroscopy** a "minimally invasive" surgical peration at which instruments are passed rough the wall of the abdomen either for e diagnosis of abnormalities of the abdom- al or pelvic organs (such as the FALLOPIAN UBES, OVARIES and UTERUS) and diagnose EN- OMETRIOSIS; or therapeutically, to reach the llopian tubes for certain ASSISTED CONCEP- ION procedures (see GAMETE INTRAFALLOPIAN RANSFER and ZYGOTE INTRAFALLOPIAN TRANS- ER). Carries the hazards of surgery (damage o internal organs, hemorrhage, infection) nd the hazards of general anesthesia.

**aparotomy** a surgical operation in which he abdomen is opened; needed for MICRO- URGERY operations on the FALLOPIAN TUBES although some operations formerly done nly during laparotomy are now possible during LAPAROSCOPY). For infertility surgery, he scar from a laparotomy is usually a low, orizontal one, just above the pubic bone. Several days in a hospital are needed; most people are off work about three weeks; some numbness or sensitivity below the scar can be expected for several months, as nerves to the skin regrow.

**large bowel** the colon (*see* BOWEL).

**last menstrual period** (LMP) the normal period immediately preceding conception. For convenience, obstetricians calculate the duration of a pregnancy as starting with this date, even though pregnancy does not truly begin until FERTILIZATION (or, some would say, IMPLANTATION).

**leuprolide** a GnRH-AGONIST manufactured by Abbott and sold as Lupron. Administered by daily injection under the skin.

**Leydig cell** cells of the TESTIS lying between the tubules in which sperm are formed (hence their other name, "interstitial cells") and responsible for the production of the male sex hormone TESTOSTERONE.

**LH** *see* LUTEINIZING HORMONE

**LH surge** a sudden and huge increase in production of LUTEINIZING HORMONE by the PITUITARY GLAND in response to sustained and substantial levels of ESTRADIOL in the blood; causes OVULATION about 36 hours after it starts (about 20 hours after its peak); if not suppressed during ASSISTED CONCEPTION (see GnRH-AGONISTS and GnRH-ANTAGONISTS) it can start before HUMAN CHORIONIC GONADOTROPIN has been given, thus spoiling the timing of egg pickup; timely production of the LH surge in adult women depends on female conditioning of the HYPOTHALAMUS and/or the PITUITARY GLAND before birth.

**linkage analysis** Because it can take lots of CHROMOSOMAL CROSS-OVERS (lots of generations) to send two genes that live as neighbors on a chromosome into different directions (they end up in different people), we can do family studies to work out how closely people are related by seeing how long the runs are of identical genes.

**LMP** *see* LAST MENSTRUAL PERIOD

**long protocol** involves use GnRH-AGONISTS for more than a week before injections of FOLLICLE STIMULATING HORMONE (FSH) start for induction of SUPEROVULATION in ASSISTED CONCEPTION programs. The advantage is that any temporary rise in LUTEINIZING HORMONE levels and PROGESTERONE levels has dissipated before the development is under way of those ovarian FOLLICLES from which eggs will be removed. The disadvantage, compared with the SHORT PROTOCOL, is that higher (hence more expensive) doses of GnRH-agonist and FSH are needed. The GnRH can be started with menstruation or during the LUTEAL PHASE of the previous cycle. *See also* ULTRASHORT PROTOCOL.

**LPD**   *see* LUTEAL PHASE DEFECT

**LUF**   *see* LUTEINIZED UNRUPTURED FOLLICLE

**Lupron**   *see* LEUPROLIDE

**lupus anticoagulant**   an antibody first noted in the disease systemic lupus erythematosus that has the ability to stop blood from clotting; also called the "lupus inhibitor"; closely related to a family of antiphospholipid antibodies, especially ANTICARDIOLIPIN ANTIBODY, and a cause of RECURRENT MISCARRIAGES.

**lupus inhibitor**   *see* LUPUS ANTICOAGULANT

**luteal phase**   the part of the ovary's cycle between OVULATION and the start of a new FOLLICULAR PHASE, therefore dominated by the presence of the CORPUS LUTEUM and the PROGESTERONE it produces; normally between 11 and 16 days in length; extended by the action on the corpus luteum of HUMAN CHORIONIC GONADOTROPIN (hCG) if IMPLANTATION of the embryo is successful; shorter cycles can interfere with implantation (a LUTEAL PHASE DEFECT).

**luteal phase defect** (LPD)   also called "luteal phase insufficiency," a LUTEAL PHASE that is shorter than optimal for a fertilized egg to undergo IMPLANTATION; very likely to occur if the luteal phase is shorter than normal (11 to 16 days), but not all luteal phases within this nor-

mal range are innocent; often caused by prior defect of the FOLLICULAR PHASE or of the development of the ovulating TERTIARY (GRAAFIAN) FOLLICLE and hence by implicatio there may be a defect of the egg itself, any which may cause infertility for the cycle or a increased chance of MISCARRIAGE; also assoc ated with the LUTEINIZED UNRUPTURED FOLLICL

**luteinized unruptured follicle** (LUF)   occu when a reasonably mature TERTIARY (GRAAFIAN) FOLLICLE receives an LH SURGE tha is enough to make it start producing PROGES TERONE but is not enough to cause it to releas its egg through OVULATION; the result is tha the egg is trapped in the follicle, which to greater or lesser extent then functions like CORPUS LUTEUM, though this stage of the folli cle's life is often short, giving rise to a LUTEA PHASE DEFECT (LPD).

**luteinizing hormone**   the hormone, or go nadotropin, produced by the PITUITARY GLAN to cause OVULATION of a mature FOLLICLE i the ovary, resulting in formation of the COR PUS LUTEUM; suppressed by GnRH-AGONISTS and GnRH-ANTAGONISTS, so that (for OVULA TION INDUCTION) an injection of HUMAN CHOR IONIC GONADOTROPIN (hCG, which acts the same way) has a predictable time course of ac tion. *See also* SERUM LH.

**macrophage**   a cell in the body (a bit like the one-celled ameba) that is able to wander about and engulf and digest a huge range of foreign material and junk (including sperm cells) that get into the body's tissues. They are present in almost every tissue in the body, more so if there is inflammation. We see them as scavenging cells, ones that do the ultimate tidying up inside the body, but they can be programmed to swallow very specific targets, metimes committing suicide for the greater od. There are normally lots of macrophages the PERITONEAL CAVITY.

**agnetic resonance imaging** see MRI SCAN

**aturation arrest** *see* AZOOSPERMIA

**edical vocabulary** *see* VOCABULARY

**edroxyprogesterone acetate** (MPA) a PRO-ESTOGEN of a type related to progesterone it-lf. Marketed as Provera (tablets) and Depo-rovera (injections) by Upjohn.

**eiosis (meioses)** a process similar to MITO-s in which two successive divisions of a PLOID cell result in four "daughter" cells, each ith a HAPLOID number of CHROMOSOMES; un-ke mitosis, each chromosome therefore du-icates just once (before the beginning of eiosis). Meiosis in humans and other higher nimals takes place only among the GERM CELLS OGONIA and SPERMATOGONIA), which will ave been multiplying by mitosis. By differen-ating into, respectively, PRIMARY OOCYTES or RIMARY SPERMATOCYTES, each with 92 chromo-omes, meiosis commences. With completion f the first meiotic division the products (in-luding SECONDARY OOCYTES and SECONDARY PERMATOCYTES) each contain 46 chromo-omes. With completion of the second meiotic ivision the haploid number (23) of chromo-omes, suitable for fertilization, is reached. In he testis, meiosis and the production of new perm cells (SPERMATOZOA) can continue hroughout life, but in the ovary all egg cells hat survive commence meiosis about 20 veeks before birth, spending the remaining ime (up to 50 years or more) locked up in OLLICLES as primary oocytes. Whereas a pri-nary spermatocyte gives rise to four haploid perm cells, a primary oocyte produces just

one secondary oocyte (the spare 46 chromo-somes are dumped into the first POLAR BODY just before OVULATION), and then one egg cell (the spare 23 chromosomes are dumped into the second polar body after FERTILIZATION). *See also* CHROMOSOMAL CROSS-OVER.

**menarche** the first natural menstrual period.

**menopause** the last natural menstrual pe-riod and thus often a retrospective diagnosis; hence "menopausal" is the natural state a woman is in after the ovaries have stopped ovulating. The normal age of menopause is between 40 and 55 years, with an average in Western societies of 50 or 51 years. *See also* ES-TRONE; PREMATURE MENOPAUSE.

**menorrhagia** traditional medical term for DYSFUNCTIONAL UTERINE BLEEDING, or, simply, heavy periods.

**menstrual abortion** *see* MENSTRUAL MISCARRIAGE

**menstrual cycle** the OVARIAN CYCLE as it is ex-pressed by the ENDOMETRIUM of the UTERUS. It consists of the MENSTRUAL PHASE, the PROLIFER-ATIVE PHASE and the SECRETORY PHASE. Like the ovarian cycle itself, it is normally 24 to 35 days in length, typically 28 days, but there are lots of normal exceptions.

**menstrual miscarriage** loss of an early em-bryo at the expected time of a period; not usu-ally noticeable without special testing levels of SERUM HUMAN CHORIONIC GONADOTROPIN.

**menstrual phase** the phase of the ENDO-METRIUM during which there is menstruation, caused by withdrawal of PROGESTERONE at the end of the ovarian LUTEAL PHASE as a new ovarian FOLLICULAR PHASE starts; in ANOVULA-TORY CYCLES or during treatment with estro-gens, menstrual bleeding can occur from withdrawal, insufficiency or downward fluc-tuations of ESTROGEN alone.

**mesonephric duct**   a duct on each side of the developing embryo that leads from the em-bryo's mesonephros, or temporary kidney. In male fetuses the duct persists as the Wolffian duct to form the RETE TESTIS, the EPIDIDYMIS, the VAS DEFERENS and the SEMINAL VESICLE. In fe-male fetuses it usually disappears completely (in favor of the paramesonephric duct, better known as the MÜLLERIAN DUCT), although por-tions of mesonephric duct can remain as harmless cysts, called "Gärtner's duct cysts."

**mesonephric duct cyst**   *see* MESONEPHRIC DUCT

**mesonephric remnant**   *see* MESONEPHRIC DUCT

**MESA**   *see* MICROEPIDIDYMAL SPERM ASPIRATION

**metaphase**   the third of four stages of MITOSIS or MEIOSIS, at which the chromosomes, at-tached in a plate-like formation to a structure in the cell called a "spindle," are easily distin-guished with a microscope and can be pho-tographed to construct a KARYOTYPE.

**metaplasia**   the metamorphosis of a tissue to take on a different form, perhaps more char-acteristic of a tissue some distance away. One of the theories of the cause of ENDOMETRIOSIS is based on metaplasia.

**Metrodin**   HUMAN MENOPAUSAL GONADOTROPIN (hMG) from which LUTEINIZING HORMONE (LH) has largely been removed, leaving FOLLICLE STIM-ULATING HORMONE (FSH) as the main active substance. METRODIN HP (FERTINEX in the U.S.) is even more purified and, unlike METRODIN, has no LH activity at all. Made by Serono.

**Metrodin HP**   Called FERTINEX in the United States, METRODIN that has been "highly puri-fied" by removing all contaminating urina proteins. Contains even less LUTEINIZING HO MONE than Metrodin, and is thus similar in a tion to RECOMBINANT FOLLICLE STIMULATIN HORMONE. *See also* SERUM ESTRADIOL.

**metroplasty**   a plastic operation on the UTER to change the shape of its cavity, usually for UTERINE SEPTUM or for a BICORNUATE UTERUS, there have been a number of miscarriages.

**metrorrhagia**   traditional medical term fc INTERMENSTRUAL BLEEDING.

**microepididymal sperm aspiration** (MESA using MICROSURGERY to dissect the EPIDIDYM or RETE TESTIS, or sometimes the tubules of th TESTIS itself, to find motile sperm cells suitabl to be aspirated, isolated and prepared for a ASSISTED CONCEPTION procedure, usually in volving SPERM MICROINJECTION, especially IN TRACYTOPLASMIC SPERM INSERTION. *See also* TES TICULAR SPERM EXTRACTION.

**microsurgery**   literally, operating on tissue under the magnification provided by an oper ating microscope; the magnification is typi cally in the range of 6x to 16x for infertilit surgery. The term also implies keeping the tis sues wet with physiological salt solution dur ing the operation; using fine, nonreactiv stitches or sutures; being meticulous abou stopping bleeding from small blood vessel straightaway; and avoiding trauma to th SEROSA. *See also* FIMBRIOLYSIS; MICROEPIDIDYMA SPERM ASPIRATION; SALPINGOLYSIS; SALPINGOS TOMY; STERILIZATION-REVERSAL (which include TUBAL ANASTOMOSIS and VASOVASOSTOMY).

**minilaparoscope**   an instrument for carrying out LAPAROSCOPY that is just a few millimeter in diameter, making it possible to perform such operations in an ambulatory setting without general anesthesia. The reliability of diagnoses made this way will need careful evaluation, especially if done to exclude ENDO-METRIOSIS, which can be difficult to find even with conventional laparoscopy.

**miscarriage** the loss of or the process of losing a pregnancy before the FETUS is viable. *See also* COMPLETE MISCARRIAGE; INCOMPLETE MISCARRIAGE; INEVITABLE MISCARRIAGE; MENSTRUAL MISCARRIAGE; MISSED ABORTION; RECURRENT MISCARRIAGES; SUBCLINICAL MISCARRIAGE; THREATENED MISCARRIAGE.

**missed abortion** a MISCARRIAGE that should have happened but did not; as a result, the pregnancy tissue in the uterus gets tougher and more difficult to remove with a uterine CURETTAGE, which is the only treatment for it. The PREGNANCY TEST may stay positive for many weeks or even months.

**missed miscarriage** *see* MISSED ABORTION

**mitochondrion (mitochondria)** a tiny structure resembling a bacterium and responsible for burning carbohydrates with oxygen to produce carbon dioxide and providing energy for the cell's use; each cell has hundreds or thousands of mitochondria. If there is a single aspect of a cell that reveals the process of aging, it is the mitochondria, which get less efficient as a person (and specifically a tissue) gets older. Mitochondrial aging in egg cells might be a reason (abnormal CHROMOSOMES is another) why eggs in women over the age of 40 so often are unable to produce healthy embryos. *See also* MTDNA.

**mitosis (mitoses)** usual process by which a cell (more strictly the NUCLEUS of a cell) divides into two; each CHROMOSOME duplicates before the beginning of mitosis, and mitosis involves separation of the resulting duplicates so that one goes into each daughter nucleus. At the third of four stages of mitosis, called METAPHASE, the chromosomes are easily distinguished with a microscope and can be photographed to construct a KARYOTYPE. *See also* MEIOSIS.

**mixed reproductive loss** repeated loss of pregnancies at different stages of development of the EMBRYO or FETUS, that is, at different stages of pregnancy.

**monoamniotic twins** identical or MONOZYGOTIC TWINS in which the split has occurred after formation of the BLASTOCYST, so that the twins share the same GESTATIONAL SAC (or amniotic cavity); there is a higher risk of complications than in the more usual situation where the twins do not share the same sac.

**monosomy** an abnormality of the CHROMOSOME complement due to a loss of one chromosome from a DIPLOID set, resulting in 45 chromosomes instead of 46. The only monosomy compatible with fetal development and continued survival is that of TURNER'S SYNDROME, the KARYOTYPE of which is 45,X (a monosomy of the SEX CHROMOSOMES).

**monozygotic twins** twins formed from the splitting of a single fertilized egg, or ZYGOTE; identical twins. *See also* MONOAMNIOTIC TWINS.

**monthly fecundity** term for the monthly chance of getting pregnant. *See also* FECUNDABILITY.

**monthly fertility** another term for the monthly chance of getting pregnant, the technical term for which is FECUNDABILITY. *See also* NORMAL MONTHLY FERTILITY.

**morula** a stage of the EMBRYO or PRE-EMBRYO that consists of a ball of cells, still enclosed by the ZONA PELLUCIDA, before the next stage of BLASTOCYST; formed from the fertilized egg, or ZYGOTE, by the process of CLEAVAGE.

**motility** the quality of movement, especially forward propulsion, shown by sperm cells and caused by effective beating of their tail, or flagellum; analyzed as part of the routine SPERM COUNT.

**MRI scan** magnetic resonance imaging is a special form of imaging the body's internal structures, taken with the person enveloped in a huge and powerful magnet; a picture is built up of any cross-section or series of cross-sections through the body, using a technique that detects and pictures structures by their different content of atoms with certain resonances to induced magnetic fields. Particularly useful for investigation of the anatomy of the PITUITARY GLAND and HYPOTHALAMUS when a tumor is suspected. More expensive and less widely available than a CAT SCAN, which gives adequate results in most cases.

**mtDNA (mitochondrial DNA)** the small amount of DNA found in the MITOCHONDRIA. mtDNA carries the genetic code for 13 genes involved in metabolism. Because mtDNA is much less stable than the DNA in the CHROMOSOMES (where the huge bulk of genetic code is stored), mutations accumulate with time at a greater rate than that for chromosomal DNA and eventually limit how well a particular cell or tissue can function with increasing age. Because all of the mtDNA you have you inherited from your mother (you derive all your mitochondria from the egg you came from), we might have explanations for why all

eggs are formed before birth (so the mitochondria do not have to keep on dividing too often and risking genetic errors) and why miscarriages and infertility become more common with age (as the egg's several thousand mitochondria begin to succumb to genetic errors).

**mucus** jelly-like secretion that is at once both sticky and slippery. *See also* CERVICAL MUCUS CUMULUS MASS.

**Müllerian duct** also called the "paramesonephric duct," the internal female sex duct, which forms on each side of a female embryo to connect the PERITONEAL CAVITY with the outside of the embryo, starting at a point close to the ovary and forming first a FALLOPIAN TUBE, then meeting its fellow from the other side to form the UTERUS, and then extending downward to form the upper part of the vagina before finally connecting with a little dimple between the urethra (in front) and the anus (behind) to reach the exterior at the vulva. Passage of eggs from the ovaries (which ovulate into the peritoneal cavity of all vertebrate species) to the outside world through this duct is how animals, including humans, reproduce. Oddities in the development of the ducts cause CONGENITAL ANOMALIES of any or all of these organs. In males the ducts do not develop because the SERTOLI CELLS of the TESTES produce ANTI-MÜLLERIAN HORMONE. *See also* MESONEPHRIC DUCT.

**Müllerian inhibiting factor** *see* ANTI-MÜLLERIAN HORMONE

**myoma** *see* FIBROID

**myomectomy** an operation to remove a myoma, or FIBROID; a myomectomy for a SUBMU-

OUS FIBROID is often possible during a HYSTEROSCOPY; a myomectomy for an intramural fibroid (located within the wall of the uterus) usually requires an open operation, or LAPAROTOMY; a myomectomy for a SUBSEROUS FIBROID may be possible during LAPAROSCOPY.

**myometrium** the muscular wall of the UTERUS, surrounding the ENDOMETRIUM. *See also* ADENOMYOSIS; FIBROID.

**nafarelin** a GnRH-AGONIST manufactured by Syntex as Synarel and administered as a nasal spray.

**naturalistic fallacy** the term coined by philosopher G. E. Moore early in the twentieth century to devalue drawing ethical conclusions from EMPIRICAL observation, that is, by moving from what *is* (facts that are observed) to what *ought* (morality). Moore felt that ethics should be intuitive, not inferred, therefore presumably DEONTOLOGICAL rather than TELEOLOGICAL. Practical ethicists find this constraint unnaturally crippling as it prevents them making a VALUE JUDGMENT.

**negative history** for a disease or symptom, means that you do not have or have not had that disease or symptom.

**negative test** In medicine generally it is usually best for tests to be negative (like tests for brain tumors or tests for sexually transmitted diseases such as HIV), but this is not always so in INFERTILITY. Infertility tests are generally better if they are positive, like the POSTCOITAL TEST, tests for OVULATION, TESTS FOR TUBAL PATENCY, and (not least) a PREGNANCY TEST. *See also* NEGATIVE HISTORY.

**NET** *see* NORETHYNODREL

**neurohypophysis** the neural (nerve-containing tissue) part of the PITUITARY GLAND, lying toward the back (the POSTERIOR PITUITARY); produces the neurohormones oxytocin, which causes contraction of the uterus, and vasopressin, which helps maintain blood pressure and conserves the body's water in the kidneys.

**NOA** *see* NONOBSTRUCTIVE AZOOSPERMIA

**nonmaleficence** the ethical principle that comes from not doing harm. *See also* BENEFICENCE; SUFFERING.

**nonobstructive azoospermia** (NOA) AZOOSPERMIA caused by low sperm production rates in the TESTIS, including maturation arrest; can often be overcome with TESTICULAR SPERM EXTRACTION followed by IN VITRO FERTILIZATION utilizing INTRACYTOPLASMIC SPERM INSERTION (ICSI).

**norethisterone** name for norethynodrel in Europe and Australia.

**norethynodrel** (NET) a PROGESTOGEN of a type weakly related to the male hormone TESTOSTERONE. Progestogens of this class are commonly found in the birth control pill. Norethynodrel acetate is marketed as Primolut N and is manufactured by Schering.

**normal monthly fertility** nature gives fertility a wide range, normally from about 7 to 45 percent per month for women in the early twenties, to about 3 to 25 percent per month for women in the early thirties; for women in the early forties, it ranges from less than 1 to about 5 percent per month. *See also* MONTHLY FERTILITY.

**NSAIDs** nonsteroidal antiinflammatory drugs, for example, aspirin, mefenamic acid

(Ponstel), naproxyn sodium (Naprosyn, or in Naprogesic in combination with dextropropoxyphene), which stop the production of PROSTAGLANDINS; useful for DYSMENORRHEA and prior to a HYSTEROSALPINGOGRAM.

**nucleus** structure within a cell that contains the CHROMOSOMES. The nonnuclear part of the cell is called the CYTOPLASM, which thus contains other cellular structures, including the MITOCHONDRIA. Genetic inheritance is mostly by way of the nucleus (with a contribution from mother and father); a small part is by way of the cytoplasm (with a contribution only from the mother). *See also* MTDNA.

**obligation** a moral compulsion for ethical action, sometimes usefully distinguished from a DUTY by its derivation from example or external enforcement; according to this distinction, obligations are derived chiefly from the considerations of TELEOLOGICAL ETHICS and UTILITARIAN ETHICS.

**OHSS** *see* OVARIAN HYPERSTIMULATION SYNDROME

**oligomenorrhea** infrequent menstrual periods; by convention, a menstrual cycle that is consistently longer than 35 days. Oligomenorrhea always reflects irregularity of hormonal events coming from the ovaries.

**oligospermia** strictly, "oligozoospermia," meaning a reduced number of sperm cells in the ejaculate (compared with AZOOSPERMIA, which means no sperm in the ejaculate); more generally, a decrease in normal, motile sperm, and more or less encompassing laborious terms such as "asthenozoospermia" (weak motility) and "teratozoospermia" (abnormal sperm), and even more laborious ones, such

as "oligoasthenoteratozoospermia," which d◦ not reward the effort of concocting them.

**oligozoospermia** *see* OLIGOSPERMIA

**oocyte** the form of the ovum, or egg, whic◦ is undergoing a halving of the number o◦ CHROMOSOMES through the process of MEIOSIS *See also* PRIMARY OOCYTE; SECONDARY OOCYTE.

**oogenesis** the multiplication by the proces◦ of MITOSIS of OVA, or eggs, in the ovaries of th◦ fetus.

**oogonium (oogonia)** the earliest recogniz◦ able form of the OVUM, or egg; present only i◦ the ovaries of fetuses; multiplies by th◦ process of MITOSIS before developing int◦ OOCYTES by the process of MEIOSIS; the mal◦ equivalent (the SPERMATOGONIUM) normally persists in the testicles until old age.

**oophorectomy** *see* OVARIECTOMY

**OPU (ovum pickup)** *see* FOLLICLE ASPIRATION

**orchidopexy** an operation to move an un◦ descended TESTIS down into the scrotum, so that it has more chance of developing normally and producing sperm cells. *See also* CRYPTORCHIDISM.

**osteoporosis** an abnormal condition of the bones, which are weakened by a loss of calcium. It is the loss of estrogen, such as after MENOPAUSE or after PRIMARY OVARIAN FAILURE (premature menopause), that eventually causes osteoporosis, with a tendency to bone fractures, especially of the wrist, thigh and backbone.

**ovarian cycle** the ordered sequence of timely development of TERTIARY FOLLICLES to maturity of a dominant follicle (the FOLLICULAR PHASE, characterized by increasing production of the estrogen, ESTRADIOL), through OVULA-

ON (when estradiol falls and PROGESTERONE arts to rise), followed by the development of e CORPUS LUTEUM and with the further pro- iction of progesterone, which then decline. ecause estradiol and progesterone control e growth and development of the EN- OMETRIUM in the uterus, the ovarian cycle etermines the MENSTRUAL CYCLE (normally sting from 24 to 35 days in length, and with typical duration of about 28 days) and also e cycle of the normal female HYPOTHALAMUS nd PITUITARY GLAND.

varian hyperstimulation syndrome (OHSS) complication of OVULATION INDUCTION with, sually, FOLLICLE STIMULATING HORMONE, espe- ially in cycles of SUPEROVULATION for ASSISTED ONCEPTION when more than one egg is to be btained. The ovaries become too large, they an be painful and there is excessive fluid re- eased into the abdomen (the PERITONEAL CAV- TY); either the production of this fluid or the ccurrence of vomiting can cause dehydra- ion, thickening of the blood and, occasion- lly, a serious thrombosis, such as a stroke; here have been deaths. Moderate to severe OHSS is treated in a hospital, with adminis- ration of fluid intravenously, sometimes in- luding albumin.

varian pregnancy an ECTOPIC PREGNANCY lo- ated within the OVARY, presumably because an gg has been fertilized while still in a FOLLICLE.

variectomy surgical removal of the OVARY. f the other ovary remains, OVULATION and MENSTRUAL CYCLES usually continue as before; also called "oophorectomy."

ovary the female organ that produces eggs; located on each side of the UTERUS.

oviduct another name for FALLOPIAN TUBE.

ovulation natural process by which a mature FOLLICLE opens to release the SECONDARY OOCYTE, or egg, enclosed in a sticky blob of mucus-like material, the CUMULUS MASS. See also HUMAN CHORIONIC GONADOTROPIN; LH SURGE: LUTEINIZING HORMONE.

ovulation induction the use of drugs to stimulate FOLLICLES in the OVARIES to undergo OVULATION, such as CLOMIPHENE, various prep- arations containing FOLLICLE STIMULATING HORMONE (FSH) and HUMAN CHORIONIC GO- NADOTROPIN (HCG). The two main situations for it are in the treatment of INFERTILITY due to ANOVULATION (typically when there is OLIGO- MENORRHEA or AMENORRHEA), and for SUPER- OVULATION in ASSISTED CONCEPTION (for ex- ample, IN VITRO FERTILIZATION and GAMETE INTRAFALLOPIAN TRANSFER). See also OVARIAN HYPERSTIMULATION SYNDROME.

ovulatory dysfunctional uterine bleeding heavy but generally regular bleeding caused either by pathology in the uterus, such as FIBROIDS, or by a generalized bleeding disor- der, such as thrombocytopenia (a low platelet count), von Willebrand's disease (may run in families) or treatment with anti- coagulant drugs. Often used synonymously with MENORRHAGIA.

ovum (ova) the female sex cell, or egg, from the earliest stage (the OOGONIUM in the fetus), through its release from the FOLLICLE (OVULA- TION) as an OOCYTE, and (to professional em- bryologists) through FERTILIZATION up to and sometimes beyond the stage of IMPLANTATION. See also BLIGHTED OVUM.

ovum pickup (OPU) see FOLLICLE ASPIRATION

Parlodel see BROMOCRIPTINE

**parthenogenesis** can occur when an egg is activated (by itself with some nonspecific stimulus or through fertilization by a sperm) and starts to divide (CLEAVAGE), but the male CHROMOSOMES are not incorporated and the egg remains HAPLOID; its further development will soon stop, probably well before IMPLANTATION.

**paternalism** a method of medical or administrative practice in which the values of the practitioner or administrator are imposed upon the person most affected by the decisions to be made, without adequately heeding that person's own values or power to make decisions that will directly affect them.

**PCB** *see* POSTCOITAL BLEEDING

**PCO** *see* POLYCYSTIC OVARIES

**PCOD (polycystic ovary disease)** *see* POLYCYSTIC OVARY SYNDROME

**PCOS** *see* POLYCYSTIC OVARY SYNDROME

**PCR** *see* POLYMERASE CHAIN REACTION

**PCT** *see* POSTCOITAL TEST

**Pergonal** mixture of HUMAN MENOPAUSAL GONADOTROPINS containing FOLLICLE STIMULATING HORMONE and manufactured by Serono; virtually equivalent to HUMEGON.

**peritoneal adhesions** *see* ADHESIONS

**peritoneal cavity** the general abdominal cavity in which lie the stomach, the intestines and the UTERUS, OVARIES and FALLOPIAN TUBES, each covered by a thin, moist, slippery surface layer, the peritoneal SEROSA, or PERITONEUM. An examination of the peritoneal cavity is called a LAPAROSCOPY. *See also* ADHESIONS.

**peritoneal serosa** the SEROSA of the PERITONEAL CAVITY.

**peritoneum** the smooth, moist lining of t[...] PERITONEAL CAVITY that forms the SEROSA of t[...] organs this cavity contains. For purists, su[...] serosa is "visceral" peritoneum, and the pa[...] of the peritoneum covering the wall of the a[...] dominal cavity away from organs is the "par[...] etal" peritoneum.

**peritubal adhesions** ADHESIONS around t[...] FALLOPIAN TUBE.

**perivitelline space** the space between the eg[...] (the vitellus) and the ZONA PELLUCIDA; sper[...] are injected into this space with SUBZONAL IN[...] SERTION, or SUZI.

**pituitary gland** gland located at the base [...] the brain and responsible for driving th[...] ovaries by way of the pituitary hormones FOL[...] LICLE STIMULATING HORMONE (FSH) an[...] LUTEINIZING HORMONE (LH), which are und[...] the influence of GONADOTROPIN-RELEASIN[...] HORMONE from the HYPOTHALAMUS. Com[...] posed of two parts, the ADENOHYPOPHYSIS, o[...] truly glandular part, in front, and the NEURO[...] HYPOPHYSIS, which is a down-growth of th[...] brain, behind.

**placenta** that part of the products of CONCEP[...] TION apart from the FETUS composed of TRO[...] PHOBLAST. Together with the membranes an[...] the umbilical cord composes the afterbirth.

**plasma glucose** a measurement of suga[...] (glucose) in the blood plasma to detect dia[...] betes, an occasional cause of RECURRENT MIS[...] CARRIAGE; usually checked a few hours after [...] meal or, more formally, with a "glucose toler[...] ance test" that involves a standard drink o[...] glucose (after prior fasting) followed by seria[...] measurements of plasma glucose over thre[...] hours.

**MS** either PREMENSTRUAL SPOTTING or PREMENSTRUAL SYNDROME (see premenstrual tension).

**MSP** *see* PREMENSTRUAL SPOTTING

**MT** *see* PREMENSTRUAL TENSION

**polar body** a tiny, compact packet of excess CHROMOSOMES discarded first by the PRIMARY OOCYTE as it becomes a SECONDARY OOCYTE just before OVULATION (the first polar body, with 6 chromosomes); and second by the secondary oocyte immediately after it is fertilized or otherwise activated (the second polar body, with 23 chromosomes). *See also* MEIOSIS.

**polycystic ovaries** (PCO) in full, "micropolycystic ovaries"; a diagnosis made on TRANSVAGINAL ULTRASOUND, with lots of medium-sized follicles visible around the rim of the ovaries; can be part of the POLYCYSTIC OVARY SYNDROME (the "cysts" are not real cysts and do not themselves need treatment).

**polycystic ovary syndrome** (PCOS) or **disease** (PCOD) POLYCYSTIC OVARIES associated with any clinical symptom or sign of too much male hormone effect: long or absent cycles (OLIGOMENORRHEA or AMENORRHEA), acne or excess body hair (HIRSUTISM).

**polymerase chain reaction** (PCR) a method of amplifying a single piece of DNA (the stuff of GENES) to get enough of it to analyze physically or chemically. A machine is used that employs alternate cycles of *high* temperature to separate DNA's two strands and *medium* temperature to combine each of the two single strands with free nucleic acids to make new complementary strands, thus doubling the amount of DNA in the machine's soup each cycle. A few hours in the machine automatically creates millions of identical DNA molecules from just one specimen. Needless to say, it is extremely important that you start with the right bit of DNA, so you are not inadvertently amplifying a bit of contamination. In the film *Jurassic Park*, PCR was used to amplify bits of dinosaur DNA recovered from the bellies of contemporary insects, which had been trapped and preserved for millions of years inside pieces of amber. A biopsy of a single cell from an embryo after IVF can, with PCR, produce enough DNA to test it for certain genes that cause serious genetic disease. *See also* PREIMPLANTATIONAL DIAGNOSIS.

**polyp** a benign growth of tissue, usually of the lining of a hollow organ such as the intestine or the uterus. The presence of a polyp of the CERVIX (cervical polyp) increases the chance that there is a polyp of the endometrium (*see* ENDOMETRIAL POLYP).

**polyploid, polyploidy** a multiple of the HAPLOID number of CHROMOSOMES in a cell other than the normal DIPLOID state. Includes TRIPLOID (three times the haploid number, or 69 chromosomes) and tetraploid (four times the haploid number, or 92 chromosomes).

**polyspermic fertilization** *see* POLYSPERMY

**polyspermy** or polyspermic fertilization; fertilization of an egg (a SECONDARY OOCYTE) by more than one sperm. In IN VITRO FERTILIZATION, more common if eggs are recovered that are either immature or overly mature; evident later, with the appearance of more than two PRONUCLEI. In natural conditions, a cause of a POLYPLOID state in the embryo. *See also* TRIPLOID.

**positive history** for a disease or symptom means that you have or have had that disease or symptom.

**positive test** In medicine, generally it is usually best for tests to be negative (like tests for brain tumors or tests for sexually transmitted diseases, such as HIV), but not so for infertility. Infertility tests, such as the POSTCOITAL TEST, tests for OVULATION, TESTS FOR TUBAL PATENCY, and (not least) a PREGNANCY TEST, are better if they are positive. *See also* POSITIVE HISTORY.

**postcoital bleeding** (PCB) bleeding after sex; typically the result of abrasion of the CERVIX (which might be abnormal and you should have a checkup and a PAP smear) or of trauma to the vagina; sometimes due to a CERVICAL POLYP.

**postcoital contraception** using a contraceptive after intercourse instead of before intercourse to interrupt implantation of the embryo. Taking two birth control pills the morning and the night after the unanticipated opportunity for pregnancy is reasonably effective, but see your doctor for details to carry this out safely.

**postcoital test** (PCT) a test of receptiveness of the CERVICAL MUCUS to sperm and sperm MOTILITY, both of which are needed for the test to be POSITIVE; it is essential that the test be done to coincide with OVULATION, tested with a URINARY LH-KIT or measurements of SERUM ESTRADIOL (high), SERUM LH (preferably high) and SERUM PROGESTERONE (still low), because the job description of the cervical mucus at other times is to be impenetrable to sperm, that is, the PCT will be negative for normal reasons.

**postimplantational embryopathy** an abnormality of the EMBRYO (or FETUS) that arises after the embryo implants in the ENDOMETRIUM, the lining of the uterus; might, sooner or late cause a MISCARRIAGE or birth abnormality.

**predecidual reaction** a partial confluence of STROMAL CELLS of the ENDOMETRIUM (lying between the endometrial glands), caused by prolonged exposure (10 days or more) to PROGESTERONE or a PROGESTOGEN. *See also* DECIDUA REACTION.

**pre-embryo** the EMBRYO or OVUM from the stage of fertilized egg up to the stage of IMPLANTATION. During this time any of the cell of the fertilized ovum can develop into whole new embryo—they are "totipotent."

**pre-embryo biopsy** a BIOPSY, or removal of one or two cells, from a PRE-EMBRYO (typically at the stage of eight cells) for PREIMPLANTATIONAL DIAGNOSIS.

**pregnancy rate** the percentage of months or treatment cycles that result in clinical pregnancy, excluding BIOCHEMICAL PREGNANCIES but including ECTOPIC PREGNANCIES, MISCARRIAGES and all potentially viable pregnancies (twins are not counted twice; stillbirths and all live births are included); less important for most patients' purposes than the TAKE-HOME-BABY RATE.

**pregnancy test** nowadays a measurement of HUMAN CHORIONIC GONADOTROPIN in SERUM or urine, usually as a simple yes-or-no test. In principle it cannot distinguish a normal pregnancy from an ECTOPIC PREGNANCY or one destined to miscarry (a MISCARRIAGE). *See also* SERUM HCG.

**Pregnyl** HUMAN CHORIONIC GONADOTROPIN (HCG) manufactured by Organon.

**preimplantational diagnosis** genetic diagnosis of an IN VITRO FERTILIZATION embryo (or,

tually, PRE-EMBRYO) before transfer, made
ossible by removing one or two cells of the
mbryo (PRE-EMBRYO BIOPSY). *See also* FLUO-
SCENT IN SITU HYBRIDIZATION (FISH); POLY-
RASE CHAIN REACTION (PCR).

**eimplantational embryopathy** an abnor-
ality of the EMBRYO or fetus that arises before
e embryo (really the PRE-EMBRYO) implants
the ENDOMETRIUM, the lining of the uterus.
ually causes MISCARRIAGE.

**emarin** a mixture of ESTROGENS in tablet
rm (from Ayerst Laboratories) with the
putation of being "natural," although in re-
ity extracted from the serum of pregnant
ares (horses); the main estrogen it contains
ESTRONE.

**remature labor** the onset of labor, leading
delivery, before 37 weeks have elapsed since
e last menstrual period; the more prema-
urely babies are born, the greater the diffi-
ulty that they have surviving, even with ex-
ert care.

**remature menopause** menopause before
e age of 40. *See also* PRIMARY OVARIAN FAILURE.

**remenstrual biopsy** *see* PREMENSTRUAL EN-
OMETRIAL BIOPSY

**remenstrual endometrial biopsy** a small
ample (or BIOPSY) is taken of the lining of the
terus (the ENDOMETRIUM) just before a pe-
iod is expected, aiming to show advanced
tages of PROGESTERONE's effect on it, in the
orm of an adequate PREDECIDUAL REACTION; a
ery sensitive test of the adequacy of the
UTEAL PHASE; can be combined with a LAP-
ROSCOPY or carried out in isolation as an of-
ice procedure; it is best to be sure that there is
o possibility of pregnancy during the cycle

the test is conducted, as occasionally the
biopsy jeopardizes a pregnancy.

**premenstrual spotting** (PMSP) also called
"premenstrual staining," a form of light intermenstrual bleeding consistently timed over a
few days to a week before the period starts
properly, although it may not happen every
month; about 80 percent of the time it signals
the presence of ENDOMETRIOSIS; about 10 percent of the time it means an abnormality of
the uterus such as FIBROIDS, an ENDOMETRIAL
POLYP or ENDOMETRITIS; the remaining 10 percent of the time there is no explanation found;
it has nothing to do with PREMENSTRUAL TEN-
SION, which if present is a coincidence.

**premenstrual syndrome** (PMS) *see* PREMEN-
STRUAL TENSION

**premenstrual tension** (PMT) a distressing
group of symptoms usually timed for the lead
up to a period, then relieved as menstruation
takes place, although many women experience
different timing; includes downheartedness or
depression (certainly an absence of well-being), aggression, fluid retention and weight
gain, painful breasts (mastalgia), headaches
and pain in the pelvis; caused by a periodic
fall in the brain's ENDORPHINS, in turn usually
precipitated by falling levels of PROGESTERONE
in the second half of the LUTEAL PHASE, although similar symptoms often accompany
the use of PROGESTOGENS, especially in older
women; can be better during SUPEROVULATION
cycles because of generally higher hormone
levels, but this is not always the case and PMT
at the end of an unsuccessful cycle of ASSISTED
CONCEPTION is particularly hard to put up
with. Usually treated (up to a point) sympto-
matically, perhaps with fluid tablets (diuret-
ics) and analgesics, although it is claimed that

the drug Prozac has a specifically beneficial effect on mood, and encouragement of endorphin release with exercise can also be useful. Because progesterone and progestogens are the culprits, an operation to remove the ovaries (plus HYSTERECTOMY to simplify ESTROGEN REPLACEMENT THERAPY without needing PROGESTOGENS) is usually curative, but drastic.

**primary amenorrhea**   AMENORRHEA when a woman has never had a spontaneous menstrual period, that is, a period not brought on by hormone treatment.

**primary follicle**   the first stage of growth or further development of the FOLLICLE, in which the egg is enclosed by a single layer of round-shaped follicle cells, which are multiplying.

**primary oocyte**   the form of the OVUM, or egg, produced in the ovaries of fetuses by OOGONIA that have begun the first part of the cell division known as MEIOSIS, by which the CHROMOSOMES will eventually halve in number; persists into childhood and adult life by containment in FOLLICLES; gives rise to a SECONDARY OOCYTE and the first POLAR BODY just before OVULATION. *See also* IN VITRO MATURATION.

**primary ovarian failure**   failure of the ovaries to produce enough FOLLICLES because of a problem in the ovary itself; and resulting in DEPLETION OF EGGS before the age of 40 (known as PREMATURE MENOPAUSE, a cause of SECONDARY AMENORRHEA), or perhaps even before the age puberty is expected (causing failure of puberty to happen, including PRIMARY AMENORRHEA). Sometimes occurs despite good numbers of PRIMORDIAL FOLLICLES that (inexplicably, so far) will not develop (the "resistant ovary" syndrome). The younger the woman, the more likely that an ANEUPLOIDY will be found if a

KARYOTYPE is done on blood or on a biopsy the ovary. ESTROGEN REPLACEMENT THERAPY prevent osteoporosis is very important.

**primary spermatocyte**   the form of t sperm cell at the first stage of SPERMATOGEN SIS, by which SPERMATOGONIA enter MEIOSIS start to reduce the number of CHROMOSOM for the more mature sperm cells that w eventuate.

**Primolut N**   NORETHYNODREL acetate (Unit States) or NORETHISTERONE acetate (Europ Australia) manufactured by Schering.

**primordial follicle**   the resting, unstimulat stage of the FOLLICLE, in which the egg is e closed by just a few thinly stretched FOLLIC CELLS. Primordial follicles persist in the ova from fetal life to the time of MENOPAUSE, d clining in number every day during this tim as some start to develop into PRIMARY FOLL CLES, most of which then are lost through th process of FOLLICULAR ATRESIA. What the stim ulus or signal is for primordial follicles to sta growing remains completely unknown.

**Profasi**   HUMAN CHORIONIC GONADOTROPI (HCG) manufactured by Serono.

**professionalism**   for this book, the practi of maximizing the involvement of a client c patient seeking the service of a professional i making decisions that will directly affe them.

**progesterone**   the ovary's second main hor mone, produced only after OVULATION an during pregnancy (first by the CORPUS LU TEUM, then by the PLACENTA); sometimes ad ministered by injection or by intravaginal pes sary to supplement natural production; se also ESTROGEN and PROGESTOGEN.

## The Fishy Side of Prolactin

Prolactin is an old hormone in the animal kingdom. It has had many and varied roles. In fish it is important in regulating water entering and leaving the tissues. In mammals, including women, prolactin is well known is well known as stimulating milk production, but prolactin produced by **decidual cells** in the **endometrium** during pregnancy seems to be important in regulating the passage of water into the **gestational sac**, a function that seems to have been inherited down the millions of years since our ancestors were fish.

---

**progestin** *see* PROGESTOGEN

**progestogen** a PROGESTERONE-like substance, usually more active when given by mouth than natural progesterone; used with an ESTROGEN in the birth control pill. Commonly used examples have a structure like progesterone itself (for example, MEDROXYPROGESTERONE ACETATE, or Provera; CYPROTERONE ACETATE, or Androcur) or have a structure distantly related to the male hormone testosterone (NORETHYNODREL and norethisterone, or Primolut N; norgestrel).

**prolactin** hormone produced by the PITUITARY GLAND to stimulate milk production in the breasts; produced in increasing amount during pregnancy, although milk secretion is postponed until levels of ESTROGEN and PROGESTERONE fall after the baby has been born.

**proliferative phase** the phase of development of the ENDOMETRIUM during which, after the MENSTRUAL PHASE, the endometrium grows to regain thickness under the influence of ESTRADIOL; therefore it corresponds in time with the FOLLICULAR PHASE in the ovary.

**pronuclear-stage transfer** (PROST) a form of ASSISTED CONCEPTION in which IN VITRO FERTILIZATION (IVF) is used to produce fertilization of one or more recovered eggs; useful if the potential fertilizing ability of sperm is in doubt; transfer is made on the day after egg pickup and IVF, before the fertilized egg divides (it is at the "pronuclear" stage); the transfer is made to the FALLOPIAN TUBE to obtain advantages similar to GAMETE INTRAFALLOPIAN TRANSFER (GIFT) and is made possible by LAPAROSCOPY (with anesthesia) or by TRANSVAGINAL ULTRASOUND (without anesthesia); synonymous with ZYGOTE INTRAFALLOPIAN TRANSFER (ZIFT). *See also* PRONUCLEUS.

**pronucleus (pronuclei)** a visible blob (or vacuole), usually two of them, inside a fertilized or otherwise activated egg and enclosing the CHROMOSOMES from the egg (the female pronucleus) and from the sperm (the male pronucleus); if three pronuclei are observed, the chances are that two sperms have entered the egg (POLYSPERMY).

**PROST** *see* PRONUCLEAR-STAGE TRANSFER

**prostaglandins** substances, first isolated from the PROSTATE GLAND's contribution to SEMEN, now known to be universally present throughout the body, being especially produced during inflammation (when they cause pain). Drugs that stop prostaglandins being produced are used as analgesics (so-called NONSTEROIDAL ANTI-INFLAMMATORY DRUGS or NSAIDs, which are useful also in minimizing contractions of the uterus in DYSMENORRHEA and PREMATURE LABOR.

**prostate gland**　the male sex gland located just below the bladder, in front of the rectum, through which the urethra runs; it contributes secretions to the SEMEN.

**Provera**　MEDROXYPROGESTERONE ACETATE, a PROGESTOGEN manufactured by Upjohn.

**pseudohermaphroditism**　synonymous with INTERSEX, except that intersex also includes TRUE HERMAPHRODISM.

**Puregon**　RECOMBINANT FOLLICLE STIMULATING HORMONE (*r*FSH) manufactured by Organon.

**pyosalpinx**　a fallopian tube obstructed at its outer end and containing pus as a result of ACUTE SALPINGITIS.

**qualitative**　something you cannot put a number on to give it its meaning or value, such as SUFFERING. *See also* HAZARD; QUANTITATIVE.

**quantitative**　something you can give meaning or value to by giving it a number, such as PREGNANCY RATE. *See also* QUALITATIVE; RISK.

**recessive inheritance**　pattern of inheritance of a characteristic (such as blue eye color) or abnormality (such as CONGENITAL ABSENCE of the VAS DEFERENS) in which two GENES or ALLELES are needed to confer the characteristic or abnormality, in contrast to DOMINANT INHERITANCE, which requires just one such gene. In the case of alleles found on X chromosomes but not on the smaller Y chromosomes, a recessive gene will be unopposed (and so will act as a

dominant gene) in males, whereas female carriers of an abnormal allele will be unaffected except in the extremely unlikely event that the inherit (or gain by mutation) a second abnormal allele; this mode of inheritance is called "sex-linked recessive inheritance" and an example is hemophilia. *See also* HOMOZYGOUS.

**recombinant follicle stimulating hormone** (*r*FSH)　FOLLICLE STIMULATING HORMONE derived from genetic engineering instead of being extracted from the urine of postmenopausal women (HUMAN MENOPAUSAL GONADOTROPIN or hMG) or from the PITUITARY GLANDS of cadavers (HUMAN PITUITARY GONADOTROPIN, or hPG). Being marketed by the two pharmaceutical companies Organon (as PUREGON) and Serono (as GONAL F) to eventually replace their hMG preparations. Has the advantage over hMG (and its purified derivatives) of being standard in biological structure and activity and not being of a human source (hPG having been implicated in transmission of Creuzfeldt Jakob disease). Shares with FORTINEX (METRODIN HP outside the U.S.) a complete absence of LUTEINIZING HORMONE (LH), which means that SERUM ESTRADIOL levels are lower in some stimulated cycles for OVULATION INDUCTION and ASSISTED CONCEPTION, especially with "ultra short" regimens of GnRH-ANALOGS.

**recombinant human follicle stimulating hormone** (*rh*FSH)　*see* RECOMBINANT FOLLICLE STIMULATING HORMONE

**rectum**　connects the large BOWEL (the colon to the anus; lies behind the vagina in women

**recurrent miscarriages**　a series of three or more consecutive MISCARRIAGES.

**relative infertility**　synonymous with "subfertilty"; INFERTILITY that is not ABSOLUTE or

COMPLETE INFERTILITY (*see also* STERILITY, as these three terms are synonyms), but nevertheless there is a reduced chance of getting pregnant each month. More or less definite causes can include OLIGOSPERMIA, POLYCYSTIC OVARY SYNDROME (and other causes of OLIGOMENORRHEA), ENDOMETRIOSIS, PERITUBAL ADHESIONS, FIBROIDS (especially SUBMUCOUS FIBROIDS) and increased age, especially of the woman. *See also* CUMULATIVE CHANCE OF PREGNANCY; MONTHLY FERTILITY.

**relative risk** the chance of having something or being affected by something compared with other people in a comparable situation. Can be given as a ratio, proportion or percentage (as in the chance of having ENDOMETRIOSIS: if your sister has it, you have a relative risk of 7:1, or seven times the risk as compared with the general population of women of the same age; your relative risk of developing cancer of the ovaries if you have accumulated 10 years on the oral contraceptive pill is 1:5, 0.2 or 20 percent). *See also* ABSOLUTE RISK.

**resistant ovary syndrome** *see* PRIMARY OVARIAN FAILURE

**rete testis** tiny ducts (about 20 in number) connecting the tubules of the TESTIS with the EPIDIDYMIS.

**retrograde ejaculation** ejaculation in which SEMEN, instead of spurting out from the penis during male orgasm, spills upward into the bladder; usually has a medically important cause, which requires investigation. Treatment can be successful by isolating sperm from the urine and carrying out some form of ASSISTED CONCEPTION, such as ASSISTED INSEMINATION or IN VITRO FERTILIZATION.

**retroverted uterus** a UTERUS that lies more toward the back than the front. Retroversion of the uterus can be normal and, of itself, this is not a cause of INFERTILITY; rarely it might repeatedly get in the way during sex and cause pain (DYSPAREUNIA), in which case there are operations available to bring it forward, out of the way. Retroversion can also develop from scarring caused by ENDOMETRIOSIS, in which case there can be pain with sex and infertility (caused by the endometriosis).

*r*FSH *see* RECOMBINANT FOLLICLE STIMULATING HORMONE

*rh*FSH *see* RECOMBINANT HUMAN FOLLICLE STIMULATING HORMONE (*rh*FSH)

**right** the reciprocal, or other side, of a DUTY or OBLIGATION, often conferred by society on the basis of equity or consistency and matched either by intuitive duties or by conferred obligations.

**risk** chance, expressed as a ratio, proportion or percentage. If the word is unqualified, it usually means ABSOLUTE RISK (the actual risk in a group of the population), in contrast to RELATIVE RISK (which measures one person's risk compared with another person's). *See also* HAZARD.

**ROSI** *see* ROUND SPERMATID INJECTION

**ROSNI** *see* ROUND SPERMATID NUCLEAR INJECTION

**round spermatid injection** (ROSI) experimental form of TESTICULAR SPERM EXTRACTION (TESE) followed by INTRACYTOPLASMIC SPERM INSERTION (ICSI) in which a round (very immature) SPERMATID is isolated for injection into the egg. Seems to be less successful than a similar procedure in which the nucleus is isolated from the spermatid and used instead (ROUND SPERMATID NUCLEAR INJECTION).

**round spermatid nuclear injection** (ROSNI) experimental form of TESTICULAR SPERM EXTRACTION (TESE) followed by INTRACYTOPLASMIC SPERM INSERTION (ICSI) in which the NUCLEUS of a round (very immature) SPERMATID is isolated for injection into the egg. Intended to be used in treating nonobstructive AZOOSPERMIA with severe maturation arrest, when more mature sperm cells are not obtainable. Animal studies show higher pregnancy rates than with ROUND SPERMATID INJECTION, but limited studies in humans still indicate very high rates of EMBRYOPATHY.

*r*-selection   a reproductive strategy where survival of a species is optimized by explosive increases in numbers of animals whenever environmental circumstances are favorable; favors small animals that reach sexual maturity quickly, which reproduce just once but with many progeny and which do not need to tend to their progeny after birth. In extreme cases (seen in many lower animals such as insects), death of the father follows impregnation and death of the mother follows parturition (giving birth). The opposite reproductive strategy to *K*-SELECTION.

**Rubin's test**   *see* TESTS FOR TUBAL PATENCY

**rudimentary horn**   the small part of a BICORNUATE UTERUS in which one side is very small; with regard to the side that is bigger (*see* UNICORNUATE UTERUS), it may be "communicating" or "noncommunicating," depending on whether it has a cavity that joins the main ENDOMETRIAL CAVITY.

**salpingectomy**   surgical removal of the FALLOPIAN TUBE (the Latin for which is *salpinx*).

**salpingitis**   inflammation of the FALLOPIAN TUBES, usually due to infection; may be ACUTE (gonorrhea, CHLAMYDIA and other infection) or chronic (persisting chlamydia, tuberculosis, various fungus infections). Leads to blockage of the tubes and ADHESIONS around the tubes if not treated promptly and effectively with antibiotics. *See also* DISTAL TUBAL OBSTRUCTION; HYDROSALPINX; PROXIMAL TUBAL OBSTRUCTION; PYOSALPINX.

**salpingitis isthmica nodosa**   a nodular ("nodosa") thickening of the fallopian tube's ISTHMUS ("isthmica"), probably due to previous SALPINGITIS. Can cause localized obstruction of the tube and, if the obstruction is partial, an ECTOPIC PREGNANCY can be caused; can be overcome with microsurgery (TUBAL ANASTOMOSIS) or by TUBAL CANALIZATION.

**salpingogram**   an X-ray of the FALLOPIAN TUBE. *See also* HYSTEROSALPINGOGRAM; SELECTIVE SALPINGOGRAM.

**salpingolysis**   MICROSURGERY to remove PERITUBAL ADHESIONS or perifimbrial adhesions sometimes carried out during LAPAROSCOPY. *See also* FIMBRIOLYSIS.

**salpingoscopy**   looking inside the FALLOPIAN TUBE with a fiber-optic instrument through its relatively wide outer FIMBRIAL END; carried out during LAPAROSCOPY or LAPAROTOMY. *See also* FALLOPOSCOPY.

**salpingostomy**   MICROSURGERY to make a permanent, new opening at the outer FIMBRIAL END of the FALLOPIAN TUBE after it has become blocked (*see* HYDROSALPINX) from SALPINGITIS or, uncommonly nowadays, from FIMBRIECTOMY. Sometimes attempted during LAPAROSCOPY, although mostly with a reduced chance of success. *See also* FIMBRIOLYSIS.

**salpingotomy** an operation involving a temporary opening along the length of the FALLOPIAN TUBE, usually for the treatment of a (tubal) ECTOPIC PREGNANCY; occasionally performed for a PYOSALPINX. Can be carried out efficiently during LAPAROSCOPY.

**secondary amenorrhea** AMENORRHEA when a woman has had at least one spontaneous menstrual period, but then menstruation stops.

**secondary follicle** the second stage of growth of the FOLLICLE, in which the egg is enclosed by a layer that is more than one cell thick of round-shaped, multiplying FOLLICLE CELLS; virtually all secondary follicles will go on to become TERTIARY FOLLICLES.

**secondary oocyte** the form of the OVUM, or egg, produced from the PRIMARY OOCYTE late in the life of the maturing FOLLICLE, just before OVULATION; the egg stays at this stage until it is fertilized by a sperm cell. *See also* MEIOSIS.

**secondary ovarian failure** failure of OVULATION along with low ESTROGEN production from the ovaries because of insufficient signaling from the PITUITARY GLAND by its hormones, the GONADOTROPINS.

**secondary spermatocyte** the form of the sperm cell in the second stage of SPERMATOGENESIS (through which the sperm cells are formed in the TESTES), produced from PRIMARY SPERMATOCYTES in the first cell division of MEIOSIS, and giving rise to SPERMATIDS, which have just half the normal cell's complement of CHROMOSOMES, through the second division of meiosis; enveloped by SERTOLI CELLS in the tubules of the testes.

**secretory phase** the phase of development of the ENDOMETRIUM during which, after the PRO-LIFERATIVE PHASE, the endometrium stops growing but starts producing secretions (which nourish an implanting EMBRYO) under the influence of PROGESTERONE (therefore it corresponds in time with the LUTEAL PHASE in the ovary).

**selective catheterization** an X-ray-directed technique for placing fine catheters in veins of the body to sample the local production of hormones from a particular gland.

**selective feticide** *see* FETAL REDUCTION

**selective salpingogram** an X-ray like a HYSTEROSALPINGOGRAM in which a catheter is passed through the cervix and uterus and then wedged into the FALLOPIAN TUBE to fill it with fluid visible on X-ray. High pressure can be applied, so some tubes that seem blocked on hysterosalpingogram (or on passing dye during LAPAROSCOPY) can be shown in fact to be open.

**semen** fluid produced by the male genital tract at ejaculation; contains SPERMATOZOA as well as many other substances, including those that make the ejaculate coagulate. Sperm cells account for only about 1 percent of the volume of the ejaculate, so it is not possible to be confident about a man's SPERM COUNT just on the basis of the volume of the semen ejaculated.

**semen analysis** *see* SPERM COUNT

**semen sperm antibodies** a test for detecting SPERM ANTIBODIES in SEMEN.

**seminal fluid** *see* SEMEN

**seminal vesicles** male sex organs that are joined to the VAS DEFERENS on each side as they enter the PROSTATE GLAND to join the urethra; once thought to act as receptacles for storing sperm, they are now known to be more important for contributing constituents of SEMEN.

**septate uterus**  *see* UTERINE SEPTUM

**septum**  Latin for a "barrier"; for example see UTERINE SEPTUM.

**serological test for syphilis**  one of a number of tests to detect previous or untreated syphilis, an important (though nowadays rare) cause of birth defects and RECURRENT MISCARRIAGES; the chance of detecting unsuspected syphilis might be very low, but the penalty for missing it is great, so it is still a routine test in early pregnancy; tests are done on serum and include the venereal disease research laboratory (VDRL) test and the WASSERMAN REACTION (WR) test.

**Serophene**  CLOMIPHENE, manufactured by Serono.

**serosa**  the delicate, one-cell-thick outside lining of an organ in the body, particularly (in this book) the organs of the PERITONEAL CAVITY. Unlike other body surfaces, such as the skin and the lining of the stomach or intestines, an ulcer (or missing part) of the peritoneal serosa always heals in eight days, however big the ulcer, or defect, is. *See also* PERITONEAL ADHESIONS; PERITONEUM.

**Sertoli cell**  cells lining the tubules of the TESTES that nurture the developing sperm cells; responsible in fetal life for the production of ANTI-MÜLLERIAN HORMONE, which stops the male fetus from developing fallopian tubes, a uterus and a vagina; a source of ESTRADIOL in men.

**serum**  that part of blood that is left after it clots; distinct from plasma, which is that part of unclotted blood that remains on top whe blood is spun down in a centrifuge (whic will still clot and leave serum unless an ant coagulant is added); various serum tests ar described below.

**serum alpha fetoprotein**  measurement ( ALPHA FETOPROTEIN (AFP) in blood serum high levels can indicate a birth abnormalit involving the brain or spinal cord, such a anencephaly or spina bifida (confirmed AMNIOCENTESIS shows high AFP levels in th amniotic fluid); low levels, especially in con junction with measurements of SERUM HCC and a metabolic product of ESTROGEN known as "estriol" can indicate an increase risk of DOWN'S SYNDROME (or trisomy 21) signaling the need for a KARYOTYPE of the fe tus's tissues by CHORIONIC VILLUS SAMPLIN( (CVS) or AMNIOCENTESIS.

**serum anticardiolipin antibody**  a test don to investigate RECURRENT MISCARRIAGES. Se *also* LUPUS ANTICOAGULANT.

**serum CA125 antigen**  measurement o CA125 ANTIGEN in serum; a test done to inves tigate, particularly, ADENOMYOSIS and cancer o the ovary. Levels can also be increased with ENDOMETRIOSIS, normal menstruation anc normal early pregnancy.

**serum copper**  a test done to screen fo Wilson's disease, in which there is abnorma retention of copper in the body, a rare cause o RECURRENT MISCARRIAGES.

**serum estradiol**  measurement of ESTRADIOL in blood serum; used especially in ASSISTEL CONCEPTION to estimate development of FOL LICLES happening naturally or in response to OVULATION INDUCTION; for this purpose the re-

It should be available within four hours. Levels are influenced mainly by FOLLICLE STIMULATING HORMONE, but normal responses also require a small amount of LUTEINIZING HORMONE, usually present naturally, and present in most preparations of HUMAN MENOPAUSAL GONADOTROPIN, including METRODIN, but absent in FERTINEX (METRODIN HP) and from preparations of rFSH.

**serum FSH** measurement of FOLLICLE STIMULATING HORMONE in serum; useful at the time of menstruation for indicating a significantly decreased number of eggs left in the ovaries in the few years leading up to MENOPAUSE (that is, indicative of impending OVARIAN FAILURE); continuously high in women after menopause.

**serum hCG** measurement of HUMAN CHORIONIC GONADOTROPIN in serum; essentially a PREGNANCY TEST, but carried out more precisely (QUANTITATIVELY) than is the case with a yes-or-no test (which is QUALITATIVE). Often carried out serially, to determine if a pregnancy is: thriving (hCG levels double every two or three days in normal early pregnancy); languishing (levels rise more slowly, seen with an ECTOPIC PREGNANCY and with an INEVITABLE MISCARRIAGE); or resolving naturally (levels that are falling).

**serum HIV antibodies** a test for HIV, the virus that causes AIDS, and which comes in two strains, type 1 and type 2; they need separate tests but both are usually done as a routine. The test looks for the development of an immune reaction against the virus; it does not look for the virus itself, so it is possible for a few weeks to have been infected (and to be infective) with the test itself still NEGATIVE.

**serum LH** measurement of LUTEINIZING HORMONE in serum; used to judge the occurrence of the LH SURGE; the result should be available within four hours for this purpose.

**serum progesterone** measurement of PROGESTERONE in serum; often done to check the occurrence of prior OVULATION; used to infer the onset of ovulation in OVULATION INDUCTION or ASSISTED CONCEPTION programs, and attaches extra significance to an apparently raised SERUM LH in judging the onset of the LH SURGE; the result should be available within four hours for these purposes. *See also* PREMENSTRUAL ENDOMETRIAL BIOPSY.

**serum prolactin** measurement of PROLACTIN in serum. An increase is called HYPERPROLACTINEMIA.

**serum 17-hydroxyprogesterone** measurement in serum of 17-hydroxyprogesterone, which is formed from PROGESTERONE in the ADRENAL GLANDS, mostly as an intermediary substance on the way to making the adrenal's main hormone, cortisol, and in the ovaries, on the way to making ANDROGENS and ESTROGENS). A congenital lack of one or other of the enzymes needed to make cortisol in the adrenal causes androgens to be made instead, in turn causing HIRSUTISM and OLIGOMENORRHEA in women, perhaps with the POLYCYSTIC OVARY SYNDROME (in mild cases) or (in severe cases) causing INTERSEX at birth; the adrenal glands enlarge in an attempt to maintain production of cortisol, hence "congenital adrenal hyperplasia" (CAH). An inappropriately high level of 17-hydroxyprogesterone in serum is diagnostic of CAH.

**serum sperm antibodies** estimation of SPERM ANTIBODIES circulating in the blood; generally not as useful as estimating SEMEN SPERM ANTI-BODIES (for men) or CERVICAL MUCUS SPERM ANTIBODIES (for women), as these fluids have more immediate contact with sperm cells.

**serum testosterone**  measurement of TESTOSTERONE, the chief male sex hormone (ANDROGEN) circulating in serum; if increased in women with OLIGOMENORRHEA or AMENORRHEA, indicative of the POLYCYSTIC OVARY SYNDROME; the FREE ANDROGEN INDEX is a more sensitive test.

**serum TSH**  measurement of THYROID STIMULATING HORMONE in serum. *See also* THYROID FUNCTION TESTS.

**serum urea and creatinine**  a test of kidney function; sometimes measured when screening for a kidney (renal) cause of RECURRENT MISCARRIAGES.

**sex**  sexual intercourse (coitus or having sex) or GENDER or relating to it (as in SEX CHROMOSOME).

**sex chromosome**  a CHROMOSOME that is either the X chromosome (a pair confers normal femaleness in a normal DIPLOID complement of chromosomes) or the Y chromosome (just one confers maleness in a normal diploid complement of chromosomes); distinct from the nonsex chromosomes, or AUTOSOMES (which are numbered from 1 to 22); ANEUPLOIDIES give rise to TURNER'S SYNDROME, KLINEFELTER'S SYNDROME, TRIPLE-X SYNDROME, EXTRA-Y-CHROMOSOME SYNDROME; examined in a test called a KARYOTYPE.

**sex-linked recessive inheritance**  *see* RECESSIVE INHERITANCE

**short protocol**  the short protocol for using GnRH-AGONISTS with injections of FOLLICLE STIMULATING HORMONE (FSH) for induction SUPEROVULATION in ASSISTED CONCEPTION programs involves starting the GnRH-agonist day or two before the injections of FSH star The advantage is one of cost: less FSH (ar less GnRH-agonist) is used compared wi the LONG PROTOCOL. The disadvantage is th LUTEINIZING HORMONE levels and PROGE TERONE levels can rise, possibly (in some cycl of treatment) spoiling optimal developme of ovarian FOLLICLES. The GnRH-agonist continued (in contrast to the ULTRASHORT PR( TOCOL) until follicles are mature and HUM/ CHORIONIC GONADOTROPIN is given to start th process of ovulation.

**Simms-Huhner test**  *see* POSTCOITAL TEST

**small bowel**  the small intestine, leading o of the stomach; narrower than the large inte: tine (or colon), to which it connects. *See al* BOWEL.

**small-for-dates**  a general term used by ot stetricians or pediatricians to refer to a FETL or newborn baby that seems smaller than should be for the assumed duration of th pregnancy so far. The three main causes are genetic abnormality of the fetus; insufficier nutrition for an otherwise normal fetus; an an incorrect calculation of the dates, perhap because OVULATION and conception took plac later than the usual two weeks after the LAS MENSTRUAL PERIOD.

**SMI**  *see* SPERM MICROINJECTION

**spastic colon syndrome**  *see* IRRITABLE BOWE SYNDROME

**sperm**  colloquial abbreviation for SPERMATO ZOON or its plural "spermatozoa"; also used i the form "sperm cell(s)."

**erm antibodies** the result of a reaction of the mune system against sperm and, by limiting e ability of sperm to show MOTILITY, a contribory or (occasionally) sole cause of INFERTILITY; n be present in SERUM, in CERVICAL MUCUS or in MEN; may be agglutinating (which make erm stick in clumps), immobilizing (which ipple sperm particularly effectively and kill em) or coating, which interfere with sperm atchment to the egg. The screening test for erm antibodies involves IMMUNOBEADS.

**erm count** semen analysis, measuring the olume of the ejaculate, the *density* of sperm . it (expressed as so many million sperm per illiliter), the proportion of sperm swiming normally (the MOTILITY), and the proortion with normal *shape*. A normal sperm ount consists of a volume of more than 1 illiliter; a density of more than 20 million er milliliter; a motility of more than 50 pernt; and normal forms of more than 50 pernt (casual examination) or more than 14 ercent (critical examination by the "strict iteria" recently advocated by the World ealth Organization).

**erm microinjection (SMI)** either INTRAYTOPLASMIC SPERM INSERTION (ICSI) or SUBONAL INSERTION (SUZI, now obsolete).

**permatid** the product of the SPERMATOCYTE hen it has completed MEIOSIS (by which the umber of chromosomes is halved, so it is in e HAPLOID state), and also enclosed in the ibules of the testis by the SERTOLI CELLS; early permatids are round-shaped, whereas late permatids closely resemble mature SPERMAOZOA. *See also* SPERMIOGENESIS.

**permatocyte** the sperm cell equivalent to e OOCYTE stage of the egg. *See also* PRIMARY

SPERMATOCYTE; SECONDARY SPERMATOCYTE; SPERMATOGENESIS.

**spermatogenesis** development of a sperm cell, in the tubules of the TESTES, from SPERMATOGONIUM and SPERMATOCYTE to maturity; the last part of this process, from SPERMATID to SPERMATOZOON, is called SPERMIOGENESIS. The process of spermatogenesis takes 56 days. At any one location in a tubule there are cells at four different stages of maturity, so mature sperm are released from a particular location every 14 days. A systematic interruption of spermatogenesis is called "maturation arrest."

**spermatogonium (spermatogonia)** the replicating phase of the sperm cell, equivalent to the OOGONIUM in the ovaries; located among the supporting cells (SERTOLI CELLS) in the tubules of the TESTIS; divides by the process of MITOSIS until it begins to undergo MEIOSIS by changing into the PRIMARY SPERMATOCYTE; unlike the oogonia, spermatogonia normally persist until old age.

**spermatozoon (spermatozoa)** the final stage of development of the maturing sperm cell, as it leaves the tubules of the TESTIS, to mature in the EPIDIDYMIS; composed of a head (including the ACROSOME), a midpiece loaded with energy and a tail for propulsion.

**spermiogenesis** the final part of the formation of a mature sperm cell, by which the SPERMATID (already HAPLOID) loses its round shape to acquire the features of the mature SPERMATOZOON, with a head, midpiece and tail.

**Spinnbarkheit** German for "ability to be spun," meaning "stretchability"; one of the measurable qualities of CERVICAL MUCUS that indicates receptiveness to sperm.

"Significant" or "Important"?

In considering **statistical significance,** we conventionally regard a one in 20 chance of an association as being safe enough not to be just a coincidence. This represents a P-value, or probability measurement, of 0.05 or less, which is represented as P < 0.05. More conservative cutoffs (for example, P < 0.02, or 1 in 50; P < 0.01, or 1 in 100) need to be used if the data accumulating as a research study continues are examined more than once, rather than just at the end of the study, or if more than one association is being looked for at the same time. For example, among the babies born from IVF in its earlier days, the frequency of birth defects of the neural tube type (such as spina bifida) appeared to be significantly increased (and cleft lip or palate appeared to be significantly decreased), but it was only because more than 100 individual birth defects were looked at, several of which you might then expect to have a one in 100 chance of being too high or too low; with more babies born, the numbers slipped into statistical insignificance.

Showing that there is a statistically significant association between one observation and another does not of itself imply cause and effect. The two observations may both be effects, with a yet-to-be-looked-for shared cause. For example, there is a statistically significant association between smoking and salpingitis (inflammation of the fallopian tubes), but no one believes that one is the cause of the other. For another example, we know that IVF is significantly associated with pre-term birth (even when the effects of multiple births are excluded), but we do not know that IVF causes premature birth: there might be a common reason for the prematurity and

---

**spontaneous abortion** *see* MISCARRIAGE

**statistical significance** a point at which STATISTICS indicate that a set of measurements or observations is regarded as different from normal (it is ABNORMAL) or from a CONTROL GROUP and that the difference is unlikely to have come about just by the effects of chance.

**statistics** the science and art of using arithmetic and probability theory to work out how likely an association between sets of measurements or between sets of observations is to have happened by chance alone. *See also* STATISTICAL SIGNIFICANCE and the box, "Significant or Important?"

**sterility** the state of ABSOLUTE INFERTILITY or COMPLETE INFERTILITY, with no chance of getting pregnant naturally without special help; causes include AZOOSPERMIA, ANOVULATION (especially PRIMARY OVARIAN FAILURE) and

## "Significant" or "Important"? (concluded)

for the need to employ IVF (various hypotheses, including pelvic adhesions or poor sperm, are under investigation).

The size of the statistical significance is quite different from the size of the actually demonstrated difference (a large sample size can make even the most trivial difference statistically significant at $P < 0.01$), although generally it is easier to show significance for a smallish sample if the difference itself is sizable! Conversely, failing to show a statistically significant difference is not the same as saying that there is no difference; the size of the sample may just have been too small to draw a safe conclusion either way.

For other reasons, too, statistical significance is not the same as "medical importance." Tall people might bump their head significantly more often than short people, but that does not necessarily mean that tall people should wear crash helmets, let alone that wearing crash helmets must for this reason become a matter of public policy (which we might distinguish as "administrative importance"). In setting our clinical policies at Sydney IVF, for example, we take more account of medical importance than statistical significance of certain outcomes, so that satisfying a probability level of 1 in 5 ($P < 0.2$) is often enough for us to change our clinical or laboratory practices (the different outcome thus becomes administratively important) if from theory the change makes sense and if other effects from making the change are likely to be trivial.

For these reasons, as medical writers who are proud of precision, we avoid the use of the word "significant," outside a statistical sense, when the word "important" will serve our purpose better.

---

blocked FALLOPIAN TUBES. (Although words like "sterility" and "sterile" sound insensitive, specially for a book like this, it is important in medicine to avoid ambiguity.)

**sterilization**    an operation designed to induce STERILITY. In men, usually carried out by removing small segments of each VAS DEFERENS (vasectomy); in women, usually carried out by removing, crushing or otherwise destroying a small segment of each FALLOPIAN TUBE, preferably close to the uterus (often called "tubal ligation"). *See also* FIMBRIECTOMY.

**sterilization reversal**    an operation involving MICROSURGERY to rejoin the healthy ends of the VAS DEFERENS or FALLOPIAN TUBE to reverse the effects of a previous STERILIZATION operation. *See also* TUBAL ANASTOMOSIS; VASOVASOSTOMY.

**STDs**    sexually transmitted diseases, such as gonorrhea, CHLAMYDIA and HIV.

**subclinical miscarriage**    an early MISCAR-RIAGE, usually within a week or two of the period that had been expected. Traditionally, no CURETTAGE was needed; these days a subclinical miscarriage is one that has not resulted in a GESTATIONAL SAC visible on TRANSVAGINAL ULTRASOUND.

**subfertility**    *see* RELATIVE INFERTILITY

**submucous fibroid**    a FIBROID (or myoma) that grows from the wall of the UTERUS inward to distort the ENDOMETRIAL CAVITY; can be a cause of menorrhagia (heavy periods), INTERMENSTRUAL BLEEDING, PREMENSTRUAL SPOTTING, INFERTILITY and MISCARRIAGE. *See also* MYOMECTOMY.

**submucous myoma**    *see* SUBMUCOUS FIBROID

**subseptate uterus**    *see* UTERINE SEPTUM

**subserous fibroid**    a FIBROID (or myoma) that grows from the outside surface of the uterus, into the cavity of the abdomen, or PERITONEAL CAVITY; the least likely of any sort of fibroid to affect reproduction, but can cause symptoms of pressure or pain should it twist or degenerate. *See also* MYOMECTOMY.

**subserous myoma**    *see* SUBSEROUS FIBROID

**subzonal insertion** (SUZI)  an IVF technique involving sperm microinjection (SMI), in which one or more sperm are injected through the ZONA PELLUCIDA into the PERIVIT-ELLINE space of the egg; now obsolete (because its efficiency is limited by sperm having to have undergone the ACROSOME REACTION) and replaced by INTRACYTOPLASMIC SPERM INSER-TION (ICSI—where the acrosome reaction is not a requirement).

**suffering**  The prevention from and alleviation of a patient's personal suffering is the doctor's ultimate DUTY and the principal pur pose of the professional practice of medicin The suffering can be physical or mental. Th ethical values of NONMALEFICENCE, JUSTICE an equity, for many thoughtful doctors, becom subordinate to the BENEFICENT duty of makin the patient better. For the infertile couple, pre vention from or relief of suffering most obv ously means the doctor helping them to hav a baby; this is not always possible, however, i which case other medical and personal strate gies need to be explored if the suffering is t be lessened.

**superovulation**    intentional induction c multiple ovulations at once, using injection of FOLLICLE STIMULATING HORMONE and HUMA CHORIONIC GONADOTROPIN, for ASSISTED CON CEPTION; inevitably there is a risk of multipl pregnancy. *See also* OVULATION INDUCTION OVARIAN HYPERSTIMULATION SYNDROME (OHSS

**Suprefact**    *see* BUSERILIN

**surrogate**    in reproductive medicine, a wo man who has a baby on another woman' behalf, often called a "gestational carrier. *See also* GESTATIONAL SURROGACY; TRADITIONA SURROGACY.

**SUZI**    *see* SUBZONAL INSERTION

**Synarel**    *see* NAFARELIN

**syngamy**    If FERTILIZATION is the "marriage between egg and sperm, then syngamy is it "consummation," as the male and female PRO NUCLEI come together for the respective HAP LOID sets of CHROMOSOMES to combine into DIPLOID set; an event of legislative importanc in the state of Victoria, Australia, after whic permission for embryo research become much harder to obtain.

**ake-home-baby rate**    the percentage of eatment months or treatment cycles that reult in the woman taking home one or more abies (although twins are not counted separately); the statistic of most interest to paents and, in an age of skepticism in the comunity, the most politically correct statistic or clinics to quote, but it is less useful for linics' quality control purposes than the CONEPTION RATE, the IMPLANTATION RATE and the iable pregnancy rate, because it excludes obtetric misadventures often beyond the conrol of the infertility clinic, and there is a long ag before it can be calculated, making results t best about 9 months old.

**eleological ethics**    in this book, a set of ethcal beliefs based on the goodness or badness f consequences, whether actual, intended or redicted; here, restricted to consequences to ndividuals, in contrast to UTILITARIAN ETHICS; open to change according to empirical observation of outcomes. *See also* DEONTOLOGICAL THICS.

**eratozoospermia**    *see* OLIGOSPERMIA

**ertiary follicle**    the third stage of growth of the FOLLICLE, in which the egg is enclosed by a hick layer of round-shaped FOLLICLE cells among which an antrum, or fluid-filled space, has formed; this antrum will come to dominate the size of the follicle; the first stage of the follicle visible with TRANSVAGINAL ULTRASOUND (when it reaches about 4 millimeters in diameter); further growth of the early tertiary follicle is determined by FOLLICLE STIMULATING HORMONE.

**TESE**    *see* TESTICULAR SPERM EXTRACTION

**TEST**    *see* TUBAL EMBRYO STAGE TRANSFER

**testicle**    diminutive of TESTIS, a word with which it is interchangeable.

**testicular biopsy**    a BIOPSY of the TESTIS to work out the reason behind an absence of sperm cells (AZOOSPERMIA).

**testicular feminization**    a state of INTERSEX in which the KARYOTYPE is male (46,XY), the GONADS are TESTES (hence also male), but the body is completely unresponsive to TESTOSTERONE and to its metabolite DIHYDROTESTOSTERONE, so it develops in the female way, with a normal vulva and vagina apparent at birth, and with normal development of the breasts at puberty. Invariably these children are raised as females, normal except for their PRIMARY AMENORRHEA and their INFERTILITY, because the testes still secrete ANTI-MÜLLERIAN HORMONE and so there is no uterus.

**testicular sperm extraction** (TESE)    dissection into the TESTIS itself, in men with AZOOSPERMIA due to maturation arrest, to recover (by "teasing out") immature sperm cells from the (often small) fraction of tubules there that still contain such cells. The sperm cells are used for IVF using INTRACYTOPLASMIC SPERM INSERTION.

**testicular tubules**    the main constituent of the TESTIS, lined by SERTOLI CELLS and containing the developing sperm cells. *See also* SPERMATOGENESIS.

**testis (testes)**    the male GONAD, located normally in the scrotum; produces the hormone TESTOSTERONE as well as the male GERM CELLS, or SPERMATOZOA. Interchangeable with "testicle."

**testosterone**    the main male sex hormone, or ANDROGEN, in the blood, where it is measured as SERUM TESTOSTERONE; secreted in large amounts by the TESTES in men and by the THECAL CELLS of the OVARIES in women. Before it acts on the tissues it is converted to DIHYDROTESTOSTERONE.

**tests for tubal patency**　tests that check if the FALLOPIAN TUBES are open, usually by passing fluid through the CERVIX to fill the ENDO-METRIAL CAVITY and then demonstrate it coming out the ends of the tubes. The most common test is to pass a blue dye during LAPAROSCOPY. The second most common is a HYSTEROSALPINGOGRAM. Once upon a time, carbon dioxide gas was used and listened for with a stethoscope (a Rubin's test); a high-tech version of Rubin's test uses ultrasound to show the gas. *See also* FALLOPOSCOPY.

**theca interna**　a layer of cells in the OVARY lying immediately around the FOLLICLE; under the influence of LUTEINIZING HORMONE it is responsible for producing the weak male sex hormone ANDROSTENEDIONE, which is then converted by the follicle cells (the GRANULOSA CELLS) into ESTROGEN, principally ESTRADIOL.

**thecal cells**　cells that make up or come from the THECA INTERNA.

**threatened miscarriage**　traditionally, any bleeding from the uterus during pregnancy while the cervix is (still) closed. Today, there would need to be a normal EMBRYO as well and, a little later, normal fetal heart movement pattern on TRANSVAGINAL ULTRASOUND to separate it from an INEVITABLE MISCARRIAGE.

**thyroid function tests**　usually two tests: a serum THYROXINE, low for underactivity, high for overactivity, and a serum THYROID STIMU-LATING HORMONE (TSH), high for underactivity based primarily in the thyroid gland, low for overactivity based primarily in the thyroid gland and low for underactivity based in the PITUITARY GLAND. As a screening test for ma function of the thyroid gland a serum TSH will generally suffice.

**thyroid stimulating hormone** (TSH)　a hormone produced by the ADENOHYPOPHYSIS (the front, glandular part of the PITUITARY GLAND that switches on the thyroid gland, causing to make and release THYROXINE. *See also* THYROID FUNCTION TESTS.

**thyroxine**　the main hormone of the thyroid gland; responsible for controlling the rate of metabolism in the body; activity of the thyroid gland is measured with THYROID FUNCTION TESTS.

**time left for conception**　one of the two most important variables that determine the chance of still getting pregnant naturally in RELATIVE INFERTILITY and unexplained infertility (the other is DURATION OF INFERTILITY). The longer the time still available the better the chance that, sooner or later, pregnancy will happen. Broadly limited by the female partner's age, but personal circumstances and ambitions within the biologically available time frame may shorten it, leading to a decision to seek treatment with ASSISTED CONCEPTION. *See also* FECUNDABILITY.

**totipotent**　*see* PRE-EMBRYO

**traditional surrogacy**　surrogacy in which the woman who is the SURROGATE for the intended pregnancy provides the eggs (through her own OVULATION); is impregnated by AS-SISTED INSEMINATION; carries (gestates) the pregnancy and gives birth and then gives up the baby to the person who commissioned the

rrogacy arrangement. Also known as "ge-
-tic-plus-gestational surrogacy." The surro-
-te is as much the biological mother of the
-ild as if she had conceived in natural cir-
-mstances, except that the male by whom
-e has been impregnated has no prior social
-lationship with her. In no countries other
-an the United States, where commercial sur-
-ogacy can be legal, has the practice been en-
-ouraged, whether for altruistic or commer-
-al reasons.

**ansvaginal ultrasound**   ultrasound imag-
-g of the pelvic organs for diagnosing abnor-
-alities of (particularly) the UTERUS and the
VARIES and for monitoring the development
-f ovarian FOLLICLES with OVULATION INDUC-
ION and ASSISTED CONCEPTION programs;
-mong the pioneers were Dr. Karl Popp, who
-sed a mechanical sector scanner vaginally in
-lamburg in 1984, and Dr. Jock Anderson,
-ho used the first vaginal linear array scanner
-n Australia at Sydney IVF in 1985, leading to
-ts widespread use subsequently in Australia
-nd the United States.

**rimester**   literally, a three-month time pe-
-iod; so the nine months of pregnancy are di-
-ided into the first, second and third
-rimesters. Most MISCARRIAGES take place in
-he first trimester (up to 12 or 13 weeks).
-regnancies that reach the third trimester (be-
-ond 27 weeks) have an increasingly good
-hance of being viable (although, with inten-
-ive care, survival has occurred from about 24
-weeks).

**riple-X syndrome**   a TRISOMY with a KARY-
OTYPE of 47,XXX, a female with an extra X
-chromosome; the old description of "super fe-

male" is misleading because fertility, if affected, is likely to be reduced; PRIMARY OVARIAN
FAILURE is more common than with a normal
chromosome complement and PREMATURE
MENOPAUSE then follows.

**triploid, triploidy**   a state of 69 chromosomes, or three times the HAPLOID number,
most commonly caused by fertilization of the
egg with two sperm; the PRE-EMBRYO that results, although a FETUS may form, is doomed
to miscarry; the TROPHOBLAST of the placenta
often undergoes hydatidiform degeneration
(resembling a HYDATIDIFORM MOLE but without the sinister consequences); the result is
often called a partial hydatidiform mole, in
contrast to the more dangerous COMPLETE HY-
DATIDIFORM MOLE.

**triptorelin**   a GnRH-AGONIST marketed in
Europe by Ipsen Biotech as Decapeptyl and
administered by monthly injection.

**trisomy**   an abnormality of the CHROMOSOME
complement in which there is an extra chromosome seen on the KARYOTYPE. The extra
chromosome can be an AUTOSOME, such as
in DOWN'S SYNDROME (trisomy 21), or a SEX
CHROMOSOME, such as in TRIPLE-X SYNDROME
(47,XXX), KLINEFELTER'S SYNDROME (47,XXY)
and    EXTRA-Y-CHROMOSOME    SYNDROME
(47,XYY).

**trisomy 21**   TRISOMY for chromosome number
21, or an extra chromosome 21. This is the
most common of the trisomies and gives rise
to DOWN'S SYNDROME, or mongolism. Research
has shown that the commonest source of the
extra chromosome is a mistake in the first division of MEIOSIS in the egg cell (during the
many years it rests as a PRIMARY OOCYTE).

**trophoblast** As the cells of the PRE-EMBRYO specialize, they soon differentiate into central ones that will form the EMBRYO or FETUS itself and peripheral ones (the trophoblast) that will be responsible for invading the mother's tissues (*see* IMPLANTATION) and will form the PLACENTA and the membranes.

**true hermaphroditism** INTERSEX when tissue typical of an OVARY and a TESTIS is found in the one person. The genital organs may appear to be normal female, normal male or somewhere in between. Intersex states in which there are either normal ovaries or normal testes (but not both) are sometimes called PSEUDOHERMAPHRODITISM.

**truth** a self-evident ethical principle that has value provided no substantial harm is done; not to be dispensed with for expediency alone.

**tubal abortion** a tubal ECTOPIC PREGNANCY that is in the process of being expelled out the FIMBRIAL END of the FALLOPIAN TUBE.

**tubal anastomosis** MICROSURGERY of the FALLOPIAN TUBES in which an area of blockage is cut out and the healthy bits of tube on each side of the blockage are sewn back together. Can be done for localized SALPINGITIS, including SALPINGITIS ISTHMICA NODOSA, and for STERILIZATION REVERSAL.

**tubal canalization** overcoming a localized obstruction of the ISTHMUS or the INTERSTITIAL SEGMENT of the FALLOPIAN TUBE by pushing a wire or a catheter through it, enabling (in some cases) the tube to be "re-canalized" and thus to remain open after being blocked; it is an attractive alternative to TUBAL ANASTOMOSIS and can be performed either during the investigation of tubal infertility with HYSTEROSCO LAPAROSCOPY and FALLOPOSCOPY or at the tin of carrying out a HYSTEROSALPINGOGRAM. B cause not all tubes that seem to be blocked a in fact blocked (sometimes a normal tube w not allow fluid to pass through it for ho monal reasons or because of a spasm), ca needs to be taken to investigate the tube proj erly before canalization is undertaken.

**tubal embryo-stage transfer** (TEST) a vari tion of ZYGOTE INTRAFALLOPIAN TRANSFER (ZIF] in which, usually a day after that on whic ZIFT (or PROST) would be carried out, clea ing PRE-EMBRYOS (at a two-cell to four-ce stage) are transferred to the FALLOPIAN TUBE part of an IN VITRO FERTILIZATION program.

**tubal ligation** STERILIZATION operation in woman involving interruption of the FALLC PIAN TUBES.

**tubal patency** *see* TESTS FOR TUBAL PATENCY

**tubule** *see* TESTICULAR TUBULES

**Turner's syndrome** the combination of PRI MARY OVARIAN FAILURE with constitutional (ge netically determined) short stature; often wit other clinical abnormalities, including "web bing" of the neck, an increased "carrying an gle" at the elbow, short fourth metacarpa (hand) and metatarsal (feet) bones, anc sometimes abnormalities of the heart and the thyroid gland. Associated with a KARYOTYPI that is 45,X (a MONOSOMY, with one SEX CHRO MOSOME missing) or with partial loss (dele tion) of one of a pair of X chromosomes.

**ultrashort protocol** a variation of the SHORT PROTOCOL for using GnRH-AGONISTS with in jections of FOLLICLE STIMULATING HORMONE

SH) for induction of SUPEROVULATION in AS-
TED CONCEPTION programs. The GnRH-ag-
ist is started with menstruation, a day or
vo before the injections of FSH start, and is
scontinued after about five days from start-
ng it (that is, often a week or more before
vulation). There are no special advantages,
hereas there is a potential disadvantage: a
uch more thorough suppression occurs of
e woman's own LUTEINIZING HORMONE (and
erhaps FSH) than if the GnRH-agonist is
ontinued, sometimes allowing ATRESIA of
OLLICLES before they are fully mature. *See also*
RUM ESTRADIOL.

ltrasound an imaging procedure like radar,
ut using high frequency sound waves; used for
iagnosis. *See also* TRANSVAGINAL ULTRASOUND.

nexplained infertility INFERTILITY for which
o obvious cause has been found after the fol-
owing tests have been done with normal re-
ults: a SPERM COUNT or POSTCOITAL TEST; a test
f OVULATION, such as a SERUM PROGESTERONE
hat is satisfactorily high; and a LAPAROSCOPY
used to show that the tubes are open and that
here is no ENDOMETRIOSIS or other obvious
BNORMALITY).

nicornuate uterus a UTERINE ABNORMALITY
hat comes about when it forms (in the EM-
BRYO) from just one MÜLLERIAN DUCT; the
terus will be a little smaller than normal
(making a MISCARRIAGE or PREMATURE LABOR
more likely) and will be connected by a FAL-
LOPIAN TUBE to just one OVARY, contributing
slightly to INFERTILITY. Reproduction and fertility, however, can be normal. Diagnosed by
HYSTEROSCOPY and LAPAROSCOPY or by HYS-
TEROSALPINGOGRAM. Often there is a simultaneous abnormality of the kidneys, such as one

kidney instead of two, diagnosable by ultrasound or, more specifically, by a special kidney
X-ray study called an intravenous pyelogram.

urinary LH kit a home test for OVULATION in
which the urine is tested for LUTEINIZING HOR-
MONE; if the urine shows a POSITIVE TEST, ovulation will usually take place within 24 to 36
hours.

uterine anomaly variation of the shape of
the UTERUS a woman is born with (it is CON-
GENITAL); some uterine anomalies or ABNOR-
MALITIES tend to cause RECURRENT MISCAR-
RIAGES, PREMATURE LABOR or breech births.

uterine curettage *see* CURETTAGE; VACUUM
CURETTAGE

uterine septum a septum or barrier separating the cavity of the UTERUS into two halves; a
cause of RECURRENT MISCARRIAGES.

uterus the womb, in which pregnancy is ges-
tated from the time of IMPLANTATION of the EM-
BRYO until delivery or MISCARRIAGE; formed
from the joining of the two MÜLLERIAN DUCTS
(in the absence of ANTI-MÜLLERIAN HORMONE);
composed of the main, upper part (the uterine
FUNDUS) and a lower neck, or CERVIX, which
connects it to the upper part of the vagina;
most of its wall is made of muscle tissue (the
MYOMETRIUM), but with an inner lining of
glands (the ENDOMETRIUM) and, on the outer
surface, a thin covering of uterine SEROSA.

utilitarian ethics a set of ethical beliefs based
on maximizing good for the greatest number
of people; for purposes here, similar to TELEO-
LOGICAL ETHICS or consequential considerations but with a community-wide reference
instead of a context of individual priority; in
modern times concerned with the equitable

## Medical Vocabulary—Sensitive, Precise and Correct?

Innocent messengers can be shot for the message they deliver! Experienced and wise messengers learn to give their message with discretion. Physicians, like other professionals, sometimes must deliver bad news. The judgment a physician uses in his or her vocabulary will affect how the information that is there to be conveyed is received. This is part of the art of medicine. The adept physician draws on a substantial vocabulary to match the message to the needs and receptiveness of the patient at the moment of the consultation, taking continuing account of how it is being understood. This flexibility is not as open to the author, who anticipates a wider and more remote audience—a readership with a wide range in interests, experience, education and emotional state.

To soften an unwelcome message the language is sometimes softened. This can happen systematically (being deaf becomes being "hearing impaired"), but in time, as the new vocabulary takes over, the realities of the message resurface, and there is the same temptation to come up with another substitute. Because this process can be at a different stage for different people in different places and at different times, the vocabulary of a book can never be right (or be to the taste of) every reader. So, however careful I am with vocabulary, I know I will never please everybody.

My priority is to be unambiguous. I take Mark Twain's advice to find the facts first and then, at leisure, to rationalize them later. So I am concerned in a book like this to deliver a precise message first and then try to anticipate your responses. Having said this, many physicians will use vocabulary among themselves that they would not (or ought not) use with patients: *habitual abortion* is seen more commonly in the medical literature than its kinder and no less precise synonym, *recurrent miscarriages*. Many stark descriptions come to us from a previous era—a time of much less communication between physicians and patients than we expect today. But as medical language comes to be shared more with lay readers, physicians have to modify their discussions. We do not want to exclude everyone without a medical education, but above all we should aim to remain exact. On the one hand this means avoiding medical jargon; on the other hand it means avoiding oversensitivity that jeopardizes clarity.

and consistent distribution of restricted public resources; open to change according to the systematic assessment of outcomes. *See also* DEONTOLOGICAL ETHICS.

**vacuum curettage** CURETTAGE in which the contents of the early pregnant uterus are sucked out using a soft plastic catheter; used in the treatment of MISCARRIAGE, in the treat-

ient of HYDATIDIFORM MOLE and to induce
BORTION.

**alue judgment** a philosophical device for
noving from what *is* to what *ought*. It bridges
vhat philosophers call the NATURALISTIC FALLACY,
iut not with the approval of all philosophers.

**'alues** *see* ETHICAL VALUES

**aricocele** a varicose vein in the scrotum,
vhich in some cases can increase the temper-
ture of the TESTIS, causing OLIGOSPERMIA;
nore common on the left side than on the
ight. One of the few treatable causes of male
nfertility (the treatment is to tie off the vein),
ilthough not all sperm counts improve.

**vas deferens (vasa deferentia)** the long duct
that transports sperm cells from the EPIDIDYMIS
to the SEMINAL VESICLES; can be missing from
birth (CONGENITAL ABSENCE OF THE VASA DEFER-
ENTIA) or blocked as a result of infection or intentional interruption (VASECTOMY).

**vasectomy** STERILIZATION operation in a man
involving surgical interruption of each VAS
DEFERENS in the upper part of the scrotum.

**vasectomy-reversal** *see* VASOVASOSTOMY

**vasovasostomy** the operation in a man for
reversing a STERILIZATION operation (a VASEC-
TOMY) involving removal of the blocked part
of each VAS DEFERENS, in the upper part of the
scrotum, and joining by MICROSURGERY one
cut end of the vas to the other cut end.

**vocabulary** *see* the box "Medical Vocabulary—Sensitive, Precise and Correct?"

**Wasserman reaction** a SEROLOGICAL TEST FOR
SYPHILIS.

**Wilson's disease** *see* SERUM COPPER

**Wolffian duct** *see* MESONEPHRIC DUCT

**ZIFT** *see* ZYGOTE INTRAFALLOPIAN TRANSFER

**Zoladex** *see* GOSERELIN

**zona pellucida** the tough but glassy-looking
membrane that starts to surround the egg
while it is still in the FOLLICLE, protects it
against sperm that have not undergone the
ACROSOME REACTION at its surface, and keeps
the cells of the early EMBRYO (PRE-EMBRYO) together until the embryo, as a BLASTOCYST,
hatches through it in preparation for IMPLAN-
TATION.

**zygote** fertilized egg up to the first CLEAVAGE
division; this stage of development of the EM-
BRYO takes about 22 hours, and for the last few
of these hours it is at the pronuclear stage. *See
also* PRONUCLEUS.

**zygote intrafallopian transfer** (ZIFT) a
form of ASSISTED CONCEPTION in which IN
VITRO FERTILIZATION (IVF) is used to produce
fertilization; transfer is made on the day after
egg pickup and IVF, before the fertilized egg
divides (the ZYGOTE or pronuclear stage); useful if the potential fertilizing ability of sperm
is in doubt; the transfer is made to the FALLO-
PIAN TUBE to obtain advantages similar to
GAMETE INTRAFALLOPIAN TRANSFER (GIFT) and
is carried out by LAPAROSCOPY (with anesthesia) or by TRANSVAGINAL ULTRASOUND (without
anesthesia); synonymous with PRONUCLEAR-
STAGE TRANSFER (PROST).

# Further Reading

Cassell, E. J. 1991. *The nature of suffering and the goals of medicine.* New York: Oxford University Press.

Dunstan, G. R. 1984. The moral status of the human embryo: A tradition recalled. *Journal of Medical Ethics* 10:38–44.

———. 1986. In-vitro fertilization: The ethics. *Human Reproduction* 1:41–44.

Gutheil, T. G., H. Bursztajn and A. Brodsky, A. 1984. Malpractice prevention through the sharing of uncertainty: Informed consent and the therapeutic alliance. *New England Journal of Medicine* 311:49–51.

Leridon, H. 1977. *Human fertility: The basic components.* Chicago: University of Chicago Press.

Morris, D. 1986. *The illustrated naked ape.* London: Jonathan Cape.

Nathanielsz, P. W. 1995. *Life before birth: The challenges of fetal development.* New York: W. H. Freeman.

Short, R. V. 1984. Species differences in reproductive mechanisms. In C. R. Austin and R. V. Short, eds., *Reproduction in mammals. Book 4: Reproductive fitness.* Cambridge: Cambridge University Press.

Silber, S. J. 1990. Why are humans so infertile? In *How to get pregnant with the new technology.* New York: Warner Books.

———. 1995. What forms of male infertility are there left to cure? *Human Reproduction* 10:503–504.

Singer, P. 1983. *The expanding circle: Ethics and sociobiology.* Oxford: Oxford University Press.

Singer, P., H. Kuhse, S. Buckle, K. Dawson, and P. Kasimba. 1990. *Embryo experimentation.* Cambridge: Cambridge University Press.

Small, M. 1993. *Female choices: Sexual behavior of female primates.* Ithaca, N.Y.: Cornell University Press.

Stone, L. 1977. *The family, sex and marriage in England, 1500–1800.* London: Weidenfeld and Nicolson.

# References

## Chapter 1

Jansen, R. P. S. 1983. Peritoneal and plasma estradiol and progesterone levels in mild and moderate endometriosis: A search for luteinized unruptured follicles. *Fertility and Sterility* 39:394.

————. 1993. Relative infertility: Modeling clinical paradoxes. *Fertility and Sterility* 59:1041–1045.

————. 1995. Elusive fertility: Fecundability and assisted conception in perspective. *Fertility and Sterility* 64:252–254.

Leridon, H., and A. Spira. 1984. Problems in measuring the effectiveness of infertility therapy. *Fertility and Sterility* 41:580–586.

Norman, R. L. 1994. Corticotropin-releasing hormone effects on luteinizing hormone and cortisol secretion in intact female rhesus macaques. *Biology of Reproduction* 50:949–955.

Norman, R. L., J. McGlone and C. J. Smith. 1994. Restraint inhibits LH secretion in the follicular phase of the menstrual cycle in rhesus macaques. *Biology of Reproduction* 50:16–26.

## Chapter 2

Jansen, R. P. S. 1994. Ovulation and the polycystic ovary syndrome. *Australian and New Zealand Journal of Obstetrics and Gynaecology* 34:277–285.

Short, R. V. 1984. Species differences in reproductive mechanisms. In C. R. Austin and R. V. Short, eds., *Reproduction in mammals—Book 4: Reproductive fitness.* (24–61). Cambridge: Cambridge University Press.

## Chapter 3

Jansen, R. P. S. 1978. Fallopian tube isthmic mucus and ovum transport. *Science* 201:349–351.

————. 1980. Cyclic changes in the human fallopian tube isthmus and their functional importance. *American Journal of Obstetrics and Gynecology* 136:292–308.

————. 1984. Endocrine response in the fallopian tube. *Endocrine Reviews* 5:525–551.

————. 1985. Endocrine response in the female genital tract. In R. P. Shearman, ed., *Clinical Reproductive Endocrinology.* Edinburgh: Churchill Livingstone.

————. 1994. Follicles in competition. *Nature* 367:10.

Jansen, R. P. S., and V. K. Bajpai. 1982. Oviductal acid mucus glycoproteins in the estrous rabbit: An ultrastructural and histochemical study. *Biology of Reproduction* 26:155–168.

————. 1983. Periovulatory glycoprotein secretion in the macaque fallopian tube. *American Journal of Obstetrics and Gynecology* 147:598–608.

Jansen, R. P. S., M. Turner, E. Johannisson, B.-M. Landgren and E. Diczfalusy, E. 1985. Cyclic changes in human endometrial surface glycoproteins: A quantitative histochemical study. *Fertility and Sterility* 44:85–91.

## Chapters 4, 5 and 6

Bowman, M., and R. Jansen. 1995. How to investigate the infertile patient. *Modern Medicine of Australia* (October):130.

DeCherney, A. H., H. Kort, J. B. Barney and G. R. DeVore. 1980. Increased pregnancy rate with oil-soluble hysterosalpingography dye. *Fertility and Sterility* 33:407–410.

Gleicher, N., D. Pratt, M. Parrilli, V. Karande and L. Redding. 1992. Standardization of hysterosalpingography and selective salpingography: A valuable adjunct to simple opacification studies. *Fertility and Sterility* 58: 1136–1141.

Handyside, A. 1992. Prospects for the clinical application of preimplantation diagnosis: The tortoise or the hare. *Human Reproduction* 7:1481–1483.

Kerin, J., R. Anderson, L. Daykhovsky, A. Stein, J. Segalowitz, M. Wade, E. Surrey and W. Grundfest. 1990. Falloposcopy: A microendoscopic technique for visual exploration of the human fallopian tube from the uterotubal ostium to the fimbria using a transvaginal approach. *Fertility and Sterility* 54:390–400.

O'Neill, C., J. P. Ryan, M. Collier, D. M. Saunders, A. J. Ammit and I. L. Pike. 1989. Supplementation of in vitro fertilisation culture medium with platelet activating factor. *Lancet* 2: 769–772.

## Chapters 7 and 8

Boué, J. G., and A. Boué, 1973. Increased frequency of chromosomal anomalies in abortions after induced ovulation. *Lancet* 1:679–680.

Illeni, M. T., G. Marelli, F. Parazzini, B. Acaia, L. Bocciolone, M. Bontempelli, D. Faden, L. Fedele, A. Maffeis and E. Radici. 1994. Immunotherapy and recurrent abortion: A randomized clinical trial. *Human Reproduction* 9:1247–1249.

Jansen, R. P. S. 1980. Abortion incidence following fallopian tube repair. *Obstetrics and Gynecology* 56:499–502.

————. 1982. Spontaneous abortion incidence in the treatment of infertility. *American Journal of Obstetrics and Gynecology* 143:451–473.

————. 1990. Infertility and abortion. In H. J. Huisjes and T. Lind, eds., *Early Pregnancy Failure*. Edinburgh: Churchill Livingstone.

Jansen, R. P. S., and P. M. Elliott. 1981. Angular intrauterine pregnancy. *Obstetrics and Gynecology* 58:167–175.

Macnaughton, M.C. 1964. The probability of recurrent abortion. *Journal of Obstetrics and Gynaecology of the British Commonwealth* 71:784.

Naylor, A. F., and D. Warburton. 1979. Sequential analysis of spontaneous abortion. II. Collaborative study data. *Fertility and Sterility* 31:282–286.

Warburton, D., and F. C. Fraser. 1961. On the probability that a woman who has had a spontaneous abortion will abort in subsequent pregnancies. *Journal of Obstetrics and*

*Gynaecology of the British Commonwealth* 68:784–788.

———. 1964. Spontaneous abortion risks in man: Data from reproductive histories. *American Journal of Human Genetics* 16:1–25.

## Chapter 9

Brahams, D. 1992. Chlorambucil infertility and sperm banking. *Lancet* 339:420.

Guillette, L. J., Jr. 1995. Endocrine-disrupting environmental contaminants and reproduction. Lessons from the study of wildlife. In D. R. Popkin and L. J. Peddle, eds., *Women's health today: Perspectives on current research and clinical practice.* London: Parthenon.

Jansen, R. P. S. 1970. Electronmicroscopic observations on the Sertoli cell in the experimentally cryptorchid rat testis. *Journal of Anatomy* 106:192.

Jansen, R. P. S., J. C. Anderson, I. Radonic, J. Smit and P. D. Sutherland. 1988. Pregnancies after ultrasound-guided fallopian insemination with cryostored donor semen. *Fertility and Sterility* 49:920–922.

Klein, R. D. 1989. *Infertility: Women speak out about their experiences of reproductive medicine.* London: Pandora Press.

Liebaers, I., M. Bonduelle, E. Van Assche, P. Devroey and A. Van Steirteghem. 1995. *Sex chromosome abnormalities after intracytoplasmic sperm injection.* Lancet 346:1095.

Lilford, R., A. M. Jones, D. T. Bishop, J. Thornton and R. Mueller. 1994. Case-control study of whether subfertility in men is familial. *British Medical Journal* 309:570–573.

Lippi, J., D. Mortimer, and R. P. S. Jansen. 1993. Sub-zonal insemination for extreme male factor infertility. *Human Reproduction* 8:908–915.

Martinez, A. R., R. E. Bernardus, F. J. Voorhorst, J. P. W. Vermeiden and J. Schoemake. 1991. Pregnancy rates after timed intercourse or intrauterine insemination after human menopausal gonadotropin stimulation of normal ovulatory cycles: A controlled study. *Fertility and Sterility* 55:258–265.

Serhal, P., and I. L. Craft. 1987. Immune basis for pre-eclampsia: Evidence from oocyte recipients. *Lancet* 2:744.

Sharpe, R. M. 1995. Another DDT connection. *Nature* 375:538–539.

Sharpe, R. M., and N. E. Skakkebaek. 1993. Are oestrogens involved in falling sperm counts and disorders of the male reproductive tract? *Lancet* 341:1392–1395.

Skakkebaek, N. E., A. Giwercman and D. de Kretser. 1994. Pathogenesis and management of male infertility. *Lancet* 343: 1473–1479.

## Chapter 10

Ellison, P. T., C. Panter-Brick, S. F. Lipson and M. T. O. O'Rourke. 1993. The ecological context of human ovarian function. *Human Reproduction* 8:2248–2258.

Frisch, R. E. 1987. Body fat, menarche, fitness and fertility. *Human Reproduction* 2: 521–533.

Handelsman, D.J., R. P. S. Jansen, L. M. Boylan, J. A. Spaliviero and J. R. Turtle. 1984. Pharmacokinetics of gonadotropin-releasing hormone: Comparison of subcutaneous and intravenous routes. *Journal of*

*Clinical Endocrinology and Metabolism* 59:739–746.

Jansen, R. P. S. 1993. Pulsatile intravenous gonadotrophin releasing hormone for ovulation induction: Determinants of follicular and luteal phase responses. *Human Reproduction* 8 (supp.2): 193–196.

Jansen, R. P. S., D. J. Handelsman, L. M. Boylan, A. Conway, R. P. S. Shearman and I. S. Fraser. 1987. Pulsatile intravenous gonadotropin-releasing hormone for ovulation induction in infertile women. I. Safety and effectiveness with outpatient therapy. *Fertility and Sterility* 48:33–38.

Jansen, R. P. S., D. J. Handelsman, L. M. Boylan, A. Conway, R. P. S. Shearman, I. S. Fraser and J. C. Anderson. 1987. Pulsatile intravenous gonadotropin-releasing hormone for ovulation induction in infertile women. II. Analysis of follicular and luteal phase responses. *Fertility and Sterility* 48:39–44.

## Chapter 11

McClure, N., D. Healy, P. A. W. Rogers, J. Sullivan, L. Beaton, R. V. Haning, Jr., D. T. Connolly and D. M. Robertson. 1994. Vascular endothelial growth factor as capillary permeability agent in ovarian hyperstimulation syndrome. *Lancet* 34:235–236.

## Chapter 12

Jansen, R. P. S. 1981. Fallopian tube secretions: Implications for tubal microsurgery. *Australian and New Zealand Journal of Obstetrics and Gynaecology* 21:140–142.

———. 1993. Medicine and surgery inside the fallopian tube. *Medical Journal of Australia* 158:799–800.

———. 1995. Ultrastructure and histochemistry of estrogen-dependent acid mucu glycoproteins in the mammalian oviduct *Microscopy Research and Techniqu* 32:29–49.

## Chapter 13

Franklin, R. R., M. P. Diamond, L. R. Malinak B. Larsson, R. P. S. Jansen, S. Ronsenber; and B. W. Webster. 1995. Reduction o ovarian adhesions by the use of Interceed *Obstetrics and Gynecology* 86:335–340.

Jansen, R. P. S. 1980. Surgery-pregnancy tim intervals after salpingolysis, unilateral salpingostomy, and bilateral salpingostomy *Fertility and Sterility* 34:222–225.

———. 1982. Pelvic surgery in young women. *Medical Journal of Australia* 1 525–526.

———. 1985. Early laparoscopy after infertility surgery [abstract]. *Fertility and Sterility* 44:8s.

———. 1985. Failure of intraperitoneal adjuncts to improve the outcome of pelvic operations in young women. *American Journal of Obstetrics and Gynecology* 153:363–371.

———. 1986. Tubal resection and anastomosis. I. Sterilization-reversal. *Australian and New Zealand Journal of Obstetrics and Gynaecology* 26:294–299.

———. 1986. Tubal resection and anastomosis. II. Isthmic salpingitis. *Australian and New Zealand Journal of Obstetrics and Gynaecology* 26:300–304.

———. 1988. Early laparoscopy after pelvic operations to prevent adhesions: Safety and efficacy. *Fertility and Sterility* 49:26–31.

———. 1988. Failure of peritoneal irrigation with heparin during pelvic operations upon young women to reduce adhesions. Surgery, *Gynecology and Obstetrics* 166: 154–160.

———. 1990. Controlled clinical approaches to investigating the prevention of peritoneal adhesions. *Progress in Clinical and Biological Research* 358:177–192.

———. 1990. Prevention and treatment of postsurgical adhesions. *Medical Journal of Australia* 152:305–306.

———. 1991. Prevention of pelvic peritoneal adhesions. *Current Opinion in Obstetrics and Gynecology* 3:369–374.

Thurmond, A. S., M. Novy, B. T. Uchida and J. Rosch. 1987. Fallopian tube obstruction: Selective salpingography and recanalization. *Radiology* 163:511–514.

## Chapter 14

Jansen, R. P. S., and P. M. Elliott. 1981. Angular intrauterine pregnancy. *Obstetrics and Gynecology* 58:167–175.

## Chapter 15

Brosens, I. A. 1993. Endometriosis—Narrow but deep—Important. *Fertility and Sterility* 60:201–202.

Brosens, I. A., J. Donnez and G. Benagiano. 1993. Improving the classification of endometriosis. *Human Reproduction* 8: 1792–1795.

Gibbons, A. 1993. Dioxin tied to endometriosis. *Science* 262:1373.

Jansen, R. P. S. 1983. Peritoneal and plasma estradiol and progesterone levels in mild and moderate endometriosis: A search for luteinized unruptured follicles [abstract]. *Fertility and Sterility* 39:394.

———. 1986. Minimal endometriosis and reduced fecundability: Prospective evidence from an A.I.D. program. *Fertility and Sterility* 46:141–143.

———. 1992. Nonpigmented endometriosis. In D. C. Martin, ed., *Atlas of Endometriosis.* London: Gower Medical Publishing.

———. 1993. Endometriosis symptoms and the limitations of pathology-based classification of severity. *International Journal of Obstetrics and Gynecology* 40 (supp.): 53–57.

———. 1993. Pathology and pathogenesis of endometriosis. In C. Sutton and M. P. Diamond, eds., *Endoscopic surgery for gynaecologists.* London: W. B. Saunders Company.

Jansen, R. P. S., and P. Russell. 1986. Nonpigmented endometriosis: Clinical, laparoscopic and pathologic definition. *American Journal of Obstetrics and Gynecology* 155:1154–1159.

Nisolle, M., F. Casanas-Roux, V. Anaf, J.-M. Mine and J. Donnez. 1993. Morphometric study of the stromal vascularization in peritoneal endometriosis. *Fertility and Sterility* 59:681–684.

Simpson, J. L., S. Elias, L. R. Malinak and V. C. J. Buttram. 1980. Heritable aspects of endometriosis. I. Genetic studies. *American Journal of Obstetrics and Gynecology* 137: 327–331.

TeLinde, R. W. 1978. The background of studies on experimental endometriosis. *American Journal of Obstetrics and Gynecology* 130:570–571.

TeLinde, R. W., and R. B. Scott. 1950. Experimental endometriosis. *American Journal of Obstetrics and Gynecology* 60: 1147–1173.

Wentz, A. C. 1980. Premenstrual spotting: Its association with endometriosis but not luteal phase inadequacy. *Fertility and Sterility* 33:605–607.

## Chapter 16

Jansen, R. P. S. 1988. Endometriosis. *Australian Prescriber* 11:2–5.

———. 1992. Principles of medical therapy for endometriosis pain. *Journal of Obstetrics and Gynaecology* 12 (supp. 2): s33–s37.

Jansen, R. P. S., and E. J. Keogh. 1991. GnRH analogues in reproductive medicine. *Medical Journal of Australia* 154:571–572.

## Chapter 17

Fraser, I. S., J.-Y. Song, R. P. S. Jansen, P. Ramsay and T. Boogert. 1995. Hysteroscopic lysis of intra-uterine adhesions under ultrasound guidance. *Gynaecological Endoscopy* 4:35–40.

## Chapter 18

Jansen, R. P. S. 1997. Intersex. In P. Russell and P. Bannatyne, eds., *Surgical Pathology of the Ovary*, 2nd ed. Edinburgh: Churchill Livingstone.

## Chapter 19

Jansen, R. P. S. 1987. Assisted conception. *Modern Medicine of Australia* (June): 36–43.

———. 1987. The clinical impact of in vitro fertilization. I. Results and limitations of conventional reproductive medicine. *Medical Journal of Australia* 146:342–353.

———. 1990. Unfinished feticide. *Journal of Medical Ethics* 16:61–65.

## Chapter 20

Asch, R. H., L. R. Ellsworth, J. P. Balmaceda and P. C. Wong. 1984. Pregnancy after translaparoscopic gamete intrafallopia transfer. *Lancet* 2:1034.

Devroey, P., J. Liu, Z. Nagy, A. Goossen H. Tournaye, M. Camus, A. Va Steirteghem and S. Silber. 1995. Pre nancies after testicular sperm extractio and intracytoplasmic sperm injection i non-obstructive azoospermia. *Human R production* 10:1457–1460.

Edwards, R. G., B. D. Bavister and P. C Steptoe. 1969. Early stages of fertilization i vitro of human oocytes matured in vitr *Nature* 221:632–635.

Edwards, R. G., P. C. Steptoe and J. M. Purd 1980. Establishing full-term human pre nancies using cleaving embryos grown i vitro. *British Journal of Obstetrics an Gynaecology* 87:737–756.

Fishel, S., S. Antinori, P. Jackson, J. Johnsor F. Lisi, F. Chiariello and C. Versaci. 199( Twin birth after subzonal inseminatior *Lancet* 335:722–723.

Fluker, M. R., C. G. Zouves and M. W. Beb bington. 1993. A prospective randomize comparison of zygote intrafallopian trans fer and in vitro fertilization–embryo trans fer for nontubal factor infertility. *Fertilit and Sterility* 60:515–519.

Jansen, R. P. S. 1988. Anaesthesia and assiste conception. In D. R. Kerr, ed., *Australasia anaesthesia*, 1988. Sydney: Faculty o Anaesthetists, Royal Australasian College o Surgeons.

———. 1989. Gamete intra-fallopian trans fer. In C. Wood and A. O. Trounson, eds. *Clinical in vitro fertilization*. Berlin Springer-Verlag.

———. 1989. In vitro fertilization: A his tory of quality assurance in Australia

1980–1989. *Australian Clinical Review* 9:27–32.

ansen, R. P. S., and J. C. Anderson. 1987. Catheterisation of the fallopian tubes from the vagina. *Lancet* 2:309–310.

———. 1993. Transvaginal versus laparoscopic GIFT: A case-controlled retrospective comparison. *Fertility and Sterility* 59:836–840.

ansen, R. P. S., J. C. Anderson, W. R. S. Birrell, R. C. Lyneham, P. D. Sutherland, M. Turner, D. Flowers and E. Ciancaglini. 1990. Outpatient gamete intrafallopian transfer: 710 cases. *Medical Journal of Australia* 153:182–188.

ansen, R. P. S., J. C. Anderson and P. D. Sutherland. 1988. Nonoperative embryo transfer to the fallopian tube. *New England Journal of Medicine* 319:288–291.

ansen, R. P. S., D. Golovsky, J. Lippi and D. Mortimer. 1993. Pregnancy from sub-zonally-microinjected epididymal spermatozoa. *Medical Journal of Australia* 158:646-647.

Lippi, J., D. Mortimer and R. P. S. Jansen. 1993. Sub-zonal insemination for extreme male factor infertility. *Human Reproduction* 8:908–915.

Lippi, J., M. Turner and R. P. S. Jansen. 1990. Pregnancies after in vitro fertilization by sperm microinjection into the perivitelline space [abstract]. *Fertility and Sterility* 54:s29.

Mickle, J., A. Milunsky, J. A. Amos and R. D. Oates. 1995. Congenital unilateral absence of the vas deferens: A heterogeneous disorder with two distinct subpopulations based upon aetiology and mutational status of the cystic fibrosis gene. *Human Reproduction* 10:1728–1735.

Mortimer, D. 1986. Comparison of the fertilizing ability of human spermatozoa preincubated in calcium- and strontium-containing media. *Journal of Experimental Zoology* 237:21–24.

Silber, S. J., Z. Nagy, J. Liu, H. Tournaye, W. Lissens, C. Ferec, I. Liebaers, P. Devroey and A. C. Van Steirteghem. 1995. The use of epididymal and testicular spermatozoa for intracytoplasmic sperm injection: The genetic implications for male infertility. *Human Reproduction* 10:2031–2043.

Silber, S. J., A. C. Van Steirteghem, J. Liu, Z. Nagy, H. Tournaye and P. Devroey. 1995. High fertilization and pregnancy rate after intracytoplasmic sperm injection with spermatozoa obtained from testicle biopsy. *Human Reproduction* 10:148–152.

Steptoe, P. C., and R. G. Edwards. 1976. Reimplantation of a human embryo with subsequent tubal pregnancy. *Lancet* 1:880–882.

Steptoe, P. C., R. G. Edwards and J. M. Purdy. 1980. Clinical aspects of pregnancies established with cleaving embryos grown in vitro. *British Journal of Obstetrics and Gynaecology* 87:757–768.

Sungurtekin, U., and R. P. S. Jansen. 1995. Profound luteinizing hormone suppression after stopping the gonadotropin-releasing hormone-agonist leuprolide acetate. *Fertility and Sterility* 63:663–665.

**Chapter 21**

Trounson, A. O., and L. Mohr. 1983. Human pregnancy following cryopreservation, thawing and transfer of an eight-cell embryo. *Nature* 305:707–709.

**Chapter 22**

Daniels, K. R. 1987. Semen donors in New Zealand: Their characteristics and attitudes. *Clinical Reproduction and Fertility* 5:177–190.

Daniels, K., and O. Lalos. 1995. The Swedish insemination act and the availability of donors. Human Reproduction 10:1871–1874.

Dunstan, G. R. 1975. Ethical aspects of donor insemination. *Journal of Medical Ethics* 1: 42–44.

Handelsman, D. J., S. J. Dunn, A. J. Conway, L. M. Boylan and R. P. S. Jansen. 1984. Psychological and attitudinal profiles in donors for artificial insemination. *Fertility and Sterility* 43:95–101.

Huerre, P. 1980. Psychological aspects of semen donation. In G. David and W. S. Price, eds., *Human artificial insemination and semen preservation*. New York: Plenum Press.

Jansen, R. P. S. 1985. Sperm and ova as property. *Journal of Medical Ethics* 11:123–126.

———. 1995. Bioethics of the spermatozoon. In J. G. Grudzinskas, J. L. Yovich, J. L. Simpson and T. Chard, eds., *Cambridge reviews in human reproduction. Volume 3. Gametes: The spermatozoon.* Cambridge: Cambridge University Press.

———. 1995. Bioethics of the oocyte. In J. G. Grudzinskas, J. L. Yovich, J. L. Simpson and T. Chard, eds., *Cambridge reviews in human reproduction. Volume 2. Gametes: The oocyte.* Cambridge: Cambridge University Press.

Rowland, R. 1983. Attitudes and opinions of donors on an artificial insemination by donor (AID) program. *Clinical Repr duction and Fertility* 2:249–259.

Sauer, M. V., and R. J. Paulson. 1990. Huma oocyte and pre-embryo donation: A evolving method for the treatment of infe tility. *American Journal of Obstetrics ar Gynecology* 163:1421–1424.

Schoysman, R. 1975. Problems of selectir donors for artificial insemination. *Journ of Medical Ethics* 1:34–35.

Templeton, A. 1991. Gamete donation an anonymity. *British Journal of Obstetrics ar Gynaecology* 98:343–350.

**Chapter 23**

Barnes, F. L., A. Crombie, D. K. Gardne A. Kausche, O. Lacham-Kaplan, A.-M Suikkari, J. Tiglias, C. Wood and A. C Trounson. 1995. Blastocyst developmen and birth after in vitro maturation of hu man primary oocytes, intracytoplasmi sperm injection and assisted hatching *Human Reproduction* 10:101–105.

Eppig, J. J., A. C. Schroeder and M. J. O'Brien 1992. Developmental capacity of mouse oocytes matured in vitro: Effects o gonadotrophic stimulation, follicular ori gin and oocyte size. *Journal of Reproduction and Fertility* 95:119–127.

Gook, D. A., M. C. Schiewe, S. M. Osborn R. H. Asch, R. P. S. Jansen and W. I. H Johnston. 1995. Intracytoplasmic sperm in jection and embryo development of human oocytes cryopreserved using 1,2-propane diol. *Human Reproduction* 10:2637–2641.

Handyside, A. 1992. Prospects for the clinical application of preimplantation diagnosis The tortoise or the hare. *Human Reproduction* 7:1481–1483.

ansen, R. P. S. 1984. Fertility in older women. *International Planned Parenthood Foundation Medical Bulletin* 18(2): 4–6.

———. 1995. Older ovaries: Ageing and reproduction. *Medical Journal of Australia* 162:623–624.

Trounson, A., C. Wood and A. Kausche. 1994. In vitro maturation and the fertilization and developmental competence of oocytes recovered from untreated polycystic ovarian patients. *Fertility and Sterility* 62: 353–362.

## Chapter 25

Freeman, E. W., A. S. Boxer, K. Rickels, R. Tureck and L. J. Mastroianni. 1985. Psychological evaluation and support in a program of in vitro fertilization and embryo transfer. *Fertility and Sterility* 43: 48–53.

Jansen, R. P. S. 1994. Self-regulation or legislation in assisted reproductive technology. In D. R. Popkin and L. J. Peddle, eds., *Women's health today: Perspectives on current research and clinical practice*. London: Parthenon.

National Health and Medical Research Council. 1985. *Embryo donation by uterine flushing: Interim report on ethical considerations*. Canberra: Australian Government Publishing Service.

## Chapter 26

Hare, R. M. 1981. *Moral thinking: Its levels, method, and point*. Oxford: Clarendon Press.

Jansen, R. P. S. 1986. Conflicts of interest and the physician entrepreneur [letter]. *New England Journal of Medicine* 314:252.

———. 1987. Ethics in infertility treatment. In R. Pepperell, C. Wood and B. Hudson, eds., *The infertile couple*, 2nd ed. Edinburgh: Churchill Livingstone.

———. 1988. Advantages and disadvantages of subspecialization. *International Journal of Obstetrics and Gynecology* 27:293–296.

———. 1994. Self-regulation or legislation in assisted reproductive technology. In D. R. Popkin and L. J. Peddle, eds., *Women's health today: Perspectives on current research and clinical practice*. London: Parthenon.

———. 1995. Ethical principles and values. In R. J. A. Trent, ed., *Handbook of antenatal diagnosis*. Cambridge: Cambridge University Press.

## Chapter 27

Huxley, A. 1946. *Brave New World*. New York: Harper & Row.

Jansen, R. P. S. 1985. A practical ethical framework for in vitro fertilization and related reproductive interventions. *Annals of the New York Academy of Science* 442:595–600.

———. 1987. The clinical impact of in vitro fertilization. II. Regulation, money and research. *Medical Journal of Australia* 146:362–366.

———. 1988. Reproductive technology: Where to now. *Healthright* 7(2): 9–15.

———. 1991. Mouse tales and embryo research. In *Proceedings of the First Annual Conference of the Australian Bioethics Association*. Melbourne: Australian Bioethics Association.

Kola, I., O. Lacham, R. P. S. Jansen, M. Turner and A. Trounson. 1990. Chromosomal analysis of human oocytes fertilized by microinjection of spermatozoa into the perivitelline space. *Human Reproduction* 5:575–577.

Reddy, P. 1992. *Saadan er Danskerne* (Danes Are Like That). Aarhus: Grevas Forlag.

Stone, L. 1977. *The family, sex and marriage in England, 1500–1800*. London: Weidenfeld and Nicolson.

**Appendices**

Lancaster, P., E. Shafir, and J. Huang. 1995. *Assisted conception: Australia and New Zealand, 1992 and 1993*. Sydney: Australian Institute of Health and Welfare National Perinatal Statistics Unit.

Society for Assisted Reproductive Technology, American Society for Reproductive Medicine. 1995. Assisted reproductive technology in the United States and Canada: 1993 results generated from the American Society for Reproductive Medicine/Society for Assisted Reproductive Technology Registry. *Fertility and Sterility* 64:13–21.

# Index

Page numbers in *italics* indicate illustrations. A page number followed by an italic letter *g* indicates the location of the word or term in the Glossary.

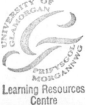